PROMOTING
TEEN
HEALTH

PROMOTING TEEN HEALTH

Linking Schools, Health Organizations, and Community

Edited by

Alan Henderson and Sally Champlin
with William Evashwick

This book was produced through the support of the FHP
Foundation and the Center for Health Care Innovation at
California State University, Long Beach.

SAGE Publications
International Educational and Professional Publisher
Thousand Oaks   London   New Delhi

For information:

SAGE Publications, Inc.
2455 Teller Road
Thousand Oaks, California 91320
E-mail: order@sagepub.com

SAGE Publications Ltd.
6 Bonhill Street
London EC2A 4PU
United Kingdom

SAGE Publications India Pvt. Ltd.
M-32 Market
Greater Kailash I
New Delhi 110 048 India

Printed in the United States of America

Library of Congress Cataloging-in-Publication Data

Main entry under title:

Promoting teen health: linking schools, health organizations, and
community / edited by Alan Henderson, Sally Champlin, and William
Evashwick.
  p. cm.
  Includes bibliographical references and index.
  ISBN 07619-0275-9 (acid-free paper)
  ISBN 07619-0276-7 (pbk. : acid-free paper)
  1. Teenagers—Health and hygiene—United States. 2. Health
education—United States—Planning. 3. Health promotion—United
States. I. Henderson, Alan C. II. Champlin, Sally. III. Evashwick,
William.
  RA564.5 .P736 1998
  613'.0433'0973—ddc21
                                97-45473

This book is printed on acid-free paper.

98 99 00 01 02 03 10 9 8 7 6 5 4 3 2 1

Acquiring Editor:	Dan Ruth
Editorial Assistant:	Anna Howland
Production Editor:	Sherrise M. Purdum
Production Assistant:	Karen Wiley
Typesetter:	Danielle Dillahunt
Designer:	Rebecca Evans
Indexer:	Paul Corrington
Cover Designer:	Candice Harman

Contents

Foreword

It should be no surprise to anyone that there are far too few teen health promotion programs in the United States and, indeed, throughout the world. This phenomenon can be attributed to several causes. A major one is that for years there was little reliable evidence that such programs had a positive effect. Today, behavioral research techniques have improved to the point that interventions can be clearly shown—by valid and reliable measures—to positively affect the health behavior of various populations, including teens.

Ironically, during wars that resulted in the drafting of young men into the military, this country realized the importance of health promotion programs and increased efforts in this direction. The reason for this was that a high percentage of young males were being rejected by the military because of health problems that were largely preventable. As soon as the wars were over, however, interest in such programs waned. Our leaders in government and in education never seemed to learn that there would be great dividends for having ongoing promotion programs.

Comprehensive school health education programs have always had to battle for a place in the curriculum. There always seems to be a larger constituency for those who argue that

"Johnny can't read, write, or calculate," and thus the traditional curriculum areas deserve the lion's share (if not all) of the school day. Some even argue that all matters dealing with health are the parents' responsibility and that schools should not play a role in promoting the health of children and youth. Those who present such an argument never seem to deal with who is going to teach the parents to assume that responsibility. Nor do they mention the fact that most parents do not assume the responsibility. Thus, we continue to see high levels of teen pregnancy and sexually transmitted diseases (including AIDS), drug and alcohol abuse, smoking, poor nutritional habits, intentional and unintentional injury, and much poor judgment in the purchase and/or use of health products and services.

Teens who are not educated in these areas stand a chance of suffering in ways that will carry into adulthood, and they likely will be prevented from enjoying a full, productive life. Through research and surveillance projects, the Centers for Disease Control and Prevention (CDC) have identified six behaviors that markedly contribute to today's major killers (e.g., heart disease, cancer, and injuries). These behaviors include tobacco use; unhealthy dietary behaviors; inadequate physical activity; sexual behaviors that may result in HIV infection, other sexually transmitted diseases, and unintended pregnancies; behaviors that may result in intentional injuries (e.g., violence and suicide) and unintentional injuries (e.g., motor vehicle crashes); and alcohol and other drug use. These behaviors generally are established during youth and then are carried into adulthood. Of great significance is that they are all preventable.

The authors of the chapters in this book collectively have the professional preparation and experience to both describe the status of teen health and provide valid/reliable techniques for promoting healthy behaviors through school and community linkages. All those employed in these efforts will find the book helpful.

PETER A. CORTESE, MPH, Dr PH, CHES
Associate Dean for Graduate Studies,
Research and Faculty Affairs (retired)
College of Health and Human Services
California State University, Long Beach
Chief, Program Development and Services
Branch (retired)
Division of Adolescent and School Health
Centers for Disease Control and Prevention
(CDC)

1

Overview of Teen Health

Susan Giarratano-Russell

About 24 million adolescents, 13 to 19 years old, live in the United States (U.S. Bureau of Census, 1992, p. 17). Nearly one third are members of an ethnic minority. Among adolescents residing in the United States, about 15% are African Americans, 12% Hispanic Americans, 4% Asian Americans, and 1% Native Americans (National Adolescent Health Information Center, 1995b, p. 1). Adolescents are diverse in their ethnicity, beliefs, and values. This diversity may play a role in determining their health status.

Adolescence is a period of turbulent transformation from childhood to adulthood, where youth undergo many physical, emotional, cognitive, and physiological changes. It is also a period of experimentation that can involve risk taking (American Medical Association, 1995, p. 3). Personal, environmental, and societal pressures put adolescents at high risk for tobacco use, substance abuse, human immune deficiency virus/acquired immune deficiency syndrome (HIV/AIDS), sexually transmitted diseases (STDs), unwanted pregnancies, violence, unintentional injuries, and mental illnesses. Some behaviors threaten current health, whereas other behaviors may have long-term health consequences, and many of these behaviors are often interrelated. A particular behavior may be both a cause and an effect of the developmental turbulence experienced by many adolescents. About 75% of all deaths among adolescents result from four major causes: motor vehicle crashes, other unintentional injuries, homicide, and suicide. Some factors that increase the likelihood of death among adolescents include not using a seat belt, driving with someone who has been drinking alcohol, carrying a weapon, drinking alcohol, and using marijuana. In the United States, 60% of all deaths and a large amount of acute and chronic morbidity result from heart disease, cancer, and stroke. Six categories of risk contributing to this morbidity and mortality include behaviors resulting in tobacco, alcohol, and other drug use; sexual behaviors that contribute to unintended pregnancy and STDs, including HIV infection; intentional injuries; unintentional injuries; dietary behaviors that result in disease; and physical inactivity (Kann et al., 1995, pp. 1-2).

Tobacco Use

Tobacco use is the single most important preventable cause of death in our society. Tobacco use causes premature mortality, jeopardizes health and well-being, and dramatically increases health care costs (Marcus,

Giovino, Pierce, & Harel, 1993, p. 20). Many adolescents do not realize the long-term effects of smoking, for example, cancer of the larynx, mouth, esophagus, kidneys, uterus, pancreas, and stomach; cerebrovascular disease; cardiovascular disease; and chronic obstructive pulmonary disease (Marcus et al., 1993, p. 20). About 90 percent of those who smoke start using tobacco when they are less than 18 years old. About 35% of adolescents currently smoke (Centers for Disease Control and Prevention [CDC], 1996c, p. 414). Those adolescents who are pregnant and smoke have an increased risk of intrauterine growth retardation, lower infant birth weight, and higher infant mortality. In 1988, maternal smoking attributed to about 2,500 infant deaths. Adolescent smokers have higher rates of respiratory problems, lower levels of physical fitness, higher levels of triglycerides, and lower levels of high density lipoproteins, compared to adolescents who do not smoke (Marcus et al., 1993, p. 20). Tobacco threatens the current and future health of today's adolescents, and it is important that we help them to understand the seriousness of the consequences of smoking—both short and long term.

Alcohol and Other Drug Use

Like tobacco, alcohol and drugs can also have devastating effects on adolescent health. Alcohol and drug use has been associated with domestic violence, abuse, and homicide. In 1987, about $185 million was spent on adolescent alcohol and drug treatment services (Gans & Shook, 1994a, p. 2). The American Medical Association has identified three realities of adolescent substance use. First, adolescents begin experimenting with alcohol and drugs at a younger age. Second, substance abuse usually proceeds in stages, beginning with tobacco and alcohol during early adolescence, marijuana during middle adolescence,

and finally cocaine during older adolescence. Third, adolescents who abuse substances often engage in other high-risk behaviors, in addition to experiencing mental and emotional disorders. Adolescents who abuse alcohol have a higher rate of suicide, mental health problems, school dropout, and delinquency (Gans & Shook, 1994a, p. 3).

Alcohol not only affects adolescents' mental health, it also dramatically affects their physical health. Over one half of the motor vehicle accidents that kill adolescents involve alcohol. Drugs and alcohol also contribute the spread of STDs and HIV, especially through sharing of contaminated needles, intravenous drug use, and impaired judgment leading to unprotected sex (Blanken, 1993, p. 25).

Sexual Behaviors Contributing to STDs, HIV, and AIDS

Adolescents account for more than 80% of the cases of STDs in the United States. Significant morbidity results from the estimated 12 million cases of STDs occurring annually among 15- to 29-year-olds and from the 20% of AIDS cases diagnosed among 20- to 29-year-olds. Today, one quarter of all new HIV infections in the United States are estimated to occur in young people between the ages of 13 and 20. And one in four new HIV infections in the United States are estimated to occur among people under the age of 20. The incubation period between infection with HIV and the onset of AIDS symptoms is about 10 years, which suggests that a large proportion of 20- to 29-year-olds who display the symptoms of AIDS were infected during adolescence (Flemming, 1996).

AIDS, STDs, and pregnancy are all consequences of unprotected sex. Nationally, about two thirds of all high school students are sexually active (CDC, 1996a, p. 66). Among those who are sexually active, more than 54% reported that they or their partner had used a condom during their last sexual intercourse. However, condom use declines with age. Slightly more than 17% of students reported that they or their partner had used birth control pills during their last sexual intercourse (CDC, 1996a, p.68).

Sexual Behaviors Contributing to Teen Pregnancy

More than 1 million adolescents become pregnant every year; the majority of pregnancies (78%) among 15- to 17-year-olds are unwanted. Young maternal age and lower socioeconomic status may increase the likelihood of adverse birth outcomes of teen pregnancies (National Adolescent Health Information Center, 1995a, p. 1).

Birth rates for adolescents in the United States declined in 1994 for the third straight year. The birth rate for 15- and 19-year-olds has dropped by 5% since 1991. Recent declines in abortion rates have also been reported. The combination of lower birth rates and lower abortion rates suggests that pregnancy rates have declined (National Adolescent Health Information Center, 1995a).

Violence

Intentional injuries caused by violence are a category of risk behavior. Violence has recently been defined as a health concern by the CDC because of its profound rise and influence on health. Adolescents are more than twice as likely as any other group to be the victim of a violent crime. Violence mortality among adolescents has reached an all-time high. Homicide rates increased 82% between 1968 and 1992 (Miller, 1996, p. 473). Among 15- to 19-year-olds, the homicide rate is 11 per 100,000. The homicide rate for African

American adolescents is 85 per 100,000. Adolescents are more likely than younger children to be victims of assault or physical, sexual, and emotional abuse. Overall, today's adolescents encounter more violence than young people in earlier generations. We live in a nation where guns have replaced fists and knives as a way of settling disputes. Children ages 12 to 15 are more than twice as likely to be the victims of violence as adults older than 24 (Gans & Shook, 1994b, p. 2).

Adolescents are not only the victims of violence, they are also the perpetrators. About 24% of all crimes that lead to arrests involve adolescents. Adolescents commit more than 40% of sexual offenses against children. About 67% of adolescent victims of violent crime reported that the offender was between 12 and 20 years old. About 18% of high school seniors claim that they have engaged in a serious fight at school or at work (Gans & Shook, 1994b, p. 2).

Physical and sexual abuse has pervasive and devastating effects on the health of adolescents, both as victims and perpetrators. Victims of abuse are at an increased risk for premature sexual activity or promiscuity, unintended pregnancy, emotional disorders, suicide attempts, confused sexual identity, drug and alcohol abuse, delinquent behavior, and eating disorders (Gans & Shook, 1994b, p. 2).

Unintentional Injuries

Unintentional injuries are another category of risk behavior, and they are the leading cause of death among those 12 to 24 years old. Accidental injuries were the leading cause of death for adolescents in 1991 (National Adolescent Health Information Center, 1995b, p. 1). Many of these injuries are preventable. Ethnicity plays a role in unintentional injury morbidity. African Americans have slightly higher death rates than whites. Native Americans and

Alaska Natives have death rates that are twice as high as those of whites. Injuries are the leading cause of potential life lost before age 65. The leading causes of death from unintentional injury are motor vehicle crashes, falls, poisonings, and drownings (Waxweiler, Harel, & O'Carroll, 1993, pp. 11-12).

Contributing to mortality from motor vehicle crashes are alcohol consumption and failure to use safety belts. Adolescents have the highest proportion of belt nonuse (83%). Unintentional poisonings are the third leading cause of unintentional injury deaths. More than 50% of these deaths are due to misuse of drugs and medication. Drowning rates are highest among children younger than 5 and among 15- to 24-year-olds. Males are five times as likely to drown as females (Waxweiler et al., 1993, pp. 11-12).

Adolescents also face high morbidity from unintentional injuries. They are at a greater risk than any other age group of sustaining a spinal cord injury. Motor vehicle crashes contribute to nearly half of all spinal cord injuries. Falls and unsafe diving also contribute to this type of injury (Waxweiler et al., 1993, pp. 11-12).

Many deaths and serious injuries suffered by adolescents are preventable. To reduce the number of adolescent deaths and injuries, certain behaviors must be practiced, including using seat belts; wearing motorcycle and bicycle helmets; not driving or riding in a car driven by someone under the influence of alcohol or other drugs; and wearing life jackets (Waxweiler et al., 1993, pp. 11-12).

Emotional Health and Eating Disorders

Adolescents commonly experience mood fluctuations and transient depression. Depression is one of the mental, emotional, and behavior disorders that can appear during adolescence. In one study, mildly depressive symptoms were found in 34% of male and 15% of female adolescents (Hamburg, 1992). In another sample, 6% had clinically significant depressive symptoms (Hamburg, 1992, pp. 190-191). The signs of depression include sadness that won't go away, hopelessness, loss of interest in usual activities, changes in eating or sleeping habits, missed school or poor school performance, aches and pains that don't get better with treatment, and thoughts about death or suicide (U.S. Department of Health and Human Services, 1996). Depression can be a precursor to suicide attempts for some adolescents. Suicide accounts for 6% of deaths among 10- to 14-year-olds, and 12% of deaths among 15- to 19-year-olds. Suicide is more common among males than females, and more common among whites than African Americans. Depression can lead to substance abuse, trouble with the law, failure in school, anxiety, and feelings of worthlessness, guilt, and shame (Hamburg, 1992, pp. 190-191).

Eating disorders, including anorexia nervosa and bulimia, are serious health concerns for today's adolescents. More common among females than males, and occurring more frequently among adolescents in upper- or middle-income families, eating disorders are a serious health threat to adolescents (Gans, 1990, p. 13). Anorexia nervosa is characterized by the individual's refusing to maintain a minimally normal body weight, by perfectionism, and by a distorted body image. Bulimia is characterized by repeated episodes of binge eating followed by purging by either self-induced vomiting, laxative abuse, diuretics, or compulsive exercising. Eating disorders may cause severe complications, and the mortality rates are among the highest for any psychiatric disorder. Estimates suggest that between 5% and 12% of adolescents suffer from eating disorders. A national survey of 8th and 10th grade students found that 32% skipped meals, 22% fasted, 7% used diet pills, 5% induced vomiting after meals, and 3% used laxatives to lose weight (CDC, 1996b, p. 4).

Factors Affecting
Teen Health Behaviors

Many of the physical, psychological, and emotional problems faced by adolescents are also influenced by personal, environmental, and societal factors. During adolescence, young people further develop their self-esteem and appear to take more risks. Families, peer pressure, the media, and community support influence the transition into adulthood.

Adolescence is a time to experience new ideas, new relationships, and new activities. The health of adolescents is dependent on their own behavior, which is heavily influenced by the environment in which they live (Friedman, 1993, p. 510). For some youth, the difficulties of this transition, combined with high-risk environments, may lead to experimentation and adoption of risky health behaviors and practices. Behavioral issues are becoming widely recognized as the key to health; many behaviors are influenced by social settings. For example, sexual intercourse may commonly begin in adolescence, as does the use of tobacco, alcohol, and other drugs (Friedman, 1993, p. 510). Adolescents whose peers were reported to engage in risk-taking behaviors were more likely to engage in risky sexual behaviors (Metzler, Noell, Biglan, Ary, & Smolkowski, 1994, p. 419).

Research indicates that before the age of 18, one in four adolescents will have engaged in behaviors that are harmful or dangerous to themselves or others. Another 25% are at moderate risk of engaging in such behaviors. This means that half of all adolescents are at risk for serious physical injuries or mental illness (Carnegie Council, 1995, p. 42).

On average, children from disrupted or never-married families are more likely to use alcohol and drugs, to become teen parents, and to achieve lower earnings and are less likely to attain a high school diploma than those from intact families with both biological parents. The majority of children brought up in single-parent families do well, with differences in well-being between those from divorced and intact families tending, on average, to be moderate to small (Carnegie Council, 1995, p. 36). Millions of adolescents are growing up under conditions that do not meet their educational, emotional, and health needs for optimal development. Today, adolescents are spending more time with their peers and less time with caring adults. Therefore, they may lack the necessary guidance from their parents and other adults. One factor responsible for decreased parental involvement in adolescents' lives is that one or more parents are now in the workplace (Hamburg, 1992, pp. 194-195).

To make the transition into adulthood more successful and healthy, it is important for the entire community (families, schools, neighborhoods, houses of worship, and youth organizations) to provide adolescents with a feeling of belonging. Today, there are more than 17,000 youth-serving organizations in the United States. These include the Boy Scouts, Girl Scouts, 4-H Clubs, YMCA, and YWCA, among others. Many offer adolescents a safe place to relax and be with friends. Some teach important life skills and provide supervision and support. The organizations, as well as youth service-learning programs, can offer experiences that can help teens build a sense of self-worth, foster cooperation, and help prepare them for a responsible future. Unfortunately, 29% of adolescents are not served by existing organizations due to limited operational hours, transportation barriers, and inadequately trained adults to provide services and supervision. Schools, too, play an important role in providing adolescents with the tools necessary for a healthy transition into adulthood. Schools must collaborate with community organizations to help adolescents become healthier and more productive community members (Carnegie Council, 1995, p. 106).

Conclusion

Adolescent use of tobacco, alcohol, and other drugs are often entangled with AIDS, STDs, pregnancy, violence, unintentional injuries, and mental illnesses. Tobacco use can lead to alcohol and other drug use, and it can cause higher rates of pregnancy complications. Alcohol and other drug abuse can affect a person's judgment, creating a higher risk for unprotected sex, suicide, violence, and other emotional problems. Violence against and by adolescents leads to higher dropout rates from school, which leads to higher unemployment, which can perpetuate more violence. As a spider spins its web and traps unsuspecting insects, many adolescents can become entrapped by their behaviors. The Carnegie Council on Adolescent Development (1995) warned that America is abandoning youth "at the most crucial turning point in their passage from childhood to adulthood." With the assistance and cooperation of schools, communities, and families, this transition from adolescence to adulthood transition can be successful.

References

American Medical Association. (1995). *Guidelines for adolescent preventive services (GAPS)*. Chicago: Author.

Blanken, A. J. (1993). Measuring tobacco use among adolescents. *Public Reports, 108*, 25-30.

Carnegie Council. (1995). *Great transitions: Preparing adolescents for a new century* (Concluding report of the Carnegie Council on Adolescent Development). New York: Author.

Centers for Disease Control and Prevention. (1996a, September 27). CDC surveillance summaries. *Morbidity and Mortality Weekly Report, 45*(SS-4), 65, 68.

Centers for Disease Control and Prevention. (1996b, June 14). Guidelines for school health programs to promote lifelong healthy eating. *Morbidity and Mortality Weekly Report, 45*(RR-9), 4.

Centers for Disease Control and Prevention. (1996c, May 23). Tobacco use and usual source of cigarettes among high school students—United States, 1995. *Morbidity and Mortality Weekly Report, 45*(20), 413-414.

Flemming, P. (1996, March). *Youth and HIV/AIDS: An American agenda—A report to the president*. Washington, DC: National AIDS Policy Office.

Friedman, H. (1993). Promoting the health of adolescents in the United States of America: A global perspective. *Journal of Adolescent Health, 14*, 509-519.

Gans, J. E. (1990). *America's adolescents: How healthy are they?* (Profiles of adolescent health series). Chicago: American Medical Association.

Gans, J. E., & Shook, K. L. (Eds.). (1994a). *Policy compendium on tobacco, alcohol, and other harmful substances affecting adolescents: Alcohol and other harmful substances*. Chicago: American Medical Association.

Gans, J. E., & Shook, K. L. (Eds.). (1994b). *Policy compendium on violence and adolescents: Intentional injury and abuse*. Chicago: American Medical Association.

Hamburg, D. A. (1992). *Today's children: Creating a future for a generation in crisis*. New York: Random House.

Kann, L., Warren, C. W., Harris, W. A., Collins, J. L., Douglas, K. A., Collins, M. E., Williams, B. I., Ross, J. G., & Kolbe, L. J. (1995, March 24). Youth risk behavior surveillance—United States, 1993. In CDC Surveillance Summaries, *Morbidity and Mortality Weekly Report, 44*(SS-1), 1-17.

Marcus, S. E., Giovino, G. A., Pierce, J. P., & Harel, Y. (1993). Measuring tobacco use among adolescents. *Public Health Reports, 108*, 20-24.

Metzler, C. W., Noell, J., Biglan, A., Ary, D., & Smolkowski, K. (1994). The social context for risky sexual behavior among adolescents. *Journal of Behavioral Medicine, 17*, 419-437.

Miller, C. A. (1996). Editorial: A contract on America's children. *American Journal of Public Health, 86*, 473-474.

National Adolescent Health Information Center. (1995a, May). *Adolescent pregnancy prevention: Effective strategies* (Division of Adolescent Medicine & Institute for Health Policy Studies: 1-4). San Francisco: Author.

National Adolescent Health Information Center. (1995b, June). *Fact sheet on adolescent demographics*. San Francisco: Author.

U.S. Bureau of the Census. (1992). *Census of population and housing: Vol. 17*. Washington, DC: Government Printing Office.

U.S. Department of Health and Human Services, Substance Abuse and Mental Health Services Administration, Center for Mental Health Services. (1996, March 14). *Major depression in children and adolescents: Fact sheet. Caring for every child's mental health: Communities together*. Washington, DC: Author.

Waxweiler, R. J., Harel, Y., & O'Carroll, P. (1993). Measuring adolescent behaviors related to unintentional injuries. *Public Health Reports, 108*, 25-30.

2

2

Preventing Unintentional Adolescent Injury

Esha Bhatia

The Adolescent Injury Problem in the United States

Deaths

Injury is the leading cause of death, hospital admission, emergency department visits, and emergency medical transport for adolescents in the United States (Schwarz, 1993). About 60% of injury-related deaths among all teenagers are unintentional (National Center for Health Statistics, 1994). These are deaths from traffic crashes (car, bicycle, pedestrian, motorcycle, etc.), from sports and other recreational activities, from working, from unintentional use of firearms, from drownings, poisonings, and from fires and burns. For youth ages 10 to 14, unintentional injury accounts for nearly three out of every four injury deaths; for 15- to 19-year-olds, unintentional injury accounts for just over half (56%) of all injury deaths (see Table 2.1). In 1991 alone, 8,856 adolescents ages 10 to 19 died as a result of unintentional injury. For 10- to 14-year-olds, deaths occur primarily as motor vehicle passengers, pedestrians, or bicyclists and from drowning and unintentional firearm injuries. For 15- to 19-year-olds, deaths occur mostly as drivers and passengers and from drowning and unintentional firearm injuries.

Nonfatal Injuries

Deaths are only part of the picture; nonfatal injuries must also be considered. For teenagers ages 13 to 19, there are 41 hospitalizations and 1,132 emergency department visits for every injury death (Gallagher, Finison, Guyer, & Goodenough, 1984). Two major causes of nonfatal injury for adolescents are sports injuries and work-related injuries.

In 1991, an estimated 10.4 million youth ages 10 to 19 required inpatient or outpatient treatment at a hospital because of an unintentional injury. The majority of nonfatal injuries consist of lacerations, contusions, and sprains, fractures, or dislocations to the upper and lower extremities. More serious injuries include traumatic brain injuries and injuries to the chest, trunk, abdomen, and pelvis.

The location of the injury varies by age. For 10- to 14-year-olds, nonfatal injuries occur mostly in outdoor areas, at school, or at home. For 15- to 19-year-olds, however, these injuries occur most often at work, in a motor ve-

TABLE 2.1. Leading Causes of Injury Fatalities in 1991 for Adolescents Ages 10 to 14 and 15 to 19

	10- to 14-year-olds		15- to 19-year-olds	
Cause of Death	Deaths	Rate[a]	Deaths	Rate[a]
Motor vehicle occupant	496	2.8	3,574	21.4
Pedestrian	258	1.5	363	2.1
Bicycle	150	0.8	73	0.4
Other motor vehicle	172	1.0	1,259	7.3
Drowning	223	1.3	453	2.6
Fire/burns	119	0.7	106	0.6
Unintentional firearm	162	0.9	324	1.9
Poisoning	42	0.2	175	1.0
Falls	48	0.3	84	0.5

SOURCE: National Center for Health Statistics, 1994.
a. Rates are deaths per 100,000 population

hicle, outdoors, and then at home and school (Lescohier & Gallagher, 1996).

Sports-Related Injuries

Sports-related injuries among children and adolescents account for 2.5 million emergency department visits and 100,000 hospitalizations annually (Davis, Kuppermann, & Fleisher, 1993). Sports are the most common cause of nonfatal injury in male and female adolescents ages 13 to 19 years (Davis et al., 1993). Forty-four percent of injuries sustained by students 14 years of age and older are caused by sports activity (Stanitski, DeLee, & Drez, 1994).

Organized team sports—football, basketball, and baseball—and roller-skating account for the largest proportion of sports injuries to teens (see Table 2.2); however, nonorganized or individual activities such as soccer, ice

TABLE 2.2. Major Causes of Sports Injuries to Adolescents

Activity	Percentage of Total Sports Injuries
Football	20
Basketball	17.4
Roller-skating	13.4
Baseball	9.4

SOURCE: Gallagher, 1993.

hockey, sledding, skiing, horseback riding, skateboarding, and track and field have a higher ratio of injuries that require hospital admission, such as concussion (Gallagher, 1993).

Most sports injuries (42%) are the result of falls, being hit by an object (28%), or overexertion (10%) (Lescohier & Gallagher, 1996). Most often, the injuries are fractures of the extremities. Hospitalizations for sports injuries account for 16% of all injury discharges with an average length of stay of 3.8 days (Lescohier & Gallagher, 1996).

Work-Related Injuries

The U.S. Department of Labor estimates that 4 million children in the United States are legally employed. At minimum, an additional 22,000 children work illegally (Butterfield, 1990). In general, U.S. child labor laws permit employment of children as young as 14 years of age, except in manufacturing, mining, and certain other occupations considered hazardous (where employment is banned for youth less than 16 years of age). Many jobs involving hazardous equipment such as use of slicing machines, baking, and commercial driving are restricted to youth 18 years of age and older. Children as young as 12 may be employed on any farm with the consent of the parent.

Work is a significant cause of nonfatal injury among adolescents. According to the National Institute for Occupation Health and Safety (NIOSH) at the CDC, each year about 70 adolescents die from injuries at work, hundreds more are hospitalized, and tens of thousands require treatment in hospital emergency rooms (U.S. Department of Health and Human Services, 1995a).

About 64,000 teenagers ages 14 to 17 were treated for work-related injuries in hospital emergency departments in 1992 (Layne, Castillo, Stout, & Cutlip, 1994). It is estimated that only one third of work-related injuries are treated in emergency departments, suggesting that about 200,000 adolescents suffer work-related injuries annually (U.S. Department of Health and Human Services, 1995a). The most common injuries to working youth are lacerations, contusions and abrasions, sprains and strains, burns, and fractures or dislocations (Layne et al., 1994). From 1980 through 1989 (see Table 2.3), the leading causes of work-related death among 16- and 17-year-olds included motor vehicles (24%), machines (17%; two thirds from agricultural machines), and electrocution (12%) (Castillo, Landen, & Layne, 1994).

In one study, 68% of 14- to 16-year-olds who sustained work-related injuries experienced limitations in their normal activities (including work, school, and play) for at least a day, and 25% experienced limitation for more than a week. More than half of these adolescents said that they had not received any training in how to prevent the injury and that a supervisor was present at the time of the injury only one fifth of the time (U.S. Department of Health and Human Services, 1995a).

There are also other health concerns for adolescent workers, related to exposure to hazardous materials and working conditions—for example, exposure to pesticides in farm work and lawn care, benzene at gas stations, lead in auto body repair, asbestos and silica in construction and maintenance work, and high noise levels in manufacturing, construction, and agriculture (U.S. Department of Health and Human Services, 1995a).

Background/Causes

Adolescents and Risk Taking

As children move from early to late adolescence, their mortality rate increases by 214% (Irwin, 1993). This increase is largely due to intentional (violence and suicide) and unintentional injuries. The rate of death from motor vehicle injuries increases by 386% and other unintentional injuries increase 75% between early and late adolescence (Irwin, 1993).

In early adolescence, teens begin to engage in a variety of behaviors that have a high probability of negative outcome—in this case, injury. Teens are less likely to use safety belts and other safety devices/protective equipment, such as helmets for in-line skating, skateboarding, and bicycling. Teens are also likely to engage in other risk-taking behaviors such as driving at high speeds, using skateboards and in-line skates recklessly, running red lights, and substance abuse (see below). The CDC's Youth Risk Behavior Surveillance System (YRBSS) reports that in 1991, only 28% of high school students said they "always" used safety belts. About 39% of high school students who rode motorcycles reported that they always wore motorcycle helmets. Among students who rode bicycles, only 1% reported that they always wore bicycle helmets. About 82% of high school students reported that they had drunk alcohol in their lifetime, with 51% reporting alcohol use in the previous 30 days. About 31% of high school students consumed five or more alcoholic drinks on at least one occasion in the previous 30 days (U.S. Department of Health and Human Services, 1992b).

TABLE 2.3. Work Associated With Large Numbers of Deaths and Serious Injuries

Kind of Work	Risk of Death and Injury
Working in or around motor vehicles • Delivering passengers and goods • Routine travel to provide home-based services such as cable repair, landscaping, appliance repair • Residential trash pickup • Road maintenance • Work at road construction sites • Work at gas stations, truck stops, and auto repair shops	Motor vehicle-related deaths accounted for 25% of job-related deaths to 16- or 17-year-olds, 1980-1989 (Castillo et al., 1994)
Operating tractors and other heavy equipment • Tractors used in farm and non-farm settings such as construction • Forklifts • Excavating machinery such as backhoes, bulldozers, steam and power shovels, and trenchers • Loaders such as bucket loaders, end loaders, and front-end loaders • Road grading and surfacing machinery such as asphalt and mortar spreaders, graders, levelers, planers, scrapers, road linemarking machinery, steam rollers, and road pavers	Machine-related deaths were the second leading cause of work-related injury death for 16- to 17-year-olds, 1980-1989 (Castillo et al., 1994)
Working near electrical hazards • Using poles, pipes, and ladders near overhead power lines during construction work, painting, and pool cleaning • Working on roofs to perform jobs such as roofing, roof maintenance, cleaning of rain gutters, installation and repair of heating and cooling equipment, installation and repair of television antennas, and cleaning of chimneys and smokestacks • Operating or contacting boomed vehicles such as bucket trucks, telescopic forklifts, and telescopic cranes • Using grain augers and moving grain elevators and irrigation pipes near power lines • Tree trimming • Wiring of electrical circuits and other work involving exposure to electrical circuitry	Electrocution was the third leading cause of work-related injury death for 16- to 17-year-olds, 1980-1989 (Castillo et al., 1994)
Working at jobs with a high risk for homicide • Working alone or in small numbers in businesses where money is exchanged with the public, for example, convenience stores, gas stations, restaurants, hotels, and motels • Working alone in contact with large numbers of people where there may be opportunities for uninterrupted assaults; for example, motel housekeeping, delivery of passengers or goods, and door-to-door sales	In 1993, assaults and violent acts accounted for one fourth of all work-related injury deaths of adolescents. Most work-related homicides are associated with robbery.
Working with fall hazards • Using ladders and scaffolds to work at heights, such as in construction, building maintenance, painting, and fruit harvesting • Working on structures or near openings in building construction • Working on roofs • Tree trimming	Falls were the fifth leading cause of work-related injury death for 16- to 17-year-olds, 1980-1989 (Castillo et al., 1994)

TABLE 2.3. *Continued*

Kind of Work	Risk of Death and Injury
Cooking and working around cooking appliances • Cooking in restaurants and other commercial settings • Servicing cooking equipment • Working near cooking appliances where workers may slip into or against equipment	Severe burns are a risk for adolescents involved in cooking. About 5,200 adolescents sought emergency room treatment for work-related burns associated with cooking from July 1992 through December 1993.
Hazardous manual lifting • Working in warehouses • Delivering furniture and appliances • Retrieving, carrying, or stocking shelves with heavy items • Working in health care settings where patients are lifted and moved • Installing or removing carpet or tile • Baling hay	From July 1992 to December 1993, adolescents were treated in hospital emergency rooms for 4,500 work-related injuries due to exertion. More than half of these injuries were attributed to lifting.
Other hazardous work • Working in petroleum and gas extraction • Commercial fishing • Many jobs that require the use of respirators • Working in sewers or sewage treatment plants • Working on industrial conveyors • Using compressed air or pneumatic tools such as nail guns • Using all-terrain vehicles in farm work • Working around many types of machines with power takeoffs or similarly rotating drivelines	Many especially hazardous jobs are prohibited by federal child labor laws. There are, however, other hazardous occupations that are not prohibited.

NOTE: Except as noted, source of information is U.S. Department of Health and Human Services, 1995a.

Other Developmental Factors

An important factor in the high number of motor vehicle-related deaths and injuries is adolescents' inexperience in operating vehicles. Teenage drivers take longer to perceive and respond to dangerous situations (Hingson & Howland, 1993) and are less likely than older drivers to know how to respond to unexpected driving conditions such as icy road conditions.

Teenage drivers perceive their risk of being in a crash as being lower than do older drivers. They view behaviors associated with a higher risk of crash involvement, such as driving in darkness, driving in rural areas, and driving on curved roads, as being less risky than do older drivers. Teenage drivers may also be overconfident about their skills and are less likely than older drivers to view safety measures, such as using lights during daylight hours

and lower blood alcohol concentration (BAC) limits for younger drivers, as helping to reduce serious crashes (Hingson & Howland, 1993).

Alcohol Use

Alcohol-related motor vehicle injuries are the leading cause of unintentional injury mortality for late adolescents. Alcohol is also a risk factor for many other unintentional injuries, including those from water sports, fires, falls, bicycles, skateboards, and other recreational activities.

Adolescents are at an especially high risk for injury involving alcohol. Among youths ages 16 to 20, 20% of drivers and 34% of pedestrians killed in fatal crashes during 1991 were legally intoxicated (U.S. Department of Transportation, 1992). In addition, 40% to 50% of young males who drowned had used alcohol prior to drowning (U.S. Department of Health and Human Services, 1992a).

All states and the District of Columbia have laws that establish the minimum drinking age at 21 years. The National Highway Traffic Safety Administration (NHTSA) estimates that these laws have reduced by 13% the number of traffic fatalities involving drivers ages 18 to 20 years and have saved about 12,360 lives since 1975 (U.S. Department of Transportation, 1992). These laws have also been linked to reductions in other types of unintentional injury and to decreases in alcohol-related suicides (Jones, Pieper, & Robertson, 1992).

Other Factors

Societal Attitudes

Despite the publicity given to alcohol-related fatalities, particularly those involving teenagers, many parents still maintain a permissive attitude toward alcohol use, often believing that alcohol is "not as bad as" other drugs and that alcohol use is a rite of passage for adolescents as they head toward adulthood.

Another factor is the belief that a teen who is old enough to obtain a driver's license should automatically be allowed to drive. Although this may relieve parents of the burden of transporting teens to and from their extracurricular activities and places of employment, it also means placing young, inexperienced drivers behind the wheel. Because of convenience, and/or the desire to give the adolescent increased responsibility, parents may not place any restrictions on the teen's driving hours or on the number of other teens he or she can have in the car, and they may not reinforce the importance of safety belt use.

Parents may not have adequate information about the teen's place of employment and the requirements that it makes of the adolescent worker. They may also be unaware of the provisions of existing child labor laws and that

certain types of jobs and job-related activities may be illegal for younger adolescents.

Parents, along with coaches and trainers, may encourage adolescents involved in school sports activities, particularly at a competitive level, to continue participating in these activities even while injured or fatigued, placing the teen at higher risk for injury. In addition, parents may encourage adolescents to participate in the more high-risk contact sports such as football. Coaches, trainers, school nurses, and others involved in school sports may not be aware of the frequency of sports-related injuries and effective prevention strategies. As a result, students may be participating in sports activities without the benefit of pre-participation physical examinations, proper conditioning and strength-building, use of appropriate safety equipment, adequate supervision and management of athletes, and adequate rehabilitation after injury.

Financial Considerations

Adolescents may lack the financial resources to purchase vehicles with state-of-the-art safety devices such as airbags and antilock braking systems. In addition, they may not have the funds to maintain their vehicles adequately and thus keep them in safe operating condition. This lack of funds may also affect their ability to purchase safety equipment such as helmets.

The expectation that adolescents earn money also means that adolescents may be driving or bicycling after dark, placing them at higher risk for injury. Furthermore, this expectation may make adolescents reluctant to question unsafe work practices for fear of losing their source of income.

Healthy Youth 2000 National Health Promotion and Disease Prevention Objectives for Adolescents

The American Medical Association's Healthy Youth 2000: National Health Promo-

TABLE 2.4. Healthy Youth 2000 Goals for Unintentional Injury Prevention

Objective Number	Objective	Baseline
9.3b	Reduce deaths among youth ages 15 through 24 caused by motor vehicle crashes to no more than 33 per 100,000 people	36.9 per 100,000 people in 1987
9.5	Reduce drowning deaths to no more than 1.3 per 100,000 people	Age-adjusted baseline: 2.1 per 100,000 people in 1987
	Special population targets	
	Men ages 15 to 34: reduce deaths to no more than 2.5 per 100,000 people	4.5 per 100,000 people in 1987
	Black males: reduce deaths to no more than 3.6 per 100,000 people	6.6 per 100,000 people in 1987
9.10	Reduce nonfatal spinal cord injuries so that hospitalizations for this condition are no more than 5.0 per 100,000 people	5.9 per 100,000 people in 1988
	Note: Adolescents ages 15 to 24 are at highest risk of spinal cord injuries, which result in life-long needs for special services and reduced potential for employment	
9.13	Increase use of helmets to at least 80% of motorcyclists and at least 50% of bicyclists	60% of motorcyclists in 1988 and an estimated 8% of bicyclists in 1984

tion and Disease Prevention Objectives for Adolescents (American Medical Association, 1990; excerpted from U.S. Department of Health and Human Services, 1991) lists four objectives that relate specifically to unintentional adolescent injury (see Table 2.4).

In addition, there are several National Health Promotion and Disease Prevention Objectives (U.S Department of Health and Human Services, 1995b) that have relevance for planning adolescent injury prevention activities (see Table 2.5) even though they are not targeted specifically to teens.

Injuries Are Not Accidents: We Can Prevent Them

Unintentional adolescent injuries are preventable. By better understanding the risk factors for each type of injury, we can develop programs and strategies that can reduce the incidence of the injury and/or the severity of any injury sustained. Injury control focuses on minimizing the impact of injury on a population group—in this case, adolescents. It encompasses

TABLE 2.5. National Health Promotion and Disease Prevention Objectives

Objective Number	Objective	Baseline
10.2f	Reduce work-related injuries to adolescent workers resulting in medical treatment, lost time from work, or restricted work activity to no more than 3.8 cases per 100,000 full-time workers	5.8 cases per 100,000 full-time workers in 1992
4.1b	Reduce deaths to people ages 15 to 24 caused by alcohol-related motor vehicle crashes to no more than 12.5 per 100,000 people	21.5 per 100,000 people in 1987

Prevention: preventing, reducing, or modifying hazards or events that can cause injury, for example, reducing the risk of head injury in a motorcycle crash (the "event") by mandating motorcycle helmet use.

Acute care: minimizing the damage done by the hazard or event by stabilizing and repairing the damage, for example, by training paramedics and emergency medical technicians in how to respond to the special medical needs of injured children and adolescents.

Rehabilitation: restoring function to the injured person, for example, by providing an injured person with physical therapy.

A comprehensive approach to injury prevention involves the three E's of injury prevention: Education, Enactment/enforcement, and Engineering. This translates into three main approaches to preventing adolescent injury:

Education: persuading people to change behaviors that put adolescents at risk, for example, through educational programs encouraging employers of teenage workers to obey child labor laws.

Enactment/enforcement: requiring behavior change by regulation or legislation, for example, by passing a zero tolerance law making it illegal for anyone under 21 to drive with any measurable amount of alcohol in his or her blood.

Engineering: providing automatic protection via product and environmental design and redesign, for example, by redesigning equipment to eliminate features that are unsafe for adolescent workers.

Historically, many injury prevention programs focused only on the first E, education. In most cases, however, significant improvements in the safety of children were not achieved without the expansion of the program to include enactment/enforcement and engineering components. One example is the North Carolina Child Passenger Safety Program (National Committee for Injury Prevention and Control, 1989).

Phase 1: Education. In 1977, the State Governor's Highway Safety Program began allocating funds for the University of North Carolina Highway Safety Research Center to educate the public about child passenger and motor vehicle safety. These activities were associated with a small decrease in death rates of child motor vehicle occupants and a 6% increase in safety seat usage rates (from 5% to 11%) for children involved in crashes from 1978 to 1981.

Phase 2: Education and engineering. In 1980, the Highway Safety Research Center began receiving additional state funds, which were used to develop child safety seat rental programs. By 1984, the number of these programs in North Carolina had increased from 10 to 125. The Highway Safety Research Center also established a toll-free hotline to answer questions about child safety seat use and to refer parents to local rental programs. Written materials were also distributed throughout the state.

Phase 3: Education, engineering, and enactment/enforcement. The program's limited impact on child safety seat usage rates led to the passage of a statewide child passenger safety law in 1982. Public education efforts were stepped up in conjunction with the law taking effect in July 1982. Between July 1982 and December 1984 child safety seat usage rates jumped from 30% to 70%.

In recent years, injury prevention programs have expanded to include public policy (enactment/enforcement) and engineering (technological/environmental) approaches in addition to education campaigns. A comprehensive program to reduce bicycle-related injury could look something like the one described in Table 2.6.

The same approach can be applied to any type of injury, for example, work-related inju-

TABLE 2.6. Model of a Comprehensive Program to Reduce Bicycle-Related Injury

Injury	Education	Enactment/Enforcement	Engineering
Bicycle-related injury	• Peer-to-peer education about bicycle-related injury in elementary, middle, and high school	• Passage of a bicycle helmet law requiring that everyone under age 21 wear a bicycle helmet when riding a bicycle	• A bicycle helmet giveaway program for low-income students
Bicycle skills-building rodeos held on school grounds		• Implementation of a school policy requiring that anyone riding a bicycle to school wear a helmet	• Building of bicycle paths to separate bicycle riders from motor vehicle traffic

ries. Here, specific risk factors can be used to develop an approach (see Table 2.7).

The remainder of this chapter will discuss strategies that schools, parents and teenagers, legislators and regulators, law enforcement, health care providers, and health departments and community agencies can implement to help reduce the number of adolescents killed and injured each year. Tools and resources to assist these groups in their activities are also discussed.

Taking Action

Strategies for Schools

Alcohol-Related Injuries

- Use school facilities to provide alcohol-free activities for teenagers in evening hours, particularly in the summer months.
- Work with the community to provide expanded public transportation opportunities for students, particularly during times of the

TABLE 2.7. Model of Comprehensive Approach to Reducing Work-Related Injuries

Factor	Education	Enactment/Enforcement	Engineering
Unsafe equipment	• Education of workers about safe and unsafe uses of equipment	• Increased penalties for employers who continue to use unsafe equipment • Implementation of an equipment inspection program • Regulations requiring that employees be trained on safe and unsafe uses of equipment	• Revised equipment design to eliminate features that are unsafe for adolescents
Exceeding maximum hours of employment	• Educating parents about child labor laws so they can monitor the number of hours that their children work	• Tightening penalties for employers who go over the maximum • Passing school policies about maximum numbers of hours worked on school nights	• Developing timecard programs keyed to age that automatically notify an employer if a teen exceeds the maximum hours of employment

school year when alcohol use may be more prevalent, such as during graduation.

- Provide training to school-based clinic and other school staff so that they can assess and refer students for alcohol and other drug use.

Unintentional Firearm Injuries

- Discuss the danger of firearms in the home with parents and adolescents.

Traffic-Related Injuries

- Require that students who bicycle or drive motorcycles or cars to school use appropriate safety equipment such as helmets and safety belts.
- Educate students and parents about traffic safety. Require that traffic safety instruction be a part of the curriculum.
- Work with helmet manufacturers, local and state SAFE KIDS coalitions, and other groups to provide inexpensive or free bicycle or other helmets to students.

Sports Injuries

- Provide participants with appropriate protective equipment.
- Require and provide instruction to participants and athletic teachers on how to minimize the risk of injury.
- Inspect and maintain playing fields and equipment such as soccer goals.
- Ensure that coaches and others supervising these activities are trained in injury prevention as well as in first aid and CPR.
- Ensure that each participant receives a thorough medical examination before participating and after any injuries and keep records on their health status. Don't allow students to participate in sports if they are currently using pain control for a previous injury.
- Implement adequate conditioning and training programs for participants.

Work-Related Injuries

- Ensure that anyone responsible for signing work permits knows the state and federal child labor laws.

- Talk to students about safety and health hazards in the workplace and students' rights and responsibilities as workers.
- Ensure that school-based work-experience programs (such as vocational education programs and School-to-Work programs) provide students with work experience in safe and healthful environments free of recognized hazards.
- Ensure that school-based work-experience programs incorporate information about workers' legal rights and responsibilities and training in hazard recognition and safe work practices.
- Consider incorporating information about workers' rights and responsibilities and occupational safety and health into high school and junior high curricula to prepare students for employment.

Strategies for Parents and Teenagers

- Treat driving as a privilege, not a right. Restrict adolescent's nighttime driving. Limit the number of passengers that the adolescent can have in the car. Suspend driving privileges for violations of rules such as not wearing a safety belt, breaking curfew, and drinking.
- Find out about the working conditions at teen's places of employment and monitor the number of hours that teens are working.
- Find out about teens' rights to work in safe and healthful work environments and about the right to refuse to work on unsafe tasks and under hazardous conditions.
- Ensure that teen workers know that they can file complaints with the U.S. Department of Labor if they feel their rights have been violated or their safety jeopardized.
- Ensure that teen workers know that they are entitled to workers' compensation if they become ill or injured on the job.
- Be clear that alcohol use is *not* permitted. Coordinate with other parents when parties are taking place to make sure no alcohol is allowed.
- Be sure teens understand that participating in sports activities while injured, sick, or ill is unsafe.
- Work with other teens to promote passage of a bicycle helmet law and to enforce motorcycle helmet laws.

- Educate younger teens about the dangers of alcohol and other substance use.
- Turn over any firearms kept in the home to a police department that melts firearms down. If firearms are kept in the home ensure that the firearms are kept unloaded and locked up separately from the ammunition. An easily accessible gun may put a teenager or other family member in danger.

Strategies for Legislators/Regulators

Zero Tolerance for Youth

It is illegal in every state for anyone under the age of 21 to purchase and be in public possession of alcoholic beverages. It should also be illegal for anyone under age 21 to drive if they have been drinking. A zero tolerance law makes it illegal for anyone under 21 to drive with any measurable amount of alcohol in their blood. As of September 1995, 27 states and the District of Columbia had set the BAC limit at .02 or lower for drivers under age 21. These laws work: an evaluation of the 0.02 law in Maryland showed an 11% decrease in the number of drivers under 21 involved in crashes who had been drinking (U.S. Department of Transportation, 1995). A study of the laws in Maine, New Mexico, North Carolina, and Wisconsin revealed a 34% decline in fatal adolescent nighttime crashes after the zero tolerance laws were implemented (U.S. Department of Transportation, 1995).

To be effective, a zero tolerance law should allow a police officer to require a breath test from a driver under the age of 21 if the officer has probable cause to believe that the driver has been drinking. These laws are needed because in 1993 alone, more than 2,300 youths ages 15 to 20 died in alcohol-related crashes. Younger drivers who have been drinking are at risk for fatal crashes at a lower BAC than older, more experienced drivers. Research suggests that zero tolerance laws leading to the loss of a driver's license can reduce alcohol-related deaths.

Graduated Driver Licensing System

States can implement a graduated driver licensing system that eases young drivers into the driving environment through more controlled exposure to progressively more difficult driving experiences or licensing states prior to full licensure.

Young drivers are twice as likely as adult drivers to be in fatal crashes because of driving inexperience and lack of adequate driving skills, excessive driving during nighttime high-risk hours, risk-taking, and poor driving judgment and decision making. The crash rate per mile for drivers 15 to 20 years of age is 20 times as high as for adults. States with nighttime driving restrictions or curfews for young novice drivers experience lower crash rates than comparison states.

To address these problems, the National Highway Traffic Safety Administration (NHTSA) and the American Association of Motor Vehicle Administrators (AAMVA) developed an entry level driver licensing system that consists of three stages: learner's permit, intermediate (provisional) license, and full license.

Each stage has recommended components and restrictions for states to consider when implementing a graduated licensing system that deals with number of people allowed in the car, restricted driving hours, and skills development.

Evaluations have shown the benefit of this system. California had a 5% reduction in crashes for drivers ages 15 to 17 (U.S. Department of Transportation, 1992), and Maryland experienced a 5% reduction in crashes and a 10% reduction in convictions for drivers ages 16 to 17 (U.S. Department of Transportation, 1992).

Motor Vehicle Injuries

Make all safety belt laws primary laws so that someone can be stopped for not wearing a safety belt. Currently, many safety belt laws are secondary laws: Someone can be ticketed for not wearing a safety belt only if the car is first stopped for some other traffic violation.

Unintentional Firearm Injuries

- Require police agencies to melt down firearms that have been confiscated or decommissioned rather than sell them.
- Establish strict licensing and storage standards for gun manufacturers, sellers, and owners.
- Establish criminal penalties for adult gun owners whose unsafe firearm storage methods result in death, injury, or firearms being taken to school.
- Mandate safety features for guns such as trigger locks and loading indicators.

Work-Related Injuries

- Pass state child labor laws that decrease the maximum hours of employment and have stiffer penalties for employers who break the law.

Strategies for Law Enforcement

- Police and the courts can implement well-publicized enforcement of laws related to driving while drinking, safety belt use, speed limits, alcohol sales to minors, and so on.
- Judges and police officers can serve as community resources for health educators and others seeking to educate adolescents and their families about injury prevention.

Strategies for Health Care Providers

- Assess and refer adolescents for alcohol and other drug use.
- Counsel adolescents and parents about injury risks. Be aware of the laws in your state. Is there a zero tolerance law or are there lower BAC limits for youth? What age groups are covered?
- Counsel parents about the safe storage of firearms kept in the home.
- Educate policymakers about legislative strategies to discourage alcohol use by youth under age 21 and to reduce the number killed and injured in alcohol-related crashes, such as zero tolerance laws and stiffer penalties

for stores that sell alcohol to youth under 21. Support lower BAC levels for youth and work with state highway safety offices to promote zero tolerance. Communicate support of these laws to the governor and state legislature. Health care professionals make compelling witnesses at hearings. Remind them of the financial costs to society of impaired driving.
- Encourage police to promote and enforce zero tolerance laws and use-lose and under 21 laws. Communicate the message that the community supports laws to prevent underage drinking and driving.

Strategies for Health Departments and Community Agencies

- Work with other agencies to prevent alcohol sales to youth under age 21. For example, in Alaska, staff at the Anchorage Health Department coordinated with police and others to:
  — Develop criteria for evaluating applications for permits to sell alcohol on municipal property
  — Establish procedures for formal review by the health department and other agencies of all applications for permits to sell alcohol in a public place
  — Enforce the existing ordinance banning the sale of alcohol in public places and delete the provision allowing this ordinance to be waived
  — Persuade nonprofit organizations that hold fund-raising events to look for sponsorship from soft drink manufacturers and other companies rather than beer manufacturers
Work with others to restrict the number of alcohol outlets and the manner in which they operate.
- Restrict alcohol advertising on state university campuses.
- Prohibit alcohol advertising on public transportation.
- Prohibit alcohol advertising within 2,000 feet of schools.
- Coordinate with other agencies that have jurisdiction over alcohol, such as the parks and recreation department, local zoning board,

and alcohol beverage licensing authority, to monitor the sale of alcohol to communities.

- Help hospitals develop alcohol data collection systems and analyze the collected data. Health departments can bring people together to facilitate linking alcohol, injury, and medical cost data.
- Educate the public, particularly parents, about child labor laws and their limitations. This may help parents assess risks faced by their teens in their work environments. It may also create public pressure to strengthen these laws and their enforcement.
- Work with schools and employers, particularly those involved in school-to-work partnerships to ensure that comprehensive health and safety education is provided to participants and that health and safety language is added to any implementation plans for the federal School to Work Opportunities Act.
- Encourage better enforcement of child labor laws.
- Purchase helmets in bulk for giveaways or for sale at low prices.
- Educate the public, particularly parents, about safe storage of firearms kept in the home.
- Educate the media about injury prevention, and work with newspapers, radio, television, and other media to educate the public.
- Educate legislators and policymakers about injury prevention and the effectiveness of legislative approaches such as bicycle helmet laws.
- Educate health care providers about how to counsel adolescents and their parents about injury prevention, substance use, and prevention of unintentional firearm injuries.

Resources and Tools

Children's Safety Network (CSN)

A network of injury and violence prevention resource centers funded by the Maternal and Child Health Bureau, Health Resources and Services Administration, Public Health Service, U.S. Department of Health and Human Services.

CSN National Injury and Violence Prevention Resource Centers
Education Development Center, Inc.
55 Chapel Street
Newton, MA 02158-1060
(617) 969-7100

National Center for Education in Maternal and Child Health
2000 15th Street North
Suite 701
Arlington, VA 22201-2617
(703) 524-7802

CSN Rural Injury Prevention Resource Center
National Farm Medicine Center
1000 North Oak Avenue
Marshfield, WI 54449
(715) 387-9298

Adolescent Health Project at the National Center for Education in Maternal and Child Health
2000 15th Street, North, Suite 701
Arlington, VA 22201
(703) 524-7802/fax (703) 524-9335

Collects, develops, and disseminates information on adolescent health development, services, programs, and training materials in support of initiatives funded by the Maternal and Child Health Bureau. This project provides information, technical assistance, and resource referrals to local, state, and national agencies, health care providers and consumers, trainers of health care professionals, and researchers.

Zero Tolerance Resources

Mothers Against Drunk Driving
(214) 744-MADD

Remove Intoxicated Drivers
(518) 372-0034

Students Against Driving Drunk
(508) 481-3568

National Highway Traffic Safety Administration (NHTSA)
(202) 366-9588

Graduated Licensing Resources

National Highway Traffic Safety Administration (NHTSA)
(202) 366-9588

American Association of Motor Vehicle Administrators (AAMVA)
4200 Wilson Boulevard, Suite 1100
Arlington, VA 22203
Contact: Mike Calvin,
    Director of Driver Services,
    (703) 522-4200/
    fax (703) 522-1553

National Association of Independent Insurers (NAII)
2600 River Road
Des Plaines, IL 60018-3286
Contact Joe Anotti, (208) 297-7800/
    fax (708) 297-5064

Alcohol Resources

Manual for Community Planning to Prevent Problems With Alcohol Availability, by Friedner Wittman, Ph.D., and Patricia Shane, M.P.H., California State Department of Alcohol and Drug Programs. Available from:

Institute for the Study of Social Change
University of California at Berkeley
2232 Sixth Street
Berkeley, CA 94710
(510) 540-4717

Alcohol Use at Community Events: Creating Policies to Prevent Problems, developed by the University of California at San Diego. Available from:

Ava Gill
UC San Diego
0176-9500 Gilman Drive
La Jolla, CA 92093-0176

Surgeon General's Workshop on Drunk Driving: Proceedings. Available for loan from:

Librarian
National Center for Education in Maternal and Child Health
2000 15th Street North
Suite 701
Arlington, VA 22201-2617
(703) 524-7802/fax (703) 524-9335

Work-Related Injury Resources

U.S. Department of Labor
Employment Standards Administration
Wage and Hour Division
200 Constitution Avenue, NW,
    Room S3510
Washington, DC 20210
(202) 219-8305

Administers and enforces the Fair Labor Standards Act (FLSA) with respect to private sector and state and local government employment. FLSA's child labor provisions are designed to protect the education opportunities of minors and prohibit their employment in jobs that are harmful to their health and well-being. Some states also have their own child labor laws, typically these are enforced by state Department of Labor investigators.

Occupational Safety and Health Administration (OSHA)
U.S. Department of Labor
200 Constitution Avenue, NW
Washington, DC 20210
(202) 249-8148

The National Child Labor Committee
1501 Broadway, Suite 1111
New York, NY 10036
(212) 840-1801

Provides technical assistance, research, and public information in several areas: helping prepare youth for adulthood, preventing the exploitation of children and youth in the labor market, and improving health and education opportunities for the children of migrant farmworkers.

References

American Medical Association. (1990). *Healthy Youth 2000: National health promotion and disease prevention objectives for adolescents.* Chicago: Author.

Butterfield, B. D. (1990, April 22). Children at work. *The Boston Globe,* pp. 1-16.

Castillo, D. N., Landen, D. D., & Layne, L. A. (1994). Occupational injury deaths of 16- and 17-year-olds in the United States. *American Journal of Public Health, 84,* 646-649.

Davis, J. M., Kuppermann, N., & Fleisher, G. (1993). Serious sports injuries requiring hospitalizations seen in a pediatric emergency department. *American Journal of Diseases of Children, 147,* 1001-1004.

Gallagher, S. S. (1993). Massachusetts: A case study of how surveillance systems work. In *Injuries in youth: Surveillance strategies* (Workshop proceedings, NIH Publication No. 93-3444, pp. 33-39). Bethesda, MD: National Institutes of Health.

Gallagher, S. S., Finison, K., Guyer, B., & Goodenough, S. (1984). The incidence of injuries among 87,000 Massachusetts children and adolescents: Results of the 1980-1981 statewide injury prevention program surveillance system. *American Journal of Public Health, 74,* 1340-1347.

Hingson, R., & Howland, J. (1993). Promoting safety in adolescents. In S. G. Millstein, A. C. Petersen, & E. O. Nightingale (Eds.), *Promoting the health of adolescents: New directions for the twenty-first century.* New York: Oxford University Press.

Irwin, C. E. (1993). Adolescence and risk taking: How are they related? In N. J. Bell & R. W. Bell (Eds.), *Adolescent risk taking.* Newbury Park, CA: Sage.

Jones, N. E., Pieper, C. F., & Robertson, L. S. (1992). The effect of legal drinking age on fatal injuries of adolescents and young adults. *American Journal of Public Health, 82*(1), 112-115.

Layne, L. A., Castillo, D. N., Stout, N., & Cutlip, P. (1994). Adolescent occupational injuries requiring hospital emergency department treatment: A nationally representative sample. *American Journal of Public Health, 84*(4), 657-660.

Lescohier, I., & Gallagher, S. S. (1996). Unintentional injury. In R. J. DiClemente, W. B. Hansen, & L. E. Ponton (Eds.), *Handbook of adolescent health risk behavior.* New York: Plenum.

National Center for Health Statistics. (1994). Data from the National Vital Statistics System, compiled by L. A. Fingerhut per special request.

National Committee for Injury Prevention and Control. (1989). Injury prevention: Meeting the challenge. Published as a supplement to the *American Journal of Preventive Medicine, 5*(3). London: Oxford University Press.

Schwarz, D. (1993). Adolescent trauma: Epidemiologic approach. *Adolescent Medicine: State of the Art Reviews, 4,* 11-22.

Stanitski, C. L., DeLee, J. C., & Drez, D., Jr. (1994). *Pediatric and adolescent sports medicine.* Philadelphia: W. B. Saunders.

U.S. Department of Health and Human Services, Public Health Service. (1991). *Healthy Children 2000: National health promotion and disease prevention objectives related to mothers, infants, children, adolescents, and youth.* Washington, DC: Author.

U.S. Department of Health and Human Services. (1992a). *Youth and alcohol: Dangerous and deadly consequences.* Washington, DC: Author.

U.S. Department of Health and Human Services. (1992b). *1991 Youth Risk Behavior Surveillance System (YRBSS).* Atlanta, GA: Author.

U.S. Department of Health and Human Services. (1995a). *Alert: Request for assistance in preventing deaths and injuries to adolescent workers.* Atlanta, GA: Author.

U.S. Department of Health and Human Services. (1995b). *Healthy People 2000: Midcourse review and 1995 revisions.* Washington, DC: Author.

U.S. Department of Transportation. (1992). *1991 alcohol fatal crash facts.* Washington, DC: Author.

U.S. Department of Transportation. (1995). *State legislative fact sheet.* Washington, DC: Author.

3

Physical Activity and Fitness

Dixie Grimmett

As a group, adolescents are not in good physical condition. They have less muscle tone, poorer endurance, and a greater percentage of body fat than the previous generation. Despite research and data supporting the health benefits of physical activity, the public has been slow to embrace physical activity as a lifelong commitment. According to the 1996 U.S. Surgeon General's report on physical activity and health, physical activity declines dramatically with age during adolescence. Sadly, this is not a new phenomenon. Concerns about the physical fitness of our youth have had a great deal of attention, albeit episodically, throughout the 20th century.

When the United States entered World War I, thousands of young men, volunteers or draftees, were not able to pass their physical examinations. This shocked policymakers and was part of the impetus behind the initiation of mandatory physical education in our schools. When the United States entered World War II, the same phenomenon occurred. There were similar experiences in the Korean and Vietnam wars. Yet, none of these experiences has yielded a sustained national, state, and local effort to promote physical activity and fitness among youth.

The current condition of youth is influenced by even more sedentary lifestyles. At

home, work, and play, Americans find themselves in physically less demanding physical environments. Physical exertion has been substantially reduced in American lifestyles, contributing to the alarming development of a generation of youth with poor physical strength, flexibility, and endurance, as well as a greater percentage of body fat at younger ages. For most Americans, including physical exertion in their daily activities, even in the mildest form, is too much effort to sustain much beyond New Year's resolutions and required physical education at school. Unfortunately, most schools do not require physical education throughout the K to 12 years.

Nearly 50% of youth ages 12 to 21 years do not vigorously participate in physical activity on a regular basis (U.S. Department of Health & Human Services, 1996). Female adolescents are much less physically active than male adolescents. Among high school students, enrollment in daily physical education classes has dropped from 42% in 1991 to 25% in 1996. Only 19% of all high school students are physically active for 20 minutes or more in physical education classes every day during the school week.

Table 3.1 briefly summarizes the overall health benefits of habitual physical activity. What the table does not capture are the cumu-

TABLE 3.1. Benefits of Regular Physical Activity

Reduces risk of dying prematurely

Reduces the risk of dying from heart disease

Reduces the risk of developing diabetes

Reduces the risk of developing high blood pressure

Reduces the risk of colon cancer

Reduces feelings of depression and anxiety

Helps control weight

Helps build and maintain healthy bones, muscles, and joints

Promotes psychological well-being

Reduces risk of developing osteoporosis

SOURCE: U.S. Department of Health and Human Services, 1996.

lative benefits—to society, the economy, and the family—of a healthy population.

Definitions

Physical fitness has many meanings. People often think of physically fit individuals as those who excel in sports: basketball players, Olympic runners, bicycle racers, gymnasts, and the like. We would like to differentiate between sports and physical fitness. For men and women athletes, physical fitness makes it possible to participate and excel in their chosen sport. Sports involve both individual and team competition within a framework of rules. Over the years, many sports participants have discovered the benefits of becoming physically fit, or systematically improving fitness, to improve training for their sport and ultimately enhance competitive performance.

Rather than competition on the athletic field, physical fitness for adolescents, as well as the rest of the population, involves several important aspects of our physical functioning:

Cardiovascular endurance: The heart, lungs, and circulatory system need to be trained to maximize efficiency and effectiveness, to strengthen the heart muscle, and to help the lungs make maximum use of their breathing capacity.

Muscular strength and endurance: How much can one push, pull, and lift things, over what length of time? Muscles need to be used consistently to be able to exert the kind of force needed in our daily activities.

Flexibility: Bending, stretching, and moving muscles and joints sustains their entire range of motion. Without consistent movement, joints lose their flexibility with a consequent loss in the range of motion.

As you will see on the following pages, to be physically fit does not require following the regimen of elite competitive athletes. Rather, fitness is something we can achieve and sustain within the range of our normal everyday activities.

The remainder of this chapter will examine the historical background of physical activity and focus specially on the adolescent population. In addition, the components and benefits of daily activity will be discussed. Also, specific examples of the types and amount of activities that schools and community organizations can use in their programs for adolescents will be identified.

History

The Greeks were the first among the ancients to embrace the concept that physical activity contributed to the development of the whole individual. The need to defend their homelands inspired the development of a high degree of physical prowess among all cultures. The Greeks included other ideals, such as grace and beauty, in their definition of sports participation. The modern Olympic Games can be traced to the ancient Greeks and their sports festivals. Under the Roman influence, sport festivals became brutal spectacles, and there was an element of professionalism in their competitions.

The Middle Ages reflected little progress beyond the contribution of the Greeks and Romans. During the centuries that followed, however, play and exercise began to be regarded as beneficial because of health values. To a great degree, the economy and social life of all civilizations depended upon strength, flexibility, and endurance. Activities that promoted physical fitness were part of daily life.

Daily life was a struggle throughout history, as it is for the majority of the world's population today. Threats from the lack of food, or its contamination, plus physical dangers from climate, work, and even home had a profound impact on longevity and health status. For example, it was only at the beginning of the 20th century that U.S. life expectancy exceeded 50 years, on average.

Compared to European countries, the United States lagged in the development of a physical education system for public schools during the 1800s. By 1900 and the onset of World War I, the United States placed more emphasis on games and sports rather than the European calisthenics type of training. The U.S. concept of using games and sports for physical development spread to school programs with the same emphasis.

During the Depression years, physical education in schools was deemphasized and, in many cases, eliminated completely. With the advent of World War II, many new training programs appeared and new physical fitness developments were supported through systematic research efforts. Despite the virtual universal participation in the war effort, there was little sustained residual effect on American society once the war concluded. Once again, physical education in school reverted to an emphasis on simple games and some sports.

In 1953, the publication of Hans Kraus and R. P. Hirshland's research comparing fitness levels of American and European children renewed interest in physical fitness. The comparative weakness of American children aroused the public and generated a resurgence of the fitness movement. Physical fitness was associated no longer with preparation for war, but with health benefits.

The creation of the President's Council on Physical Fitness in the 1960s, during the Kennedy administration, resulted in the development of systematic physical fitness testing in public schools throughout the nation. Nevertheless, in recent years, there has been a decline in physical education requirements and participation in America's schools. This occurred despite numerous research reports and policy statements calling for renewed efforts to improve the fitness of American youth.

With the publication *Physical Activity and Health* (U.S. Department of Health and Human Services, 1996), a renewed emphasis on physical fitness for youth in American society may be upon us. Although the life expectancies of today's youth will most certainly continue to increase, it is quite possible that they will not be able to fully enjoy the benefits of a long life. Today's challenge to all who participate in the lives of youth is to develop physical activities that are fun to do and will lead to fitness.

Being Physically Fit in Contemporary Society: A Challenge

The problems noted above, such as youth who are heavier and fatter than the previous generation, are genuine public health issues requiring thoughtful and coordinated efforts to resolve. Many societal changes are thought to contribute to the current concern over the fitness levels of youth. These include the following:

- Lack of physical challenges in the lives of youth
- Diets, including total caloric intake, fats, and simple sugars
- More demands on time, leaving less discretionary time
- Youth fitness activities typically thought to be in the context of organized sports

- Changing family structures, with a substantial number of latchkey kids
- Less time for play, with leisure time spent in sedentary pursuits such as video games
- Concern over personal safety, keeping kids indoors after school
- Socioeconomic status, which inhibits planned as well as unplanned physical activity
- Decreased time in the school day for exercise, and many physical education classes that are too large, making effective instruction difficult
- Difficulty in establishing habitual physical activity as part of lifestyle: physical exertion as a negative phenomenon
- Perception that physical fitness means participation in a competitive individual or team sport
- Lack of access to parks, recreational areas, and sidewalks
- Residual negative feelings toward exercise from prior school or organized sport experiences, that is, exercise as punishment
- School and work patterns that limit participation, such as students being bused across town for school, which inhibits their participation in unorganized and organized after-school activities.

Prevention and Promotion Goals

The challenges to helping youth develop a physically fit lifestyle can be seen as daunting. Nevertheless, progress cannot be measured by attempting to eliminate or reduce all of these barriers to fitness. Many are impervious to individual effort. Rather, the focus should be on working with youth, families, and communities to improve opportunities for recreation and play among children and to promote fitness through examples set by those who participate in the lives of our youth: parents, other family members, friends, school authorities, community organization leaders, and church leaders.

In recognizing some of the problems listed above, the Surgeon General's report, *Healthy People 2000* (U.S. Department of Health and Human Services, 1991), developed fitness objectives for the nation. Table 3.2 presents objectives created for youth in the publication *Healthy Children 2000.*

To achieve these objectives, youth and adults must participate in habitual moderate physical activity on a daily basis. This does not mean that an individual has to join a gym or purchase expensive clothing and shoes to prepare to run in a 10-kilometer race or a marathon. The emphasis is on moderate physical activity that the individual finds enjoyable and that fits into daily life. The amount of activity is a function of duration, intensity, and frequency. Benefits can accrue from longer sessions of moderate activities, such as brisk walking, as well as shorter sessions of more strenuous activities.

Examples of moderate amounts of activity from the Surgeon General's report on Physical Activity and Health, which will lead to fitness, include the following:

Washing and waxing a car for 45 to 60 minutes
Washing windows or floors for 45 to 60 minutes
Playing volleyball for 45 minutes
Playing touch football for 30 to 45 minutes
Gardening for 30 to 45 minutes
Wheeling self in wheelchair for 30 to 45 minutes
Walking 1 3/4 miles in 35 minutes (20 minutes per mile)
Basketball (shooting baskets) for 30 minutes
Bicycling 5 miles in 30 minutes
Dancing fast (social) for 30 minutes
Pushing a stroller 1 1/2 miles in 30 minutes
Raking leaves for 30 minutes
Walking 2 miles in 30 minutes (15 minutes per mile)
Water aerobics for 30 minutes
Swimming laps for 20 minutes
Wheelchair basketball for 20 minutes
Basketball (playing a game) for 15 to 20 minutes
Bicycling 4 miles in 15 minutes
Jumping rope for 15 minutes
Running 1 1/2 miles in 15 minutes (10 minutes per mile)
Shoveling snow for 15 minutes
Stairwalking for 15 minutes

TABLE 3.2. Healthy People 2000 Fitness Goals for Youth

Objective Number	Objective
1.3	Increase to at least 30% the proportion of people age 7 and older who engage regularly, preferably daily, in light to moderate physical activity for at least 30 minutes per day
1.4	Increase to at least 20% the proportion of people age 18 and older and to at least 75% the proportion of children and adolescents ages 6 through 17 who engage in vigorous physical activity that promotes the development and maintenance of cardiorespiratory fitness 3 or more days per week for 20 or more minutes per occasion
1.5	Reduce to no more than 15% the proportion of people age 6 and older who engage in no leisure-time physical activity
1.6	Increase to at least 40% the proportion of people age 6 and older who regularly perform physical activities that enhance and maintain muscular strength, muscular endurance, and flexibility
1.7	Increase to at least 50% the proportion of overweight people age 12 and older who have adopted sound dietary practices with regular physical activity to attain an appropriate body weight
1.8	Increase to at least 50% the proportion of children and adolescents in 1st through 12th grade who participate in daily school physical education
1.9	Increase to at least 50% the proportion of school physical education class time that students spend being physically active, preferably engaged in lifetime physical activities

U.S. Department of Health and Human Services, 1991.

Prevention and Intervention Strategies

Given the conditions that have helped create the fitness problems described above, the task of developing successful interventions is daunting. Much needs to be done to develop a culture that prizes physical activity as a daily part of our lives. As a nation, we are fortunate to have a large cadre of specialists in physical fitness, exercise, sports, medicine, and public health. Many of these experts are in our communities working in school settings, youth-serving organizations such as the YMCA, corporate fitness programs, sports programs, and gyms and workout centers. Most colleges and universities have academic programs in physical education that offer programs to the public and have faculty who are expert in developing programs and conducting research.

The major difficulty to employing this considerable expertise is the fragmentation of programs and services. Heretofore, there has been an emphasis on individual programs and sports, rather than an overall view of contributions of physical fitness and activities to the nation's health. Coalition building and collaborative activities have not been a part of the effort to bring public attention to this vital public health need, aside from the federal Council on Physical Fitness and state-level Governor's Councils on Physical Fitness. As public as these bodies are, there is a need to be able to make connections between available expertise and those who participate in the lives of our youth.

Community leaders must create opportunities for young people to play and exercise. Communities lacking in parks and recreational facilities should work with businesses and schools to create such facilities. Where personal safety is a concern, parents and community organizations can join together to provide supervision so that young people can play in a safe environment. Schools, which often have excellent facilities for physical activities, can be opened earlier and closed later so that youth and those involved in their lives can participate in activities. Many shopping malls open before store hours to allow walkers to keep their activity level up in a safe and comfortable environment. Businesses with their own facilities may wish to donate their unneeded equipment and make their facilities available to their surrounding communities. In sum, creativity is needed by a coalition of concerned citizens to help address this issue.

Rarely is there a need for sophisticated equipment and extensive training schedules to establish useful fitness programs for youth. Physical activities can be developed on a simple and routine basis: walking instead of driving, taking the stairs instead of an elevator, and participating in children's play, as appropriate. It is important that such activities be introduced early and often to youth. Social support for moderate as well as vigorous activities and games is essential if children and adolescents are to adopt healthy lifestyles. Positive approaches are needed that place less emphasis on competitiveness and more emphasis on mastery, skill development, and personal enjoyment.

Summary

To make exercise and fitness activities fun and consistent within the lives of children and youth is our challenge. It is easier to adapt to a sedentary lifestyle rather than to be physically active. Poor fitness results in poorer health later in life. It is up to us to develop opportunities for children and to encourage them by setting good examples. It is also our challenge to work together to make this possible. There may be no greater challenge in health promotion than to develop patterns of habitual physical activity in youth. For the benefit of the future, we need to take on this challenge.

References

Kraus, H., & Hirshland, R. P. (1953). Muscular fitness and health. *Journal of Health, Physical Education, and Recreation, 24,* 17-19.

U.S. Department of Health and Human Services. (1991). *Healthy People 2000.* Washington, DC: Government Printing Office.

U.S. Department of Health and Human Services. (1996). *Physical activity and health: A report of the surgeon general.* Washington, DC: Government Printing Office.

4

◦

Nutrition for Teens

Gail Frank

An overriding concern about nutrition during the teenage years is the general ignorance about two concepts—first, that eating behavior influences health, and second, that eating behavior in childhood and adolescence initiates adult eating patterns. The independence among teens creates a daily eating environment where teens are the major decision makers about the food they eat. Some parents and other adults share the responsibility for the foods served to teens. Ideally, all players would understand and acknowledge the benefits of sound nutrition for the long-term health of the teen, for example, prevention of cancer, heart disease, obesity, and osteoporosis, but the major nutrition challenge in most families, schools, and community-based organizations serving teens is their immediate short-term health and immediate food satisfaction.

Youth face short-term risks resulting from their daily eating behavior and the long-term chronic disease risks reflecting years of eating habits. Primary prevention efforts for chronic disease are more effective if youth are identified who are at high risk for chronic disease. Lifestyle changes early in life can affect the course of disease. It is assumed that changes may be easier to achieve at young ages, before lifelong habits are established.

Anatomical data from youth dying violent deaths have strengthened the argument for a low-fat eating pattern in youth (Strong, 1995). The percentage of atherosclerotic lesions in both the aorta and the right coronary artery had a positive association with serum LDL cholesterol and a negative association with serum HDL cholesterol. Smoking was strongly associated with raised lesions in the abdominal aorta. After adjusting for lipoprotein levels and smoking, African Americans had more extensive lesions (Wissler et al., 1990). Primary prevention efforts are fueled by another important finding, that risk factors for heart disease tend to remain or track in the same relative rank within a population. Youth at high cardiovascular risk are earmarked for adult disease (Berenson et al., 1980; Webber, Cresanta, Voors, & Berenson, 1983).

Tracking data indicate that specific teens who will continue to have abnormal levels of risk factors can be identified. Specific primary preventive measures can be taken to meet the unique needs of these teens as stated in *Healthy People 2000,* which sets the nutrition agenda for teens (U.S. Department of Health and Human Services, 1990).

Healthy People 2000 Objectives for teens include nutrition objectives focusing on both acute problems and chronic diseases (see Table

TABLE 4.1. Healthy People 2000 Nutrition Objectives for Teens

Number Objective Baseline

2.3 Reduce overweight to a prevalence of no more than 20% among people ages 20 and older and no more than 15% among adolescents ages 12 to 19
(Baseline: 26% for people ages 20 through 74 in 1976-1980, 24% for men and 27% for women; 15% for adolescents ages 12 through 19 in 1976-1980)

Note: For people ages 20 and older, overweight is defined as body mass index (BMI) ≤ 27.8 for men and ≤ 27.3 for women. BMI is calculated by dividing weight in kilograms by the square of height in meters

2.5 Reduce dietary fat intake to an average of 30% of energy or less and average saturated fat intake to less than 10% of energy among people ages 2 and older

2.6 Increase complex carbohydrate and fiber-containing foods in the diets of adults to five or more daily servings for vegetables (including legumes) and fruits, and to six or more daily servings for grain products

2.7 Increase to at least 50% the proportion of overweight people age 12 and older who have adopted sound dietary practices combined with regular physical activity to attain an appropriate body weight

2.8 Increase calcium intake so at least 50% of youth ages 12 through 24 and 50% of pregnant and lactating women consume three or more servings daily of foods rich in calcium, and at least 50% of people ages 25 and older consume two or more servings daily

2.17 Increase to at least 90% the proportion of school lunch and breakfast services and child care food services with menus that are consistent with the nutrition principles in the Dietary Guidelines for Americans

2.19 Increase to at least 75% the proportion of the nation's schools that provide nutrition education from preschool through 12th grade, preferably as part of quality school health education

4.6 Reduce the proportion of young people who have used alcohol in the past month, as follows:

Substance/Age	*1988 Baseline*	*2000 Target*
Alcohol/ages 12 to 17	25.2%	12.6%
Alcohol/ages 18 to 20	57.9%	29.0%

4.7 Reduce the proportion of high school seniors and college students engaging in recent occasions of heavy drinking of alcoholic beverages to no more than 28% of high school seniors and 32% of college students (Baseline: 33% of high school seniors and 41.7% of college students in 1989)

Note: Recent heavy drinking is defined as having five or more drinks on one occasion in the previous 2-week period as monitored by self-reports

8.9 Increase to at least 75% the proportion of people ages 10 and older who have discussed issues related to nutrition . . . alcohol . . . with family members on at least one occasion during the preceding month

13.1 Reduce dental caries (cavities) so that the proportion of children with one or more caries (in permanent or primary teeth) is no more than 35% among children ages 6 through 8 and no more than 60% among adolescents age 15
(Baseline: 53% of children ages 6 through 8 in 1986-1987; 78% of adolescents age 15 in 1986-1987)

	Special Population Targets	
Dental Caries Prevalence	*1986-1987 Baseline*	*2000 Target*
13.1d American Indian/Alaska Native adolescents age 15 in permanent teeth in 1983-1984	93%	70%

13.2 Reduce untreated dental caries so that the proportion is no more than 15% among adolescents age 15
(Baseline: 23% of adolescents age 15 in 1986-1987)

SOURCE: Reprinted from U.S. Department of Health and Human Services, 1991a.

4.1). The nutrition objectives address reducing weight; improving eating behavior—reduced fat and increased complex carbohydrates and calcium; reducing dental caries; decreasing alcohol consumption; and improving meals at school.

Adult gatekeepers, for example, health educators, middle and high school teachers, school and health administrators, social workers, and community-based organization staff, should know the nutrition needs of teens and integrate these needs and health-promoting

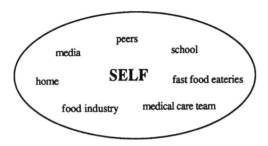

Figure 4.1. Multiple Environments of Youth That Influence Their Daily Living and Eating Behavior

TABLE 4.2. Age and Gender-Specific (85th percentile) Body Mass

Age	Indices (wt/ht²) Defining Overweight Teens	
	Boys	Girls
12-14	> 23	> 23
15-17	> 24	> 26
18-19	> 26	> 26

SOURCE: National Health and Nutrition Examination Survey II, 1976-1980.

eating recommendations into creative ways they present meals, snacks, and nutrition education (Frank, 1994a). Only with the availability and consistent ingestion of a variety of healthy foods can teens experience the benefits of good nutrition.

Good nutrition contributes to positive feelings and an energetic nature. Healthy teens have improved athletic performance, mental prowess, and physical attractiveness. They have good skin and hair quality and body leanness complemented with a small amount of body fat.

Teens identify with desirable role models, for example, athletes and entertainers, and the eating patterns they project. Teens who practice unhealthy eating habits are negative role models. Overemphasis on lean bodies with no fat may lead students to distorted body perceptions, lack of interpersonal trust, and bizarre weight control methods.

Hunger, on the other hand, still exists, especially among low-income families. Teens who experience hunger face additional pressures in school due to their high-risk status, that is, lack of alertness, illness, and absenteeism.

The eating patterns and nutritional well-being of teens are influenced by the multiple environments of their daily living (see Figure 4.1). This means that the home and family, school with teachers and food services, all forms of media, the health care setting, fast food establishments, and peer groups all influ-

ence what a teen chooses to eat. The effect can be positive or negative on the overall health of the teen (Frank, 1994a, 1994b).

Growth and Development

Nutritional health depends on the foods ingested and how the body uses them. Recommended daily nutrient intakes may or may not be achieved with the meal and snack choices of youth.

During the teen years, growth and development are continuous and monitored by two common nutritional indicators, height and weight. Many teens exist at one of the extremes, that is, either too heavy or too light for age or height. Teens exceeding their recommended weights by 15% and 20% are overweight and obese, respectively. About 25% of school-age children are overweight. Excess weight predisposes teens to high blood cholesterol and sets them on a track for chronic disease (Berenson et al., 1980). The overweight guidelines for teens are outlined in Table 4.2.

At the other extreme, underweight and malnourished teens present a different mosaic of nutritional problems, many of which began during infancy and preschool years (Frank, 1994b). The lack of access to food greatly influences growth and development. A 1991 survey of childhood hunger in the United States did not assess hunger specifically for teens. Key findings were as follows (Food Re-

TABLE 4.3. Recommended Dietary Allowances (RDA) for Teens, National Academy of Sciences, National Research Council

Sex/Age	Vitamin A (RE)	Vitamin D (ug)	Vitamin E (mg)	Vitamin C (mg)	Thiamin (mg)	Riboflavin (mg)	Niacin (mg eq)	Calcium (mg)	Iron (mg)	Zinc (mg)
Males										
11-14	1,000	10	10	50	1.3	1.5	17	1,200	12	15
15-18	1,000	10	10	60	1.5	1.8	20	1,200	12	15
19-24	1,000	10	10	60	1.5	1.7	19	1,200	10	15
Females										
11-14	800	10	8	50	1.1	1.3	15	1,200	15	12
15-18	800	10	8	60	1.1	1.3	15	1,200	15	12
19-24	800	10	8	60	1.1	1.3	15	1,200	15	12

SOURCE: National Academy of Sciences, 1989.

TABLE 4.4. The Dietary Guidelines for Americans

1. Eat a variety of foods
2. Balance the food you eat with physical activity—maintain or improve your weight
3. Choose a diet with plenty of grain products, vegetables, and fruits
4. Choose a diet low in fat, saturated fat, and cholesterol
5. Choose a diet moderate in sugars
6. Choose a diet moderate in salt and sodium
7. If you drink alcoholic beverages, do so in moderation

SOURCE: U.S. Department of Agriculture/U.S. Department of Health and Human Services, 1995.

search and Action Center, 1991): about 5.5 million youth under 12 years are hungry, and an additional 6 million are at risk of hunger. Compared to children from nonhungry low-income families, hungry children generally are two to three times more likely to have suffered from individual health problems, such as unwanted weight loss, fatigue, irritability, headaches, and inability to concentrate.

Youth with any treatable health problem, for example, colds, flu, diarrhea, headaches, and nausea, are absent from school almost twice as many days as those not reporting specific health problems. In some ways, the problems are accentuated by newer, problematic habits, for example, alcohol intake.

Recommended Dietary Allowances

For proper growth and development, teens need an array of nutrients on a daily basis. The Recommended Dietary Allowances (RDAs) are one set of standards used to evaluate nu-tritional adequacy of foods teens consume (Food and Nutrition Board, 1989). RDAs are set for energy, protein, 10 vitamins, and seven minerals (see Table 4.3). Minimum requirements are set for sodium, chloride, and potassium. Meal planning for school meals is based on achievement of one third of the RDAs at lunch and one quarter of the RDAs at breakfast (U.S. Department of Agriculture, 1983). Additional standards for teen nutrition are the Dietary Guidelines for Americans (Table 4.4) and the National Cholesterol Education Program, Step 1 Eating Pattern (Table 4.5).

Calcium and iron intakes are of special concern for teens (Frank, 1980; Frank, Berenson, Schilling, & Moore, 1977). The 1987-1988 National Food Consumption Survey (NFCS) data indicate that 20% of adolescent boys and 40% of adolescent girls did not drink milk on the day of the survey (Wotecki, 1992). Chan studied 164 healthy Caucasian youth and found that those consuming 1000+ mg of calcium per day had a higher bone mineral con-

TABLE 4.5. The National Cholesterol Education Program, and Step 1/Step 2 Eating Pattern

	Recommended Intake	
Nutrient	Step 1 Diet	Step 2 Diet
Total fat	Average of no more than 30% of total calories	Same
Saturated fatty acids	Less than 10% of total calories	< 7% of total calories
Polyunsaturated fatty acids	Up to 10% of total calories	Same
Monounsaturated fatty acids	Remaining total fat calories	Same
Cholesterol	Less than 300 mg/day	< 200 mg/day
Carbohydrates	About 55% of total calories	Same
Protein	About 15-20% of total calories	Same
Energy	To promote normal growth and development and to reach or maintain desirable body weight	

SOURCE: U.S. Department of Health and Human Services, 1991b.

tent compared to youth with < 1000 mg intakes (Chan, 1991). The higher bone mineral content is especially crucial for girls to prevent osteoporosis later in life.

During adolescence, there is an increased demand for iron to compensate for the increased hemoglobin level with growth (Johnson, 1990). National surveys report that adolescent girls 12 to 19 years old have the highest iron deficiency anemia prevalence rates, that is, between 6% and 14%. These adolescents become our mothers of tomorrow (Wotecki, 1992).

A Typical Eating Pattern

A typical eating pattern of youth might be as follows:

- Many teens skip meals. In a sample of U.S. 4th to 8th graders, more have skipped breakfast (57%) than lunch (41%), followed by dinner (17%) (National Center for Nutrition, 1991a). The most common reasons are dislike of particular meals or snacks, lack of time, or forgetting to take food to school.

- Students who don't eat breakfast and have a morning snack are about three times more likely to meet all food group recommendations than youth eating nothing in the morning (Bidgood & Cameron, 1992). Youth who eat breakfast exhibit other healthful habits

such as brushing teeth and taking vitamin/mineral supplements. Those skipping breakfast are significantly more tired and hungry when they arrive at school, yet no significant social and emotional behavior problems have been noted (Lindeman & Clancy, 1990). Breakfast skippers may have significantly higher total cholesterol levels. This was shown in one study where serum cholesterol was 172 mg per deciliter for nonbreakfast eaters compared to eaters with 160 mg per deciliter. Skippers reported higher intake of high-fat snacks (Resnicow, 1991).

- Nutrient-rich foods are not popular. In food group analysis from the 1982-1983 Hispanic Health and Nutrition Examination Survey (HHANES) of 3,356 Mexican American children, fruits and vegetables were consumed less often than the other food groups. Children choose their calories instead from the meat, dairy, and breads/cereals groups (Murphy, Castillo, Martorell, & Mendora, 1990). Of 407 Los Angeles Latinos, 3% consumed four servings a day, which is comparable to HHANES reporting 3% of 11- to 15-year-olds eating four a day (Palmer & Johnson, 1991).

- Eighty-seven percent of teens are responsible for cooking or preparing some of their own meals, with 80% making their own breakfast and 57% involved in buying food for meals or snacks (National Center for Nutrition, 1991a).

• Students eat at least three times a day, and more than 50% eat five or more times a day. Two thirds have an afternoon snack, and 58% eat an evening snack. Only 15% have a morning snack.

• Total daily food intake averages 111% of the Recommended Dietary Allowance for food energy commonly referred to as *calories*. Males have 17% and females have 4% more calories than recommended. Students from families below the poverty level average 129% of the energy RDA. Apparently, many foods these teens eat have excess fat and sugar, yielding extra calories and promoting weight gain.

• Vitamin and mineral intake for boys of all ages exceed the RDA. This is not the case for adolescent girls. Calcium intake is relatively low, for example, 80% of recommended level for 15- to 18-year-olds and 87% of recommended level for 11- to 14-year-olds (Burghardt & Devaney, 1993).

• Students who do not eat school lunch consume more sweets and sweet drinks, and they purchase food that is often nutritionally empty–calorie foods from a vending machine, school store, or "à la carte" service in the cafeteria.

Overall eating patterns average 34% of calories from fat and 13% from saturated fat. Students from low-income families have higher fat intakes than students from higher-income households. Carbohydrates average 53% of the calories, and sodium averages 4,800 mg; strikingly high caloric and sodium intakes are reported for boys (Burghardt & Devaney, 1993). The foods these teens choose or have available at home are again high in fat and sugar and low in nutrients, for example, fried foods like French fries, inexpensive cold cuts, burgers and chips, pastries, and candy.

Overall, the eating pattern of teens reflects their living environment and becomes the basis of their health status. Each component of the living environment has an impact on both their current and long-term health.

The School Environment

The School Nutrition Dietary Assessment Study (SNDA) is the most recent survey of a nationally representative sample of schools ($n = 545$) and students ($n = 3,350$) (Burghardt & Devaney, 1993). Data show that boys eat school lunch more often than girls, and more students in rural than in urban and suburban schools eat school lunch. Students in the Northeast and West choose school lunch less than students in the Southeast, Southwest, and Mountain states. If students are allowed to leave school at lunchtime, participation declines (Burghardt & Devaney, 1993).

Over 50% of school menus offer a choice of entree daily, and about 50% of high schools have a food bar once a week. Many offer salad bars more frequently. Desserts are not required in the U.S. Department of Agriculture's reimbursable meal pattern, but 39% of lunch menus offer dessert.

The SNDA reported the following low nutrient intakes in lunch meals: iron for 11- to 18-year-old females, zinc for 11- to 18-year-old males, and calories and vitamin B6 for 15- to 18-year-old males. The average percentage of calories from total fat is 38% and from saturated fat is 15%. Sodium in National School Lunch Program (NSLP) lunches averages 1,479 mg (no more than 2,400 mg recommended per total day) and cholesterol averages 88 mg (no more than 300 mg recommended per total day).

Schools providing lunches with less than 32% of calories from fat offer ground-beef entrees less often, poultry and meatless entrees more often, fewer vegetables with added fat, and fruit and fruit juice more often. Two percent milk is usually replaced with 1% or nonfat milk. Salad dressing, cakes, and cookies are replaced with low-calorie dressings and low-fat desserts, such as yogurt and pudding made from skim milk. When fat content goes below 32%, participation declines (Burghardt & Devaney, 1993).

The School Breakfast Program (SBP) is available to slightly more than 50% of the nation's students, but less than 20% participate. Students likely to participate are those certified for free and reduced-price meals, those from low-income families, and those who are younger, male, African American, and rural. Breakfasts average 31% fat and 14% saturated fat. Cholesterol averages 73 mg; carbohydrate and sodium average 57% and 673 mg, respectively.

Comparing these figures with recommended levels in Table 4.5, one can see that breakfast is only slightly higher in fat, saturated fat, and sodium than recommended. The concern is that many teens skip breakfast, or if they eat breakfast, it provides less than one fourth of their overall food intake. The impact of a fairly healthy breakfast is then lost. As shown above, lunches average 38% of calories from fat and greatly increase the saturated fat intake. When teens skip breakfast and begin their "foods for the day" with lunch, they often begin with a higher fat, saturated fat, and sodium exposure.

The Home and
Leisure Time Environment

Parents control more of the eating environment when children are young; they control fewer food choices as children age and peers gain more influence. In addition, the home and leisure time environment of the teen may either complement or contradict any nutrition knowledge, positive attitude, or healthy eating behavior they have acquired in the school environment (Frank, 1994a).

Kirk and Gillespie (1990) identified two new roles of parents that influence teen food choices, the *meaning creator* and the *family diplomat*. In other words, parents give a meaning to eating, which is usually "for health of the teen," but they also play a mediator role

to encourage teens to choose healthy foods and make wise food choices.

Typically, mothers function as the nutritionist, economist, and *manager-organizer* for food preparation in the home. Today's contemporary mother has limited food preparation time. She may cater to the individual preferences of teens to ensure their acceptance, but by doing so, she may not offer foods meeting their nutritional needs.

Even though the parents' role in food behavior declines during the teen years, some teens seem to mimic the "all or nothing" attitude of their parents. Many teens identify foods as good or bad; in fact, 73% of 4th to 8th graders surveyed in a national sample worried about fat and cholesterol. About 85% felt they should avoid all high-fat foods, whereas 77% felt they should never eat high-sugar foods. It is better to teach teens how to fit all foods into a healthy eating pattern.

About one half of the youth eat with their family every day; 89% eat with their family three to five times per week. Students who give themselves the best nutrition rating eat more frequently with their family (National Center for Nutrition, 1991b).

The Teen's Personal
Risk-Taking Eating Environment

Alcohol

Alcohol supplants nutrient-rich foods and sets a teen on a dangerous nutrition and accident-prone track (Frank, 1994b). About 45% of Caucasian and 48% of Native American high school students in Michigan reported using alcohol, with almost one half of Caucasian, Native American, and Hispanic male users reporting heavy alcohol use (Bachman et al., 1991). Prevalence may be higher among school dropouts.

The Youth Risk Behavior Survey (YRBS) of 9th to 12th graders in 1990 reported 88% of youth consuming alcohol during their life, with 59% drinking at least once during the past 30 days. Males were more likely to drink than females, 62% and 55%, respectively, and 12th graders were more likely than 9th graders to drink. About 37% of males assessed by YRBS consumed more than five drinks at least once during the past 30 days (CDC, 1991a).

Caffeine

Caffeine is a nervous system stimulant and not generally viewed as a negative dietary component; however, caffeine lowers calcium absorption and increases heart rate and respiration. A lower calcium intake in adolescence reduces bone mass. For girls, this increases their risk of osteoporosis later in life. For boys and girls, the stimulating effect of caffeine may set a stage for needing stimulation, even in beverages.

Caffeine is classified as a drug, but society is very accepting of this stimulant and has not considered it a nuisance. Clearly, it may become the "new generation" drug by the year 2000. Arbeit and colleagues (1988) reported that caffeine intake per kilogram of body weight of Caucasian children 10 to 15 years old equalled that of adults, 2.5 versus 2.6 mg/kg. Caffeine sources for youth are carbonated beverages, chocolate candy, chocolate pudding and ice cream, and tea (Arbeit et al., 1988).

Inactivity and Obesity

Obesity, that is, being 20% above a healthy body weight, has been shown to track from childhood into adulthood (Kolata, 1986). It is estimated that 40% of children who are obese at 7 years of age carry their obesity into adulthood; about 70% to 80% of adolescents retain their obesity. Two large surveys of physical activity among U.S. youth, the National Children and Youth Fitness Study (NCYFS I) and the YRBS, profiled physical activity. NCYFS I reported that youth will participate in about 1 to 2 hours of moderate to vigorous physical activity per day as an average over a year. This includes, however, about 20% to 30% of students who spend less than one half hour a day. YRBS data with 11,319 teens in the 8th to 10th grades show that about 50% of boys and 75% of girls do not have moderate to vigorous activity three or more times a week (Pate, Dowdy, & Ross, 1990; Ross & Gilbert, 1985).

A major health concern is that physical activity has been shown to be inversely associated with adiposity (Pate et al., 1990; Suter & Hawes, 1993). An inactive lifestyle in youth sets the stage for inactivity in adulthood and the propensity for obesity (Pate, 1993). A number of controlled primary prevention studies show that by increasing physical activity, one can modestly slow the rise in adiposity in obese youth. Increasing physical activity alone is not as effective as coupling activity with dietary changes and behavior modification. Including parents of obese youth in the combined physical activity and eating behavior change strategies yields the greatest impact on weight loss (Epstein et al., 1990; Sasaki, Shindo, & Tanaka et al., 1987).

The prevalence of obesity has increased 54% among children 6 to 11 years old and 39% among 12- to 17-year-olds. Therefore, a focus on combining physical activity and food energy or total calories consumed is relevant. Hispanic children are among those experiencing as much as a 120% increase in the prevalence of obesity over the past 20 years. The excess intake of high fat and low complex carbohydrate foods along with minimal physical activity can place youth at a 38% increased risk for obesity (Kolata, 1986; Muecke, Morton-Simons, Huang, & Parcel, 1992; Schlicker, Borra, & Regan, 1994).

Television

Youth who watch more TV than their peers have greater prevalence of obesity, and super-

TABLE 4.6. Diagnostic Criteria for Four Types of Eating Disorders

Type	Diagnostic Criteria
Anorexia nervosa	There are two subtypes: restricting and binge eating/purging. In the restricting type, the person does not regularly binge, use self-induced vomiting, or misuse laxatives or diuretics. In the binge eating/purging type, the person regularly engages in these behaviors.
Bulimia nervosa	Two subgroups exist. In the purging type, the person regularly engages in self-induced vomiting or the misuse of laxatives, diuretics, or enemas. The nonpurging type involves other inappropriate compensatory behaviors, such as fasting or excessive exercise, but no regular self-induced practices of vomiting or enemas.
Binge disorder	This disorder involves recurrent episodes of binge eating and at least three of the following: eating much more rapidly than normal and until feeling uncomfortably full, eating large amounts of food when not feeling physically hungry, eating alone because of being embarrassed by how much one is eating, and feeling disgusted with oneself, depressed, or very guilty after overeating.
Eating disorder not specified	This is a transient behavior and may occur among individuals having regular menses, a normal weight, binging less than twice a week, eating small amounts of food and then self-inducing vomiting, and regular chewing and spitting food out without swallowing.

obesity, for example, 100 pounds over a healthy body weight, which replicates adult studies (Gortmaker, 1987; Tucker & Bagwell, 1991). During prime-time TV programs and commercials, references to food focus on low-nutrient beverages and sweets consumed as exciting, acceptable snacks. Emphasis is on "good taste" and "fresh and natural" with minimal attention given to foods consistent with healthy guidelines for youth (Story & Faulkner, 1990). Data from NHANES II and III found a 2% increase in the prevalence of obesity for each additional hour of television viewing. These findings remained after controlling for prior obesity status, region of the United States, season, population density, ethnicity, and socioeconomic status (Dietz & Gortmaker, 1985).

Eating Disorders

About 1 million adolescents are affected by anorexia nervosa and bulimia, which are thought to occur for a variety of reasons, including poor self-concept, body shape and size, pressure to be thin, depression, and biological errors in organ function or structure. As many as 10% of these adolescents may die prematurely as a result of the disorder. The American Psychiatric Association delineates diagnostic criteria for four types of eating disorders (American Psychiatric Association, 1994), as shown in Table 4.6.

The age of onset for anorexia seems to peak between 14 and 18 years of age and for bulimia about 18 years of age. Individuals in a middle to upper socioeconomic level who are high achievers are prone to develop an eating disorder. Situations or highly competitive sports that promote food restrictions and diet regulating may be antecedents to eating disorders, for example, ballet and gymnastics (Hsu, 1990b).

The YRBS (CDC, 1991b) of 9th to 12th graders reported that 69% of male students considered themselves at the right body weight, and 17% thought they were underweight, compared to females at 59% and 7%, respectively. Black students considered themselves less overweight than white or Hispanic students. About 44% of the girls were trying to lose weight, but only 15% of the boys reported this intent. Even 27% of girls who considered themselves at the right weight reported currently trying to lose weight by exercise, skipping meals, taking diet pills, or inducing vomiting, which they reported significantly more often than boys.

Desmond, Price, Hallinan, and Smith (1989) administered a 22-item questionnaire on weight perceptions to inner-city African American and Caucasian teens, 12 to 17 years old. About 40% of heavy black females perceived themselves as overweight compared to 100% of heavy white females, and the trend was similar for heavy males. Girls obtained their weight control information from television, family, friends, and magazines. Boys used the TV, family, and athletic coaches for advice.

Shisslak, Crago, and Neal (1990) implemented a program to educate high school students, staff, and teachers about eating disorders and found more questions about eating disorders answered correctly by participants than by controls. Larson (1991) reported that 454 Caucasian girls 14 to 19 years old who responded that their guardians "always" lectured them about food had significantly higher scores on the *drive for thinness* and *ineffectiveness* subscales. Students who responded that their guardians were unaware of their problems also had higher scores on the *ineffectiveness* and *interpersonal distrust* subscales. In another study, females identified more emotional concerns about being overweight or the need to lose weight compared with boys (Balentine, Stitt, Bonner, & Clark, 1991).

Therapy for teens with eating disorders involves a team approach including a psychiatrist and registered dietitian among others. Individual and group eating behavior sessions with clients focus on restoration of normal eating patterns, often integrating medical nutrition therapy or liquid foods and supplements with servings of real food (American Dietetic Association, 1994; Mitchell & Eckert, 1987). The outcome is highly variable and ranges from chronic symptoms and relapses to full remission at follow-up (Rorty, Yager, & Rossotto, 1993). Rates of recovery range from

13% to 60% (Reiff & Reiff, 1992; Vandereycken, Depreitere, & Probst, 1987).

Teen Pregnancy

In 1985, 1,031,000 teenagers became pregnant, and 477,710 teenagers gave birth to an infant. Of those becoming pregnant, 10,000 were 15 years of age or younger (Story, Heald, & Dwyer, 1991; Ventura, Taffel, & Mosher, 1995). Unless the teen's growth at the time she conceives is completed, there will be a greater demand for food energy and nutrients to support her own and her baby's growth. Most teens who become pregnant after age 16 do not have an increased nutrient need for growth; however, eating patterns of teens reflect a high consumption of fast foods, frequent snacking, independence of food choice, chronic dieting (i.e., about 14% skipping of meals), and preoccupation with physical appearance (Story, 1990). These habits create a health risk for the pregnant teen, because during pregnancy the nutritional needs for the fetus are met before the needs of the mother are met.

Strategies to Improve the Nutritional Health of Youth

The Pediatric Panel Report of the National Cholesterol Education Program (NCEP) underscores the Healthy People 2000 objectives for teens by recommending maintenance of a healthy body weight and a salutogenic or health-promoting eating pattern such as a Step 1 pattern: less than 30% of total energy as fat and 10% as saturated fat and less than 300 mg of cholesterol/day (National Cholesterol Education Program, 1991).

Data from the 1977-1978 and the 1987-1988 Nationwide Food Consumption Survey showed that the total average dietary fiber intake of all youth decreased. Vegetables and fruits were the major source of dietary fiber in

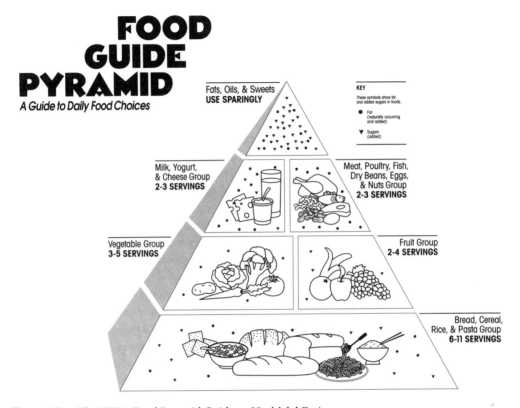

Figure 4.2. The USDA Food Pyramid Guide to Healthful Eating

the 1977-1978 data; a decade later, bread and cereal were the two major dietary fiber sources. Those who ate breakfast consumed more fiber than those who did not (Carroll, Abraham, & Dresser, 1983; Frank, 1980). The recommended formula of "AGE + 5 grams" allows youth to 18 years of age to grow into their fiber requirements as a natural way of eating (Fulgoni & Mackey, 1991).

A standard that can be used to evaluate the healthfulness of a teen eating pattern is whether they eat the recommended number of servings from each group in the USDA Food Guide Pyramid (FGP). The FGP is a visual presentation of the dietary guidelines using foods (U.S. Department of Agriculture, 1989, 1992), as shown in Figure 4.2. Fats, oils, and sweets are at the tip followed by low-fat meat and dairy products. Whole grain starches, breads and cereals, fruits, and vegetables form the bottom seg-

ments, signifying that more servings of these make for a healthier food pattern. Three overall concepts conveyed in the Pyramid Guide are: balance foods higher in nutrients with those lower in nutrients, choose a variety of foods each day, and have moderate portions of foods.

School Nutrition as a Component of Comprehensive School Health

Comprehensive School Health Education (CSHE) is a primary prevention strategy for teaching disease prevention and health promotion life skills to children, parents, and future parents (Harris, 1988). CSHE is based on a planned, sequential pre-K through 12th-grade curriculum that addresses the physical, mental, emotional, and social dimensions of the child (Allensworth & Kolbe, 1987).

Health status and health risk of teens result from multiple factors; therefore, researchers believe that multiple interventions are needed to effect behavioral, environmental, or social changes (Dryfoos, 1990). Ten content areas are essential for a comprehensive program:

- Community health
- Consumer health
- Environmental health
- Family life
- Growth and development
- School nutrition and food service
- Personal health
- Prevention and control of disease
- Safety and accident prevention
- Substance use and abuse

Common content areas required by state mandates include drug and alcohol abuse prevention in 29 states, tobacco use prevention in 20 states, and nutrition in 19 states (National Health Education Organization, 1989). School nutrition and food service is one of the 10 major comprehensive school health components. School cafeterias are a primary prevention arena—a learning laboratory for children where demonstration and education studies can be conducted to evaluate menu changes and student acceptability (Frank, Nicklas, Forcier, Webber, & Berenson, 1989a, 1989b; Frank, Vaden, & Martin, 1987). With national efforts to legislate comprehensive school health in our schools, support for this initiative strengthens each component, for example, child nutrition or physical education, and their respective programs.

Strengthening comprehensive school health education for all children (Allensworth, 1994; Cortese & Middleton, 1993; Jackson, 1994) is a first-time strategy to improve the nutritional well-being of youth. Enhancing complementary physical activity and child nutri-tion programs at schools provides a second strategy. Assessing the readiness for change of both students and teachers is a third and essential strategy before programs are planned and implemented. Youth-driven programs provide a fourth strategy, and by incorporating the family, the various living and eating environments of adolescents, and the community, a fifth strategy to achieve nutritionally healthy and fit youth by the year 2000 is identified (National Association of State Boards of Education, n.d.).

The National Commission on the Role of the School and the Community in Improving Adolescent Health has called the nation to action to address the problems of youth. In *CODE BLUE: Uniting for Healthier Youth,* the commission proclaims that the situation is an emergency and that life-threatening events are occurring in the lives of U.S. youth. These events threaten the very survival and healthy functioning of adolescents, the future of the children birthed by adolescents, and the viability and competitiveness of the American workforce in general. All sectors of society are involved, and their dedication is needed to redirect the future of this generation (National Association of State Boards of Education, n.d.). The following nutrition priorities should be addressed:

- Schools should ensure that their policies allow all teens access to reduced-price or free meals to reduce hunger or inadequate food intake.

- Physical activity programs should be blended with healthy eating behavior strategies to alter the obesity trend.

- Factors that trigger disordered eating should be identified and pertinent questions answered, such as

  Do advertising and the media promote thin bodies and extreme eating behavior?

Are specific groups of teen dieters at greater risk for developing eating disorders?

Is there an association between physical activity and food restriction in initiating and perpetuating anorexia nervosa? (Dodd & Bessinger, 1993)

• School nutrition professionals should be permanent staff with the responsibility to empower teens with skills for healthy eating. These might include learning to read food labels, analyzing their own intake and showing the difference between what they eat and what they should eat, and practicing food preparation methods for nutrient-dense foods and snacks they like.

• An operational framework should be set up to develop an action plan. Addressing predisposing, enabling, and reinforcing factors in schools can promote positive healthy eating (Green, Kreuter, Deeds, & Partridge, 1980):

Predisposing factors are the demographic and population norms often beyond the scope of a program and usually nonmodifiable; however, increasing fruit and vegetable intake to "5-A-Day" in the population would establish a new, preferred norm.

Enabling factors concern availability and accessibility in the school, such as the cafeteria, vending machines, campus stores, and fast food eateries near schools.

Reinforcing factors address attitudes and behaviors of peers, teachers, administrators, and media that either support or discourage behavioral change.

• Building teams should be appointed in schools and communities to work together for school policies that improve the nutritional health of students. This action builds capacity within a community to respond to the nutrition and health needs of teens. Only with such a combined effort can we alter the morbidity and improve the health and well-being of our youth.

Other ways to target positive change in the eating environment in schools include the following (Frank, 1994b):

USDA school meals initiative for healthy children. This initiative will take effect by the 1998-1999 school year. It will dramatically update the nutrition standards for meal planning by requiring a Nutrient Standard Menu Planning, called *NuMenuS* to provide a one-week assessment of meals to reflect nutrient content (American School Food Service Association, 1994).

Time allocation for meals. Students may have 12 to 25 minutes to obtain their meal, find a place to sit, eat, socialize, and discard waste. The rushed eating period should be extended to a minimum of 30 minutes.

Acceptability of menu. Plate waste can be lowered by developing healthy potato, salad, and sandwich bars as enticements and by organizing youth advisory groups to bring students into the planning, tasting, and decision-making process (American School Food Service Association, 1990). Foods that reflect the multicultural environment should be served.

Training of food service personnel. Plan continuing education for employees to address sanitation, safety, meal planning, health promotion, and point-of-choice nutrition information (POCNI) that focuses on marketing (Cinciripini, 1984; Schmitz & Fielding, 1986). POCNI can be placed adjacent to foods on the serving line and complement health, science, and physical education curriculum. For example, a POCNI label could read "Tossed Salad with flaked tuna: 1 and 1/2 cup, 144 calories, 241 RE vitamin A, 36 mg vitamin C," or "Hamburger on Whole Wheat Bun: 266 calories, 41% fat, 362 mg sodium" (Dodd &

Bessinger, 1993) This guides students in making healthy food choices by comparing foods and nutrients.

Implementing high-risk youth programs. Low-fat food choices matched with ample opportunities for continuous physical activities and sport participation are needed. Dedicated school staff and faculty to champion the cause must be identified. Parental involvement in the program should be garnered to build self-esteem, reinforcement of positive behavior change, and identification of barriers for obese youth and their families. The SHAPE-DOWN program is a secondary prevention program for obese adolescents. The approach has produced significant long-term outcomes among these adolescents and may provide the foundation for a school-based program (Mellin, Slinkard, & Irwin, 1987).

Community partnerships. Developing partnerships with the community may begin with the formation of a community advisory group of 8 to 12 people, possibly a community leader, a local pediatrician, a grocery store owner, a restaurant owner, an American Heart Association representative, and a newspaper/radio or TV reporter. The advisory group can respond to the needs of teens by recommending and supporting programs.

Guidelines for Adolescent Preventive Services. The American Medical Association has developed a comprehensive set of recommendations or a framework for community organizations, which can serve as the potential content of preventive health services. It is called *Guidelines for Adolescent Preventive Services* (GAPS). GAPS addresses the problems common to youth of all ethnic groups and provides a blueprint for the delivery of services.

GAPS emphasize health guidance and prevention of behavioral and emotional disorders. A series of annual health visits is recommended for all youth between the ages of 11 and 21 years. Teens who have initiated health-risk nutrition behaviors can be identified. If they are at early stages of physical or emotional disorders, opportunities for communication and support can be formed (American Medical Association, 1992).

Guidelines for school health programs to promote lifelong healthy eating (U.S. Department of Health and Human Services, 1996). In 1996, the CDC issued seven recommendations that focus on ways to ensure quality nutrition programs within a comprehensive school health program. The recommendations are

Policy: Adopt a coordinated school nutrition policy that promotes healthy eating through classroom lessons and a supportive school environment.

Curriculum for nutrition education: Implement nutrition education from preschool through secondary school as part of a sequential, comprehensive school health education curriculum designed to help students adopt healthy eating behaviors.

Instructions for students: Provide nutrition education through developmentally appropriate, culturally relevant, fun, participatory activities that involve social learning strategies.

Integration of school food service and nutrition education: Coordinate school food service with nutrition education and with other components of the comprehensive school health program to reinforce messages on healthy eating.

Training for school staff: Provide staff involved in nutrition education with adequate preservice and ongoing in-service training that focuses on teaching strategies for behavioral change.

Family and community involvement: Involve family members and the community in supporting and reinforcing nutrition education.

Program evaluation: Regularly evaluate the effectiveness of the school health programs in promoting healthy eating, and change the programs as appropriate to increase effectiveness.

TABLE 4.7. Major Intervention Studies to Alter the High-Risk Status of Youth, National Institutes of Health

Study	Year Begun	Sample	Objectives
Dietary Intervention Study of Children (DISC)	1986	8-10 year olds, 45% female, elevated LDL	To assess feasibility in children; acceptability, efficacy, and safety of diet
NHLBI Growth and Health Study (NGHS)	1985	Youth, 51% African American girls, 9-10 years old	To assess the occurrence of obesity and its association with various risk factors for heart disease
Child and Adolescent Trial of Cardiovascular Health (CATCH)	1987	12,000 3rd, 4th, 5th graders, all ethnic groups	To measure and compare the effects of school-based interventions to promote lifelong behaviors to reduce cardiovascular disease
The Framingham Heart Offspring Study	1971	Adults	To study coronary heart disease among offspring of the original cohort
Coronary Artery Risk Development in Young Adults (CARDIA)	1983	18-30 years old, 52% African American, 55% women	To study precursors and determinants of risk factors including lifestyle for heart disease

National Institute of Health (NIH) interventions. Several major intervention studies have been funded by the NIH to alter the high-risk status of youth (NIH, 1994). Results may have implications for future health policy and medical practice for teens. A brief description of these studies is provided in Table 4.7.

At the end of 6 months of intervention, in the Dietary Intervention Study of Children (DISC), the percentage of energy from total fat and saturated fat was reduced by 5.1%, $p = 0.004$ and 2.9%, $p < 0.001$ (Van Horn et al., 1993). The children will be followed until the year 2000.

The National Growth and Health Study (NGHS) is an obesity study of young women. Dietary and physical activity, socioeconomic status, and lifestyle variables are assessed. The Child and Adolescent Trial of Cardiovascular Health (CATCH) includes classroom curricula, family-focused dietary modifications, physical activity, and tobacco use. The Coronary Artery Risk Development in Young Adults (CARDIA) is a prospective observational study to monitor young adults over time for health risk and the onset of heart disease.

The Framingham Heart Study identified high blood cholesterol, high blood pressure, and cigarette smoking as the three major risk factors for heart disease. In addition, smoking was identified as a significant independent variable for stroke, and obesity was identified as a major independent risk factor for coronary heart disease. The Framingham Offspring Study reports that children have slightly lower blood cholesterol and blood pressure levels than their parents. Children of parents with hypertension have higher blood pressures than other children. Smoking among men has decreased to half that of their fathers, but women smoke more than their mothers.

Conclusion

The eating patterns and nutritional well-being of teens are influenced by the multiple environments in which they live. The home, family, school, health care system, peers, fast food establishments, and media can have either a positive or a negative effect.

Nutrition guidelines for teens exist, but implementation in each environment is challenging. Teens themselves may not believe they are at a nutritional risk or that their eating patterns can affect their current or future health. A coordinated effort involving teens, their families, and the community in which they live must occur if Healthy People 2000 objectives are to be achieved for our teenage population.

References

Allensworth, D. D. (1994). The research base for innovative practices in school health education at the secondary level. *Journal of School Health, 64*(5), 180-187.

Allensworth, D. D., & Kolbe, L. J. (1987). The comprehensive school health program: Exploring an expanded concept. *Journal of School Health, 57*(10), 311.

American Dietetic Association. (1994). Position of the ADA: Nutrition intervention in the treatment of anorexia nervosa, bulimia nervosa, and binge eating. *Journal of the American Dietetic Association, 94*(8), 902-907.

American Medical Association. (1992). *Guidelines for adolescent preventive services.* Chicago: Author.

American Psychiatric Association. (1994). *Diagnostic and statistical manual* (4th ed.). Washington, DC: Author.

American School Food Service Association. (1990). *Youth Advisory Council—at the starting line.* Alexandria, VA: Author.

American School Food Service Association. (1994, August). New CN program regs proposed. *Journal of the American School Food Service Association,* pp. 12-13.

Arbeit, M. L., Nicklas, T. A., Frank, G. C., Webber, L. S., Miner, M. H., & Berenson, G. S. (1988). Caffeine intakes of children from a biracial population: The Bogalusa Heart Study. *Journal of the American Dietetic Association, 88,* 466-470.

Bachman, J. G., Wallace, J. M., O'Malley, P. M., Johnston, L. D., Kurth, C. L., & Neighbors, H. W. (1991). Racial/ethnic differences in smoking, drinking, and illicit drug use among American high school seniors, 1976-89. *American Journal of Public Health, 81,* 372-377.

Balentine, M., Stitt, K., Bonner, J., & Clark, L. (1991). Self-reported eating disorders of black, low-income adolescents: Behavior, body weight perceptions, and methods of dieting. *Journal of School Health, 61,* 392-396.

Berenson, G. S., McMahan, C. A., Voors, A. W., Webber, L. S., Srinivasan, S. R., Frank, G. C., Foster, T. A., & Blonde, C. V. (1980). *Cardiovascular risk factors in children—the early natural history of atherosclerosis and essential hypertension.* New York: Oxford University Press.

Bidgood, B. A., & Cameron, G. (1992). Meal/snack missing and dietary adequacy of primary school children. *Journal of the Canadian Dietetic Association, 53,* 164-168.

Burghardt, J., & Devaney, B. (1993). *The school nutrition dietary assessment study—summary of findings.* Princeton, NJ: Mathematica Policy Research.

Carroll, M. D., Abraham, S., & Dresser, C. M. (1983, March). *Dietary intake source data: United States 1976-1980* (Vital and Health Statistics, Series II, 231 USDHHS, PHS, NCHS, DHHS Publ. No. 83-1681). Washington, DC: National Center for Health Statistics.

Centers for Disease Control. (1991a). Alcohol and other drug use among high school students-United States. *Journal of the American Medical Association, 266,* 3266-3267.

Centers for Disease Control. (1991b). Body weight perceptions and selected weight-management goals and practices of high school students-United States. *Journal of the American Medical Association, 266,* 2811-2812.

Chan, G. M. (1991). Dietary calcium and bone mineral status of children and adolescents. *American Journal of Diseases of Children, 145,* 631-634.

Cinciripini, P. M. (1984). Changing food selections in a public cafeteria. *Behavioral Modification, 8,* 522-539.

Cortese, P., & Middleton, K. (Ed.). (1993). *The comprehensive school health challenge: Promoting health through education.* Santa Cruz, CA: ETR Associates.

Desmond, S. M., Price, J. H., Hallinan, C., & Smith, D. (1989). Black and white adolescents' perceptions of their weight. *Journal of School Health, 59,* 353-358.

Dietz, W. H., Jr., & Gortmaker, S. L. (1985). Do we fatten our children at the television set? Obesity and television viewing in children and adolescents. *Pediatrics, 75,* 807-812.

Dodd, J. M., & Bessinger, C. (1993). Societal issues and nutrition (ADA Research Conference Proceedings). *Journal of the American Dietetic Association, 93*(1), 77-85.

Druss, R. G., & Silverman, J. A. (1979). Body image and perfectionism of ballerinas. *General Hospital Psychiatry, 2,* 115-121.

Dryfoos, J. (1990). *Adolescents at risk: Prevalence and prevention.* New York: Oxford University Press.

Epstein, L. H., Valoski, A., Wing, R. R., & McCurley, J. (1990). Ten-year followup of behavioral, family-based treatment for obese children. *Journal of the American Medical Association, 264,* 2519-2523.

Food and Nutrition Board, National Academy of Sciences, National Research Council. (1989). *Recommended dietary allowances* (10th ed.). Washington, DC: National Academy of Sciences.

Food Research and Action Center. (1991). *Community childhood hunger identification project.* Washington, DC: Author.

Frank, G. C. (1980). Dietary studies of infants and children. In G. S. Berenson et al. (Eds.), *Cardiovascular risk factors in children—The early natural history of atherosclerosis and essential hypertension* (pp. 289-307). New York: Oxford University Press.

Frank, G. C. (1994a). Assessing diets of children: Environmental influences on dietary data collection methods with children. *American Journal of Clinical Nutrition, 59*(Suppl), 207s-211s.

Frank, G. C. (1994b). Nutrition issues. In P. Cortese & K. Middleton (Eds.), *The comprehensive school health challenge* (pp. 373-411). Santa Cruz, CA: ETR Associates.

Frank, G. C., Berenson, G. S., Schilling, P. E., & Moore, M. C. (1977). Adapting the 24-hr. dietary recall for epidemiologic studies of school children. *Journal of the American Dietetic Assocation, 71,* 26-31.

Frank, G. C., Nicklas, T., Forcier, J., Webber, L., & Berenson, G. S. (1989a). Cardiovascular health promotion of children: The Heart Smart School Lunch Program, Part I. *School Food Service Research Review, 13*(2), 130-136.

Frank, G. C., Nicklas, T., Forcier, J., Webber, L., & Berenson, G. S. (1989b). Cardiovascular health promotion of children: Student behavior and institutional foodservice change, Part II. *School Food Service Research Review, 13*(2), 137-145.

Frank, G. C., Vaden, A., & Martin, J. (1987). School health promotion: Child nutrition programs. *Journal of School Health, 57*(10), 451-460.

Fulgoni, V. L., & Mackey, M. A. (1991). Total dietary fiber in children's diets. In C. L. Williams & E. L. Wynder (Eds.), Hyperlipidemia and the development of Atherosclerosis. *Annual of the New York Academy of Science, 623,* 369-379.

Gortmaker, S. L. (1987). Increasing pediatric obesity in the *American Journal of Diseases in Children, 141,* 535-541.

Green, L. W., Kreuter, M. W., Deeds, S. G., & Partridge, K. B. (1980). *Health education planning—A diagnostic approach.* Palo Alto, CA: Mayfield.

Halmi, H. K. (Ed.). (1992). *The psychology and treatment of anorexia nervosa and bulimia nervosa.* Washington, DC: American Psychiatric Press.

Harris L. (1988). *An evaluation of comprehensive health education in American public schools.* New York: Metropolitan Life Foundation.

Hsu, L. K. (1990a). Clinical features. In *Eating disorders* (pp. 22-24). New York: Guilford.

Hsu, L. K. (1990b). Epidemiology. In *Eating disorders.* New York: Guilford.

Jackson, S. A. (1994). Comprehensive school health education programs: Innovative practices and issues in standard setting. *Journal of School Health, 64*(5), 177-179.

Johnson, A. A. (1990). Iron deficiency: Pediatric epidemiology. In C. Enwonuw (Ed.), *Functional significance of iron deficiency* (Annual Nutrition Workshop Series, Vol. 3, pp. 57-65). Nashville, TN: Meharry Medical College.

Kirk, M. C., & Gillespie, A. H. (1990). Factors affecting food choices of working mothers with young families. *Journal of Nutrition Education, 22,* 161-168.

Kolata, G. (1986). Obese children: A growing problem. *Science, 232,* 20-21.

Larson, B. (1991). Relationship of family communication patterns to eating disorder inventory scores in adolescent girls. *Journal of the American Dietetic Association, 91,* 1065-1067.

Lindeman, A. K., & Clancy, K. L. (1990). Assessment of breakfast habits and social/emotional behavior of elementary schoolchildren. *Journal of Nutrition Education, 22,* 226-231.

Mellin, L. M., Slinkard, L. A., & Irwin, C. E. (1987). Adolescent obesity intervention: Validation of the SHAPEDOWN program. *Journal of the American Dietetic Association, 87*(3), 333-338.

Mitchell, J. E., & Eckert, E. D. (1987). Scope and significance of eating disorders. *Journal of Consulting Clinical Psychology, 55,* 628-634.

Muecke, L., Morton-Simons, B., Huang, I. W., & Parcel, G. (1992). Is childhood obesity associated with high-fat foods and low physical activity? *Journal of School Health, 62,* 19-23.

Murphy, S. P., Castillo, R. O., Martorell, R., & Mendora, F. S. (1990). An evaluation of food group intakes by Mexican-American children. *Journal of the American Dietetic Association, 90,* 388-393.

National Academy of Sciences. (1989). *Recommended dietary allowances,* 10th ed. Washington DC: National Academy Press.

National Association of State Boards of Education, National Commission on the Role of the School and the Community in Improving Adolescent's Health. (n.d.). *CODE BLUE: Uniting for healthier youth.* Alexandria, VA: Author.

National Center for Nutrition and Dietetics & International Food Information Council. (1991a). *Kids at the table: Who's placing the orders?* Chicago: American Dietetic Association.

National Center for Nutrition and Dietetics & International Food Information Council. (1991b). *Where do kids get nutrition information?* Chicago: American Dietetic Association.

National Cholesterol Education Program, National Heart Lung and Blood Institute, National Institutes of Health. (1991, April). *Pediatric Panel Report* (Population panel report). Washington, DC: Author.

National Health Education Organization. (1989). The limitations to excellence in education. *Journal of School Health, 54*(7), 256-257.

National Institute of Health. (1994, Fall). *Heart memo.* Bethesda, MD: Author.

Palmer, R., & Johnson, A. (1991). *Los Angeles County Unified School District data.* Los Angeles: University of Southern California.

Pate, R. R. (1993). Physical activity in children and youth: Relationship to obesity. *Contemporary Nutrition, 18*(2), 1-2.

Pate, R. R., Dowdy, M., & Ross, G. (1990). Associations between physical activity and physical fitness in American children. *American Journal of Diseases in Children, 144,* 1123-1129.

Reiff, D. W., & Reiff, K. K. L. (1992). *Eating disorders— Nutrition therapy in the recovery process.* Gaithersburg, MD: Aspen.

Resnicow, K. (1991). The relationship between breakfast habits and plasma cholesterol levels in schoolchildren. *Journal of School Health, 61,* 81-85.

Rorty, M., Yager, J., & Rossotto, E. (1993). Why and how do women recover from bulimia nervosa? The subjective appraisals of 40 women recovered for a year or more. *International Journal of Eating Disorders, 14*(3), 249-260.

Ross, J. G., & Gilbert, G. G. (1985). The national children and youth fitness study: A summary of findings. *Journal of Physical Education, Recreation, and Dance, 56,* 45-50.

Sasaki, J., Shindo, M., Tanaka, H., et al. (1987). A long-term aerobic exercise program decreases the obesity index and increases the high density lipoprotein cholesterol concentration in obese children. *International Journal of Obesity, 11,* 339-345.

Schlicker, S. A., Borra, S. T., & Regan, C. (1994). The weight and fitness status of U.S. children. *Nutrition Reviews, 52*(1), 11-17.

Schmitz, M. F., & Fielding, J. E. (1986). Point-of-choice nutritional labeling: Evaluation in a worksite cafeteria. *Journal of Nutrition Education, 18,* S65-S68.

Shisslak, C. M., Crago, M., & Neal, M. E. (1990). Prevention of eating disorders among adolescents. *American Journal of Health Promotion, 5,* 100-106.

Sloan, R. (1994). Developing an awareness of eating disorder: Identifying the high-risk client. *On the Cutting Edge, 15*(6), 21-22.

Story, M. (1990). Nutrient needs during adolescence and pregnancy. In M. Story (Ed.), *Nutrition management of the pregnant adolescent: A practical reference guide* (pp. 21-28). Washington, DC: National Clearinghouse.

Story, M., & Faulkner, P. (1990). The prime time diet: A content analysis of eating behavior and food messages in television program content and commercials. *American Journal of Public Health, 80,* 738-740.

Story, M., Heald, F., & Dwyer, J. (1991). Adolescent nutrition: Trends and critical issues for the 1990s. In C. O. Sharbaugh (Ed.), *Call to action: Better nutrition for mothers, children, and families* (pp. 169-189). Washington, DC: National Center for Education in Maternal and Child Health.

Strong, J. P. (1995). National history and risk factors for early human atherogenesis. *Clinical Chemistry, 41*(1), 134-138.

Suter, E., & Hawes, M. R. (1993). Relationship of physical activity, body fat, diet, and blood lipid profile in youths 10-15 years old. *Medical Science and Sports Exercise, 25,* 748-754.

Tucker, L. A., & Bagwell, M. (1991). Television viewing and obesity in adult females. *American Journal of Public Health, 81,* 908-911.

U.S. Department of Agriculture. (1983). *Menu planning guide for school food service* (Program Aid 1260). Washington, DC: Author.

U.S. Department of Agriculture/U.S. Department of Health and Human Services. (1989). *Nutrition and your health: Dietary guidelines for Americans* (2nd ed.). Washington, DC: Author.

U.S. Department of Agriculture. (1992). *The pyramid food guide.* Washington, DC: Author.

U.S. Department of Agriculture/U.S. Department of Health and Human Services. (1995). *Nutrition and your health: Dietary guidelines for Americans* (4th ed.). Washington, DC: Author.

U.S. Department of Health and Human Services. (1990). *Healthy people 2000.* Washington, DC: Author.

U.S. Department of Health and Human Services. (1991a). *Healthy people 2000: National health promotion and disease prevention objectives* (Public Health Service Publication 91-50212). Washington, DC: Author.

U.S. Department of Health and Human Services. (1991b). *NCEP report of the expert panel on blood cholesterol levels in children and adolescents* (NIH Publication No. 91-2732). Washington, DC: Author.

U.S. Department of Health and Human Services. (1996). *Guidelines for school health programs to promote lifelong healthy eating.* Atlanta, GA: Centers for Disease Control and Prevention.

Vandereycken, W., Depreitere, L., & Probst, M. (1987). Body-oriented therapy for anorexia nervosa patients. *American Journal of Psychotherapy, 41*(2), 252-259.

Van Horn, L. V., Stumbo, P., Moag-Stahlberg, A., Obarzanek, E., Hartmuller, V. W., Farris, R. P., Kimm, S. S., Frederick, M. N., Snetselaar, L., & Kiang, L. (1993). The Dietary Intervention Study in Children (DISC): Dietary assessment methods for 8- to 10-year-olds. *Journal of the American Dietetic Association, 93*(12), 1396-1403.

Ventura, S. J., Taffel, S. M., & Mosher, W. D. (1995). *Monthly vital statistics report: Trends in pregnancies and pregnancy rates, estimates for the United States, 1980-1992.* Washington, DC: U.S. Department of Health and Human Services.

Webber, L. S., Cresanta, J. L., Voors, A. W., & Berenson, G. S. (1983). Tracking of cardiovascular disease risk factor variables in school-age children. *Journal of Chronic Diseases, 36*(9), 647-660.

Wissler, R. W., Robertson, A. L., Cornhill, J. F., McGill, H. C., McMahan, C. A., & Strong, J. P. (1990). Relationship of atherosclerosis in young men to serum lipoprotein cholesterol concentrations and smoking. *Journal of the American Medical Association, 264*(23), 3018-3024.

Wotecki, C. E. (1992). Nutrition in childhood and adolescence—Parts 1 and 2. *Contemporary Nutrition, 17*(2), 1-2.

5

Tobacco Use and Adolescents

Dale W. Evans

Almost all current adult tobacco users initiated their habit as adolescents. It is estimated that about 3,000 youth begin smoking each day (U.S. Department of Health and Human Services, 1994). The U.S. death total from tobacco-related health problems exceeds 400,000 annually (CDC, 1995). Smoking is the leading cause of avoidable, premature death (CDC, 1995). Preventing our youth from beginning to use tobacco should be the primary focus of prevention efforts.

This chapter will examine the historical background of tobacco use and focus specifically on adolescent use of cigarettes and smokeless tobacco. In addition, the chapter will discuss characteristics of successful tobacco use control programs. Finally, specific examples of successful school and community tobacco use programs from across the country will be identified.

History

Could Christopher Columbus have predicted that his strange first sight of a San Salvadoran native "swallowing smoke" would evolve into a habit of 50 million New World residents some 500 years later? The sordid history of tobacco use includes efforts both to promote the medicinal use and to ban the product completely. During the 1500s and 1600s, the voices in opposition to this new habit were muffled by those promoting the cultivation and marketing of this product throughout the colonies. Technology was on the side of tobacco users in the late 1800s, with the development of the first cigarette-making machine and matches. Prior to that time, most tobacco was either chewed, smoked in a pipe, or smoked as individually rolled cigarettes. Smokers who rolled their own cigarettes smoked less than five per day. With the advent of mass-produced cigarettes and matches, many smokers increased consumption to more than 15 per day.

As the 20th century began, the temperance movement, which focused primarily on the reduction of alcohol use, also resulted in scattered prohibition of tobacco sales. Those controls came to a sudden halt when the U.S. government endorsed tobacco use by including tobacco in soldiers' rations during World War I. "Smoke them, if you've got them" became a popular phrase during World War II. During the 1950s and 1960s, the mounting

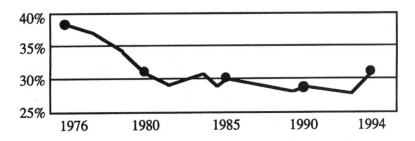

Percent of High School Seniors Who Report Smoking in Past 30 Days

Figure 5.1. Smoking Trends of Teens
SOURCE: Johnston et al., 1995.

evidence about the negative effects of tobacco culminated with the release of the first U.S. Surgeon General's report in 1964, linking tobacco use to cancer, heart disease, and other illnesses. In 1966, warning labels were required on cigarette packs, and in 1971, advertisements for cigarettes were banned on radio and TV. During the 1970s and 1980s, scientific evidence on the harmful effects of tobacco use expanded dramatically. Research that identified secondhand smoke as dangerous confirmed that smoking was much more than just a social irritant. During this time period, the number of adult smokers continued to decline. By the mid-1990s, only about 25% of U.S. adults or 50 million people were currently smokers. Most experts have recognized that tobacco use is the most preventable cause of premature death (CDC, 1995).

Over the past 25 years, tobacco manufacturers have experienced increasing criticism of both the product and the methods used to promote tobacco use. Tobacco companies fought back vigorously through the legal system, media, and other forms of marketing and public awareness. In 1991, the Tobacco Institute distributed *Tobacco: Helping Youth Say No*. According to the document, this publication was the "third in a series of booklets designed to increase communication between parents and children and to raise the levels of mutual re-

spect and trust." In 1995, the National Smokers Alliance placed full-page advertisements in major newspapers, which focused upon the concept that defending smokers' rights protects everyone's rights. In that same year, Philip Morris announced a 10-point program created to prevent cigarette sales to minors. Full- or double-page announcements in major newspapers across the country touted Action to Access: "The Best Way to Keep Kids Away from Cigarettes Is to Keep Cigarettes Away from Kids."

In 1995, President Clinton announced a plan to focus on the reduction of adolescent smokers. He noted that each day, about 3,000 teens begin smoking. His plan estimated that about half of those new smokers will eventually die from health problems related to smoking. In 1995, the number of teenage smokers was at its highest since 1985. (For trends in smoking among teens, see Figure 5.1.) This is important because almost all current smokers began when they were adolescents. Although there has been some progress in reducing the number of adult tobacco smokers, we have been less successful preventing the initiation of teen smoking. One of President Clinton's proposals suggested that because nicotine is a drug, the Federal Drug Administration (FDA) should have regulatory control of its distribution. It was not totally surprising to anti-tobacco forces that within a few days of Clinton's announcement, several tobacco manufacturers filed a lawsuit charging that under Clinton's plan, the FDA would be overstepping its statutory mandates. Surprisingly, in March 1996, the Liggett Group, the nation's fifth largest tobacco company, agreed to withdraw from the industry's battle against the FDA. The agreement was part of a more comprehensive settlement of a class-action suit by five states, seeking reimbursement for Medicaid spending on tobacco-related illnesses. The ramifications of this agreement are yet to be determined. In the broader issue of proposed expanded FDA regulations, both sides seem optimistic about the final outcome.

Current Status of Tobacco Use

The Leading Cause of Preventable Death

Although fewer adult Americans were smoking in the 1990s, estimates of yearly deaths continued to exceed 400,000 (U.S. Department of Health and Human Services, 1994). A further analysis of annual deaths caused by tobacco use reveals

- More than 120,000 deaths from lung cancer
- 30,000 other cancer deaths (mouth cancer, etc.)
- More than 200,000 deaths from cardiovascular diseases
- Over 80,000 deaths from respiratory diseases such as emphysema and bronchitis
- 2,500 deaths of infants attributed to mother's smoking
- 1,500 deaths in fires caused by smoking (CDC, 1995; Institute for Health Policy, 1993; U.S. Department of Health and Human Services, 1989)

Most experts would agree that these deaths are the result of smoking behaviors initiated

some 20 or 30 years ago. Do the current reports of an increase in adolescent smoking foretell deaths caused by smoking in 2030?

Health Consequences of Smoking

Smoking increases the mortality and morbidity of both men and women. According to *Reducing the Health Consequences of Smoking–25 Years of Progress* (U.S. Department of Health and Human Services, 1989), a causal relationship has been shown between smoking and coronary heart disease, atherosclerotic peripheral vascular disease, lung cancer, oral cancer, esophageal cancer, chronic obstructive pulmonary disease, intrauterine growth retardation, and low birth weight babies. In addition, there is mounting evidence that smoking is a contributing cause for increased infant mortality, chronic bronchitis, emphysema, peptic ulcer, and cancers of the bladder, pancreas, and kidney.

Secondhand Smoke

Secondhand smoke or Environmental Tobacco Smoke (ETS) is the inhalation by nonsmokers of air containing smoke. Many nonsmokers have recognized secondhand smoke as a social irritant. By the 1990s, numerous studies reported the health risks of secondhand smoke on the nonsmoker. In 1993, the Environmental Protection Agency (EPA) classified secondhand smoke as a Group A carcinogen (EPA, 1993). The EPA also reported increased risk of asthma, lower respiratory infections in children, low birth-weight babies, and increased heart attacks in nonsmokers married to smokers, and nonsmoking wives married to smoking husbands had increased risk of developing lung cancer. Finally, the EPA estimated that secondhand smoke is responsible for about 3,000 lung cancer deaths each year in nonsmoking adults.

Smokeless Tobacco

In 1996, about 6.8 million Americans were estimated to be current users of smokeless tobacco, and more than 90% of those users were males (U.S. Department of Health and Human Services, 1997). Some users mistakenly believe that smokeless tobacco is a safe alternative to smoking. Several studies have identified a causal link between the use of smokeless tobacco and oral cancer (U.S. Department of Health and Human Services, 1992). Two early signs of possible precancerous oral changes are leukoplakia (white lesions) and erythroplakia (red lesions). A more common oral health problem is the development of periodontal disease, which may result in loss of teeth, damage to tooth enamel caused by abrasion, and more tooth decay from sugar added to the tobacco during processing.

Cessation

Various studies have reported that over 80% of current adult smokers have tried unsuccessfully to stop (U.S. Department of Health and Human Services, 1989). As a group, former smokers in the United States may include as many as 37 million people. Formal smoking cessation programs have not been very successful. Most evidence suggests that as many as 90% of former smokers quit on their own, without a formal cessation program. Almost three fourths of 12- to 18-year-olds reported they had thought seriously about quitting, and almost two thirds had tried to quit smoking (English & Austin, 1995, Vol. 1). Although cessation programs for adolescents and for those attempting to stop smokeless tobacco use have shown very mixed results, such efforts are an important component of a comprehensive tobacco use control program. What is clear is that the major focus should be on implementing tobacco use prevention programs and limiting access to tobacco products, rather than waiting to implement cessation programs.

Tobacco Advertising

- Marlboro is the most advertised brand
- 69% of teen smokers smoke Marlboro
- 24% of adult smokers smoke Marlboro

It is estimated that $6 billion is spent annually to advertise and promote tobacco use in the United States (CDC, 1995). That is more than $11,000 per minute. Many advertising experts marvel at the success of tobacco advertising. It has been said that tobacco advertisers created a market that had not existed. Young people continue to be an important market for the tobacco industry. It should be noted that by the mid 1990s, several cigarette manufacturers had published official policies opposing access to cigarettes by youth. Many antismoking groups have questioned those statements in light of past and current advertising efforts. Children and adolescents are exposed to tobacco messages in the print media, outdoor advertising, entertainment events, and the sponsorship of sporting events. A recent and creative marketing approach involves the distribution of speciality items such as clothing. It seems clear that the creative marketing of tobacco products reaches our youth daily.

Cigarette advertisements generally focus on images rather than information to promote the attractiveness and function of smoking. An analysis of current advertisements reveals people smoking unlit cigarettes with no ashes or smoke. Common messages that appeal to adolescents include: independence, adventure, seeking, and healthful outdoor life. Advertisements often take advantage of the differences between ideal and self-image and promote smoking as a vehicle to close that gap. Finally, advertisements affect adolescents' perceptions of the pervasiveness, image, and function of smoking.

The Joe Camel advertising campaign, initiated in 1988, is but one example of a successful marketing program. Prior to the campaign, the 1986 market share of Camel's among 17- to 24-year-olds was less than 3%. By 1993, the market share for the same group rose to 13%. Joe Camel, a cool character, was found everywhere, on outdoor billboards, race cars, and promotional clothing offered for Camel Cash. In late 1995, the manufacturer of Camel's announced that the Joe Camel promotional campaign would be temporarily suspended. Furthermore, the suspension of the campaign had nothing to do with public criticism of this approach. By the spring of 1996, Joe Camel had prominently reappeared in both advertisements and promotional materials.

There is much debate about whether to expand the restriction of tobacco advertisements from television and radio to include other venues. Should print and outdoor advertisements for tobacco products be eliminated or restricted? What would be the impact of restricting promotional advertising at sporting and entertainment events? Although there is some disagreement, even among antitobacco groups, about further control or elimination of advertisements, there seems to be a consensus that advertisements and promotional events should not be aimed at youth.

Adolescent Tobacco Use

Patterns of tobacco use by adolescents have been monitored for more than 20 years. The National Household Survey of Drug Abuse (NHS) and the Monitoring the Future Survey (MTF) have reported on drug use patterns since the 1970s. Since 1991, the Youth Risk Behavior Survey (YRBS) has provided a third source of data regarding tobacco use. Each of these sources surveyed over 10,000 people. In addition, many states, communities, school districts, and health organizations such as the American Cancer Society have conducted various surveys and interviews to determine current tobacco use trends. Although it is difficult to make precise comparisons of findings because of different survey methods, questions, and so on, tobacco use trends among adolescents have been established.

Tobacco Use Among Adolescents

- About 25% of 11th and 12th grade students are regular smokers
- At least 3.1 million adolescents are current smokers
- Tobacco use begins early in adolescence, by age 16
- At least 80% of first use of tobacco occurs in adolescents
- Whites are most likely to use all forms of tobacco
- Although smoking declined in the 1970s, the decline slowed in the 1980s
- From 1991 through 1995, smoking by adolescents increased
- Both genders are equally likely to smoke
- Use of smokeless tobacco increased between the 1970s and the mid-1980s (CDC, 1995; English & Austin, 1995, Vol. 1; U.S. Department of Health and Human Services, 1994)

Many reports about the health consequences of tobacco use focus on life-threatening health problems that most often occur in middle or older age. The Surgeon General's report on *Preventing Tobacco Use Among Young People* (U.S. Department of Health and Human Services, 1994) reported that cigarette smoking during adolescence produces a number of significant health problems including: increased respiratory illnesses, decreased physical fitness, and unfavorable lipid profile. Smokeless tobacco use is associated

TABLE 5.1. Goals for Healthy People 2000, Tobacco Use Prevention Objectives

Objective Number	Objective
3.4	Reduce cigarette smoking to a prevalence of no more than 15% among people age 18 and older
3.5	Reduce the initiation of cigarette smoking by children and youth so that no more than 15% have become regular cigarette smokers by age 20
3.6	Increase to at least 50% the proportion of cigarette smokers age 18 and older who stopped smoking cigarettes for at least one day during preceding year
3.7	Increase the smoking cessation during pregnancy so that at least 60% of women who are cigarette smokers at the time they become pregnant quit smoking early in pregnancy and maintain abstinence for the remainder of pregnancy
3.8	Reduce to no more than 20% the proportion of children age 6 and younger who are regularly exposed to tobacco smoke at home
3.9	Reduce smokeless tobacco use by males ages 12 through 24 to a prevalence of no more than 4%
3.10	Establish tobacco-free environments and include tobacco use prevention in the curricula of all elementary, middle, and secondary schools, preferably as a part of quality (comprehensive) school health education
3.11	Increase to at least 75% the proportion of worksites (such as schools) with a formal smoking policy that prohibits or severely restricts smoking at the workplace
3.12	Enact in 50 states comprehensive laws on clean indoor air that prohibit or strictly limit smoking in the workplace and enclosed public places (such as schools)

SOURCE: U.S. Department of Health and Human Services, 1991.

with early indicators of periodontal disease. In addition, smokeless tobacco users are much more likely than nonsmokers to become cigarette smokers.

Among all addictive behaviors, smoking is the one most likely to become established during adolescence. Tobacco is usually the first drug used by youth, who initiate a sequence that may include tobacco, alcohol, marijuana, and other illegal drugs. Furthermore, tobacco use is associated with a number of health-compromising behaviors, including higher-risk sexual behavior, violence, and use of alcohol and other drugs. (Federal goals for changing these behaviors are listed in Table 5.1.)

Prevention Strategies: Community Mobilization

According to *Strategies to Control Tobacco Use in the United States* (U.S. Department of Health and Human Services, 1991, p. 218), although national and state tobacco control initiatives are critical, the most effective interventions are at the local level. Two practical ways to implement tobacco control programs at the local level are described as *social action* and *locality development*. The social action plan involves the mobilization of the most interested and committed local groups to demand change in the social structure. Locality development extends participation to include a broader base of individuals and groups with the goal of developing a coalition working toward tobacco control. Although coalition building is a time-consuming and complex process, the potential results can be significant. The synergy of the media, schools, health care professionals, and government working toward a common goal of reducing tobacco use can have dramatic results. Table 5.2, adapted from a table found in *Strategies to Control Tobacco Use in the United States* (U.S. Department of Health and Human Services, 1991), suggests tobacco control activities that involve a variety of local groups working together.

TABLE 5.2. Examples of Local Tobacco Control Activities

Channel	Activity	Responsibility
Media	Promote Great American Smokeout	B, C, D, E, F, H
	Advertise cessation services	
	Publish or broadcast antitobacco PSAs	
	Establish communications network among tobacco control advocates	All groups
Health care sector	Provide cessation programs for clients	B, C, D, E
	Recruit and train health care providers to be advocates	B, C, D, E
	Lobby to promote mandated insurance coverage for cessation programs and discounts for non-tobacco users	A, B, C, D, E, F, H
	Conduct community tobacco control programs	All groups
Worksite	Conduct employee assistance cessation programs	B, C, D, E
	Implement incentive program for successful quitters	B, D, H
	Support health insurance discounts for nonusers	A, B, C, D, G
	Disseminate educational information on value of not smoking	A, B, E, F
Schools	Initiate programs to train teachers to implement tobacco education curricula	B, E, F
	Conduct survey of staff and students to document tobacco use trends	B, E, F
	Initiate a smoke-free campus	All groups
	Implement comprehensive school health education program	B, E, F, G

SOURCE: Adapted from U.S. Department of Health & Human Services, 1991.
NOTE: Local groups A = Business groups (Chamber of Commerce), B = Voluntary health agencies, C = Health professional organizations, D = Health care facilities, E = Universities, medical/dental/nursing schools, F = K to 12 schools, G = Government, H = Community organizations.

Prevention of Tobacco Use Among Adolescents

Most Americans, including smokers, support various efforts to prevent tobacco use among our youth, including educational programs in schools, restrictions on promotions and advertisements, bans on all tobacco use on school grounds, prohibition of sales to minors, and increased taxes, which would then be designated to support either health-enhancing or antitobacco efforts. Although tobacco manufacturers may not support each of these efforts, most now publicly say that tobacco products should be restricted for minors. Illegal sales of tobacco products are very common. Increased enforcement efforts and educational programs are needed to restrict the illegal sales of tobacco products to youth. The cost of cigarettes is related to cigarette smoking trends; that is, as the price of cigarettes increases the incidence of smoking decreases (Consumers Union, 1995).

A review of the stages of smoking initiation among children and adolescents was presented in *Preventing Tobacco Use Among Young People: A Report of the Surgeon General* (U.S. Department of Health and Human Services, 1994). An analysis of each stage provides valuable insights for educators seeking to develop a tobacco use control program for schools (see Figure 5.2).

Characteristics of Effective School Tobacco Use Educational Programs

Because the vast majority of tobacco users begin as adolescents, it would seem that schools are in an ideal position to implement educational programs to prevent and reduce tobacco use. Those who might argue that it is unreasonable to expect schools to become involved in this issue need only to look at the facts. Tobacco use is the leading cause of preventable deaths, and most users initiate their

Psychosocial risk factors include:

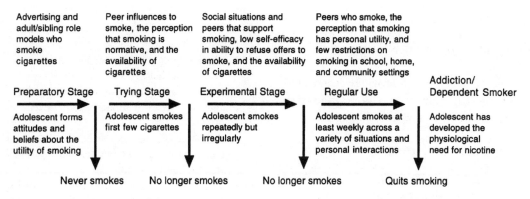

Figure 5.2. Stages of Smoking Initiation Among Children and Adolescents
SOURCE: U.S. Department of Health and Human Services, 1994, p. 126, adapted from Flay, 1993

tobacco journey in their youth. *Guidelines for School Health Programs to Prevent Tobacco Use Addiction* (CDC, 1994) and Volume 2 of the *Guide to Tobacco Use Among California Youth* (English & Austin, 1995) highlight the most current knowledge available about the most effective antitobacco use prevention strategies to improve school efforts. Many of the suggestions move well beyond the classroom and have implications for a total community effort.

Recommendation 1. Provide prevention education each year, Grades K to 12. However, when choosing to provide a less extensive program, provide comprehensive core programs in the early years with booster lessons each year thereafter.

- Tobacco education should be an integral part of comprehensive school health education.
- The NCI recommends at least five tobacco use prevention lessons in each grade, K to 12.
- Short-term programs have short-term effects.
- Ideally, tobacco use prevention programs will begin in elementary grades.
- Instruction should be especially intensive in middle school or junior high.

- Follow-up and booster lessons should continue through high school.

Recommendation 2. Emphasize social factors that influence the onset of tobacco use, normative expectations, and the consequences of tobacco use most relevant to youth.

- Investigate how peers and family influence onset of tobacco use.
- Analyze the methods and the messages used by tobacco manufacturers.
- Tobacco users are a minority; expose the myth that "all or most kids use tobacco."
- Youth are optimistic, and many believe they will live forever. Long-term effects of tobacco use seldom influence youth. Focus on short-term consequences such as the odor surrounding a smoker, bad breath, and decreased stamina.

Recommendation 3. Base tobacco use prevention programs on developing refusal skills and social skills.

- Programs that focus on a skill-based approach to tobacco use prevention have been found to be most effective.
- Curricula that help students develop resistance skills, such as refusal skills, have been found to be key components of successful programs.

- Development of social skills such as problem solving and decision making have shown potential as effective not only for tobacco use prevention programs but also for reducing other risky health behaviors.

Recommendation 4. Provide adequate training, ongoing support, and monitoring of program implementation.

- Expand teacher training and support, especially for those instructional strategies with which teachers may not be as comfortable (refusal skills, role playing, etc.).
- Train teachers using other effective teachers as teaching role models.
- Provide opportunities for classroom observations and formal feedback to teachers.
- Monitor teacher compliance and fidelity with curricular components, guidelines, and so on.

Recommendation 5. Involve students as assistants in program delivery.

- Peer education is gaining increased acceptance for inclusion within school curricula.
- Peer leaders often are perceived as more credible than adults.
- Using older students to assist in educating younger students about tobacco use has shown promise.
- Selecting, training, and monitoring peer leaders is a complex process.
- Peer leaders view the experience as beneficial and positive.

Recommendation 6. Collaborate with the community and families to expand prevention activities beyond the school.

- An effective community-wide tobacco use prevention effort involves government, official and voluntary health organizations, businesses, religious groups, and the families and schools.
- Involving parents through classroom assignments, parent-teacher organizations, and advisory groups will assist in a more uniform and consistent no-use message.

Recommendation 7. Develop and enforce a school tobacco policy consistent with the prevention program.

- A school policy on tobacco use must be consistent with federal, state, and local laws.
- A no-use school environment policy reflects and supports the tobacco use prevention program.
- Policy development should be a collaborative effort involving students, teachers, parents, and community groups.
- The policy should be communicated to students, staff, parents, visitors, and the community.

Recommendation 8. Support cessation efforts among students and all school staff who use tobacco.

- Access to cessation programs is a logical partner to a no-use tobacco policy in schools and to tobacco use prevention programs.
- Cessation programs may be available through local voluntary health agencies such as the American Cancer Society, American Heart Association, American Lung Association, or the public health department.
- Initiation of health promotion activities for students, teachers, and staff promotes healthy lifestyles and health-enhancing alternatives to tobacco use.

Strategies for the Classroom Teacher

Many experts in health education and curriculum development believe a K to 12 comprehensive school health education program holds the greatest promise for dealing with the complex health-related problems of adolescents. Although some schools have wisely chosen this comprehensive approach, others have identified specific health topics (such as tobacco, alcohol, and other drugs) to be covered at certain grade levels. Ideally, the guidelines presented in the previous section would provide the foundation for the development of a tobacco use prevention curriculum. A state department of education, school, or individual teacher could develop a tobacco curriculum specific to the unique needs of the local area or community. As an alternative, one might select a curriculum or educational resource developed by voluntary health agencies or a group advocating tobacco control. A number of these resources are identified in the last section of this chapter. In addition, numerous books, curriculum guides, and lesson plans that focus on tobacco use prevention are widely available.

Ideas for a Lesson

Each of the following is a core idea around which a classroom lesson can be developed. These ideas can be modified for use with elementary, middle, and high school students.

- Have each student bring examples of tobacco advertisements. Analyze each for method and message. What are the dominant themes? Do students think advertising is effective?
- Participate in the Great American Smokeout (GAS). GAS is the third Thursday in November. Educational materials and resources are available from the American Cancer Society.
- Infuse health into history (and other classes). Investigate the historical significance of tobacco to the economy. Identify what events may have influenced tobacco use trends.
- Integrate health into mathematics. Calculate the cost of smoking one pack of cigarettes per day for a year. How much money could be saved if one didn't smoke?
- Correlate the tobacco use prevention program with language arts. Initiate a writing campaign such as "Letter to the Editor" regarding the elimination of advertisements aimed at youth or the elimination of tobacco subsidies.
- Develop a peer tobacco use prevention program for younger students. Have students present the program to either the middle or elementary school.

- Critique an educational tool (film, CD-Rom, game, etc.) designed to deter tobacco use by teens. Have students evaluate both the methods and message for effectiveness.
- Have students create a cartoon or poem about teen use of tobacco. Submit the entries to the school newspaper or community newspaper for publication.
- Using a role-play scenario, have students demonstrate refusal skills when offered tobacco products.

Summary

Interest in tobacco by individuals, the medical and legal professions, and governmental agencies gained momentum during 1996 and 1997. By 1997, individual states and the federal government had some major successes with legal action against the tobacco industry. Although a federal court ruled that tobacco could be regulated as a drug by the FDA, it also said that the FDA could not regulate tobacco advertising. In what some might consider a major breakthrough, the Liggett Group settled a suit with 22 state attorneys, which will protect the company from further litigation in return for admitting tobacco is addictive, providing evidence implicating other tobacco companies, and agreeing to pay a large sum. Even more startling are the preliminary discussions by federal officials with the major tobacco manufacturers, which could also protect these companies from legal action while the companies agree to pay some $300 billion for health care costs incurred by the government for tobacco-related illnesses and provide some funding for tobacco use prevention programs. Although many anticipate the positive aspects of these developments, others are not optimistic the result will be a reduction in tobacco use by adolescents.

Tobacco use is clearly the leading cause of preventable premature death. Almost all tobacco users begin during adolescence. The 3,000 youth who begin smoking each day are important to the tobacco industry because they replace an increasing number of people who quit, and over 1,000 who die each day. To maximize the potential for preventing tobacco use by our youth, we must stand together as a united force. The school is but one important participant in many community antitobacco use efforts. If we as a society are to be successful, the strengths of voluntary health organizations, official health agencies, parents, schools, and youth must be focused toward the common goal of a tobacco-free future for all.

Linking Strategies: Effective Community Programs to Control Youth Access to Tobacco

A number of antitobacco community programs have shown promise in efforts to control youth access to tobacco. Collaborative programs involving government, schools, and community groups seem to be the most effective. The following list is an example of major tobacco use prevention programs and organizations available in many communities.

American Cancer Society–Contact your local office

Sponsors the Great American Smokeout each November, the most expansive antismoking awareness event. Provides educational materials on tobacco for both the community and schools. A new curriculum for upper elementary grades and middle school, *Do It Yourself: Making Healthy Choices,* was introduced in 1995.

American Heart Association–Contact your local office

Promotes a tobacco-free life as part of cardiovascular health. Distributes a variety of resources for school and community groups. Save A Sweetheart is an antismoking program that reaches adolescents through the school but outside the classroom.

American Lung Association–Contact your local office

Advocates for clean air, local offices disseminate and promote various educational resources that focus on tobacco use prevention programs. Unpuffables is a 4-week home-based course designed to help adolescents and their parents discuss the issue of preventing tobacco use.

California Department of Health Services, Tobacco Control Section, Sacramento, CA (916) 327-5427

A culturally diverse multimedia campaign to deglamorize tobacco use. Creative TV spots, in several languages, include music video and rappers. Funded by Proposition 99, the California Tobacco Tax Initiative.

Centers for Disease Control and Prevention, Office on Smoking and Health, Atlanta, GA (404) 488-5701

Governmental leader, planner, consultant, and so on in the prevention and cessation of tobacco use and protection of the nonsmoker. Assists communities and organizations develop smoking control programs.

Gloucester Prevention Network, Stop Using Nicotine (SUN) Coalition, Gloucester, MA (508) 281-0311

A grassroots effort initiated by four 7th-grade students to restrict cigarette vending machines. Eventually the city council passed a local ordinance to control vending machines.

Join Together, Boston, MA (617) 437-1500

A national resource for communities fighting substance abuse. Publishes daily electronic summaries of newspaper articles on tobacco issues through Join Together Online.

Operation SCAT, Student Coalition Against Tobacco, Springfield, MA (413) 732-7828

In 1993, a group of students who were successful in initiating a smoke-free policy for their school district began spreading their message nationally. Their experiences will be helpful for those mobilizing teens.

Smoke-Free Class of 2000–Contact the organizations locally

A joint effort of the American Cancer Society, American Heart Association, and American Lung Association began in 1988 when students were 1st graders. The goal of this project is that these students have a tobacco-free life when they graduate from high school in 2000. To date, over 2 million students have been reached.

Stop Teenage Addiction to Tobacco (STAT), Springfield, MA (413) 736-5251

Conducts training programs and consultation to prevent adolescent access to tobacco. Publishes various tobacco-related materials, of particular interest: *Tobacco-Free Youth Reporter.*

References

Centers for Disease Control and Prevention. (1994, February 25). Guidelines for school health programs to prevent tobacco use and addiction. *Morbidity and Mortality Weekly Report, 43*(No. RR-2), 1-18.

Centers for Disease Control and Prevention. (1995). *Protecting youth from tobacco addiction: Restricting access and appeal of tobacco products to children and adolescents.*

English, J., & Austin, G. (1995). *Guide to tobacco use prevention among California youth* (3 vols.). Los Alamitos, CA: Southwest Regional Laboratory.

Environmental Protection Agency. (1993). *Respiratory health effects of passive smoking* (fact sheet). Washington, DC: Author.

Institute for Health Policy. (1993). *Substance abuse: The nation's number one health problem, key indicators for policy.* Princeton, NJ: Author.

Johnson, L. D., Bachman, J. G., & O'Malley. (1995). *Monitoring the future.* Ann Arbor: Institute for Social Research, University of Michigan.

U.S. Department of Health and Human Services. (1989). *Reducing the health consequences of smoking: 25 years of progress* (A report of the surgeon general). Washington, DC: Author.

U.S. Department of Health and Human Services. (1991). *Strategies to control tobacco use in the United States: A blueprint for public health action in the 1990s.* Washington, DC: Author.

U.S. Department of Health and Human Services. (1992). *Smokeless tobacco or health: An international perspective* (Smoking and Tobacco Control, Monograph 2). Washington, DC: Author.

U.S. Department of Health and Human Services. (1994). *Preventing tobacco use among young people: A report of the surgeon general.* Washington, DC: Author.

U.S. Department of Health and Human Services. (1997). *Preliminary estimates from the 1996 national household survey on drug abuse.* Washington, DC: Author.

6

Drug Abuse

Jill English

Drug use and abuse by adolescents has been a national concern since the 1970s, when the use of alcohol and other drugs predominately on college campuses began to spread into neighborhood schools. The tracking of use, as well as the development of drug prevention programs, began about this time and has continued to evolve. The purpose of this chapter is to discuss the extent of drug use by adolescents, strategies for drug prevention, and promising approaches, with the hope of providing the practitioner with guidance on improving the health of adolescents through the prevention of drug abuse.

Extent of the Problem

There are two main sources of national data on drug use among adolescents. The first, *Monitoring the Future* (MTF) survey, is funded by the National Institute on Drug Abuse and conducted with youth in Grades 8, 10, and 11. The other is the *Youth Risk Behavior Surveillance* (YRBS), funded by the CDC and conducted with youth in Grades 9 through 12. These surveys have provided health educators and others with information about trends in adolescents' attitudes about and use of alcohol and other drugs. A look at current reports

from these surveys, as well as trends over the past 20 years, provides insight into extent of use, attitudes about, and perceptions of alcohol and other drugs.

Drug Use Among Secondary Students

In both of the national surveys, students provide self-reports of their use of various drugs within several periods of time, generally within their lifetime, within the 30 days prior to completing the survey, weekly, and daily. From this data, researchers can begin to draw conclusions about the drugs most commonly used by adolescents and the frequency of use. Table 6.1 provides data from the MTF survey for the past 3 years, noting prevalence during lifetime, annual, 30 days prior to the survey, and daily. Other highlights from recent reports of these surveys include the following:

- The proportion of 8th graders taking any illicit drug in the 12 months prior to the survey has almost doubled since 1991, from 11% to 21% (Johnston, O'Malley, & Bachman, 1995).
- Fewer than 1 in 100 8th graders use marijuana daily, yet nearly 1 in 20 12th graders is a daily marijuana user (Johnston et al., 1995).

TABLE 6.1. Drug Use Among 8th, 10th, and 12th Graders (percentage)

	8th Graders			10th Graders			12th Graders		
	1993	*1994*	*1995*	*1993*	*1994*	*1995*	*1993*	*1994*	*1995*
Marijuana/hashish									
Lifetime	12.6	16.7	19.9	24.4	30.4	34.1	35.3	38.2	41.7
Annual	9.2	13.0	15.8	19.2	25.2	28.7	26.0	30.7	34.7
30-day	5.1	7.8	9.1	10.9	15.8	17.2	15.5	19.0	21.2
Daily	0.4	0.7	0.8	1.0	2.2	2.8	2.4	3.6	4.6
Inhalants									
Lifetime	19.4	19.9	21.6	17.5	18.0	19.0	17.4	17.7	17.4
Annual	11.0	11.7	12.8	8.4	9.1	9.6	7.0	7.7	8.0
30-day	5.4	5.6	6.1	3.3	3.6	3.5	2.5	2.7	3.2
Daily	0.3	0.2	0.2	0.2	0.1	0.1	0.1	0.1	0.1
Hallucinogens									
Lifetime	3.9	4.3	5.2	6.8	8.1	9.3	10.9	11.4	12.7
Annual	2.6	2.7	3.6	4.7	5.8	7.2	7.4	7.6	9.3
30-day	1.2	1.3	1.7	1.9	2.4	3.3	2.7	3.1	4.4
Daily	0.1	0.1	0.1	0.1	0.1	a	0.1	0.1	0.1
Cocaine									
Lifetime	2.9	3.6	4.2	3.6	4.3	5.0	6.1	5.9	6.0
Annual	1.7	2.1	2.6	2.1	2.8	3.5	3.3	3.6	4.0
30-day	0.7	1.0	1.2	0.9	1.2	1.7	1.3	1.5	1.8
Daily	0.1	0.1	0.1	0.1	0.1	0.1	0.1	0.1	0.2
Crack cocaine									
Lifetime	1.7	2.4	2.7	1.8	2.1	2.8	2.6	3.0	3.0
Annual	1.0	1.3	1.6	1.1	1.4	1.8	1.5	1.9	2.1
30-day	0.4	0.7	0.7	0.5	0.6	0.9	0.7	0.8	1.0
Daily	0.1	a	a	a	a	a	0.1	0.1	0.1
Heroin									
Lifetime	1.4	2.0	2.3	1.3	1.5	1.7	1.1	1.2	1.6
Annual	0.7	1.2	1.4	0.7	0.9	12.1	0.5	0.6	1.1
30-day	0.4	0.6	0.6	0.3	0.4	0.6	0.2	0.3	0.6
Daily	a	0.1	a	a	a	a	a	a	0.1
Stimulants									
Lifetime	11.8	12.3	13.1	14.9	15.1	17.4	15.1	15.7	15.3
Annual	7.2	7.9	8.7	9.6	10.2	11.9	8.4	9.4	9.3
30-day	3.6	3.6	4.2	4.3	4.5	5.3	3.7	4.0	4.0
Daily	0.1	0.1	0.2	0.3	0.1	0.2	0.2	0.2	0.3
Alcohol[b]									
Lifetime	55.7	55.8	54.5	71.6	71.1	70.5	80.0	80.4	80.7
Annual	45.4	46.8	45.3	63.4	63.9	63.5	72.7	73.0	73.7
30-day	24.3	25.5	24.6	38.2	39.2	38.8	48.6	50.1	51.3
Daily	1.0	1.0	0.7	1.8	1.7	1.7	3.4	2.9	3.5
Cigarettes (any use)									
Lifetime	45.3	46.1	46.4	56.3	56.9	57.6	61.9	62.0	64.2
30-day	16.7	18.6	19.1	24.7	25.4	27.9	29.9	31.2	33.5
Daily	8.3	8.8	9.3	14.2	14.6	16.3	19.0	19.4	21.6
1/2 pack + per day	3.5	3.6	3.4	7.0	7.6	8.3	10.9	11.2	12.4
Steroids									
Lifetime	1.6	2.0	2.0	1.7	1.8	2.0	2.0	2.4	2.3
Annual	0.9	1.2	1.0	1.0	1.1	12.2	1.2	1.3	1.5
30-day	0.5	0.5	0.6	0.5	0.6	0.6	0.7	0.9	0.7
Daily	0.1	a	a	a	0.1	0.1	0.1	0.4	0.2

a. Indicates less than 0.05%.
b. Starting in 1993, the question was changed slightly to indicate that a "drink" meant "more than a few sips."

- Beliefs about the harmfulness of various drugs, important determinants of use, have continued to decline, especially for marijuana and cocaine (Johnston et al., 1995).
- Peer disapproval of drug use, also considered an important determinant of use, continued to decline. Yet, most students in Grades 8 (71%), 10 (60%), and 12 (57%) disapprove of trying marijuana (Johnston et al., 1995).
- About 30% of students in Grades 9 through 12 had five or more drinks of alcohol on at least one occasion during the 30 days preceding the survey (CDC, 1993).
- About 13% of students in Grades 9 through 12 had smoked cigarettes on school property during the 30 days preceding the survey (CDC, 1993).
- Over 25% of students in Grades 8, 10, and 12 say it is fairly easy or very easy to get any drug, with the perceived ease of availability of marijuana by 12th graders at over 88% (Johnston et al., 1995).
- Despite national attention to the use of drugs such as cocaine, inhalants, and amphetamines, the drugs of choice among adolescents clearly continue to be alcohol, tobacco, and marijuana, with 30-day prevalence rates for 12th graders at 51%, 34%, and 21%, respectively (CDC, 1993; Johnston et al., 1995).

Despite public perceptions, regular drug use among adolescents, defined here as 30-day prevalence of use, has remained relatively steady over the past 20 years, as depicted in Tables 6.2A and B. With the exception of the use of alcohol, tobacco, and marijuana, over 85% of 12th graders have not used drugs in the 30 days prior to the survey (Johnston et al., 1995). This is good news for health educators and others working to continue preventing drug use among adolescents.

Drug Use Among Special Populations

The public has generated perceptions about the extent of use among special populations. The common perception is that drug use among minority populations is more prevalent than among whites and that drug use is more prevalent among males than females. Data from the national surveys do not support these public perceptions.

Minorities

Although the focus of national attention has been on drugs such as crack, cocaine, amphetamines, and inhalants, the drugs used most frequently and most heavily by adolescents continue to be alcohol, tobacco, and marijuana. For this reason, attention will be focused on these three drugs. Data from the national surveys have been analyzed by racial and ethnic groups to produce the following patterns (Austin & Pollard, 1993; Bachman et al., 1991; CDC, 1993):

- Alcohol: Native American, white, and Hispanic adolescents had higher rates of current use of alcohol, with blacks and Asians having the lowest rates.
- Tobacco: Whites had the highest rates for 30-day prevalence of cigarettes, with blacks having the lowest rates.
- Marijuana: Native Americans reported the highest levels of marijuana use. Thirty-day prevalence of marijuana use was similar among whites, blacks, and Hispanics.

A summary of drug use by race/ethnicity and gender, summarized from the Youth Risk Behavior Surveillance, is provided in Table 6.3.

Gender

The Youth Risk Behavior Surveillance (CDC, 1993) analyzed drug use by gender. Some interesting findings for alcohol, tobacco, and marijuana use include the following:

- Regular cigarette use is almost identical among males and females, regardless of race or ethnicity.
- Current use of alcohol is almost identical among white females and males (49% vs. 51%), with use by females being lower than

males for blacks (37% vs. 48%) and Hispanics (47% vs. 55%).

- Fewer females are current marijuana users, regardless of race or ethnicity.

Out-of-School Youth

Surveys of drug use among youth are frequently conducted in schools, leaving out the large number of youth who are not in school, perhaps underrepresenting the extent of substance use. Recently, a survey was conducted of out-of-school youth, ages 15 to 17, in California (Horowitz, 1993). The findings from this study show a dramatically higher prevalence of drug use among out-of-school adolescents. Some of the highlights of the study include the following:

- There was little difference between the two populations on prevalence of lifetime use.
- Daily use rates were much higher for adolescents out of school than those in school, especially for marijuana/hashish (16% vs. 3%) and beer (9% vs. 1%).
- Lifetime use of crack and ice were dramatically higher for out-of-school adolescents (18% and 21%, respectively) than in-school youth (4% and 5%,, respectively).
- The age of first use was relatively comparable between the two populations (alcohol, 11 years; alcohol intoxication, 13 years; drug use, 13 years).
- Out-of-school adolescents were much more likely to have engaged in multiple substance use than adolescents in school (52% vs. 21%).

Summary

For the past 20 years, adolescent use of alcohol and tobacco, two of the traditional gateway drugs and the drugs most frequently used by adolescents, has remained relatively high and unchanged. Marijuana use, although it fluctuates more than alcohol use, still remains high. The data indicate a definite need to keep the nation's attention focused on the prevention of use of these three drugs, with less attention focused on the drugs

glamorized by the media as highly used, such as crack, amphetamines, and inhalants. In addition, efforts need to include those youth who are not reached through typical school-based programs.

National Strategies for Drug Prevention Among Adolescents

Drug abuse prevention became a major federal priority in 1986 with the passage of PL99-570, the Anti-Drug Abuse Acts and 1988 PL100-690. These laws continue to provide financial assistance to local communities and school districts to prevent drug use among youth. Through the U.S. Department of Education, entitlement money is given to each school district throughout the nation to devise and implement drug prevention activities. The Office of Substance Abuse Prevention, housed within the U.S. Department of Health and Human Services and now called the Center for Substance Abuse Prevention, provides competitive grants to agencies proposing a variety of strategies to prevent substance use among youth.

In addition, other federal agencies, such as the CDC, the National Institute on Drug Abuse, and the National Institute on Alcohol Abuse and Alcoholism, among others, provide support for efforts to curb drug use among adolescents throughout the nation.

In 1990, the U.S. Department of Health and Human Services published a report, *Healthy People 2000: National Health Promotion and Disease Prevention Objectives,* offering a vision for the upcoming century. The report was a cooperative effort of schools, community agencies, and health care providers, among others, launching a national initiative to improve the health of all Americans significantly in the next 10 years through a coordinated and comprehensive push toward prevention. Among the report's 298 objectives were 10 objectives for improving adolescent health re-

TABLE 6.2A. Long-Term Trends in 30-Day Prevalence of Use of Various Types of Drugs for 12th Graders (From the Class of 1975 to the Class of 1985)

						Percentage who used in past 30 days					
	Class of 1975	Class of 1976	Class of 1977	Class of 1978	Class of 1979	Class of 1980	Class of 1981	Class of 1982	Class of 1983	Class of 1984	Class of 1985
Approximate N =	9,400	15,400	17,100	17,800	15,500	15,900	17,500	17,700	16,300	15,900	16,000
Any illicit drug	30.7	34.2	37.6	38.9	38.9	37.2	36.9	32.5	30.5	29.2	29.7
Any illicit drug other than marijuana	15.4	13.9	15.2	15.1	16.8	18.4	21.7	17.0	15.4	15.1	14.9
Marijuana/hashish	27.1	32.2	35.4	37.1	36.5	33.7	31.6	28.5	27.0	25.2	25.7
Inhalants	—	0.9	1.3	1.5	1.7	1.4	1.5	1.5	1.7	1.9	2.2
Inhalants, adjusted	—	—	—	—	3.2	2.7	2.5	2.5	2.5	2.6	3.0
Amyl/butyl nitrites	—	—	—	—	2.4	1.8	1.4	1.1	1.4	1.4	1.1
Hallucinogens	4.7	3.4	4.1	3.9	4.0	3.7	3.7	3.4	2.8	2.6	2.5
Hallucinogens, adjusted	—	—	—	—	5.3	4.4	4.5	4.1	3.5	3.2	3.8
LSD	2.3	1.9	2.1	2.1	2.4	2.3	2.5	2.4	1.9	1.5	1.6
PCP	—	—	—	—	2.4	1.4	1.4	1.0	1.3	1.0	1.6
Cocaine	1.9	2.0	2.9	3.9	5.7	5.2	5.8	5.0	4.9	5.8	6.7
Crack	—	—	—	—	—	—	—	—	—	—	0.3
Other cocaine	—	—	—	—	—	—	—	—	—	—	2.3
Heroin	0.4	0.2	0.3	0.3	0.2	0.2	0.2	0.2	0.2	0.3	0.2
Other opiates	2.1	2.0	2.8	2.1	2.4	2.4	2.1	1.8	1.8	1.8	2.3
Stimulants	8.5	7.7	8.8	8.7	9.9	12.1	15.8	10.7	8.9	8.3	6.8
Crystal meth. (ice)	—	—	—	—	—	—	—	—	—	—	—
Sedatives	5.4	4.5	5.1	4.2	4.4	4.8	4.6	3.4	3.0	2.3	2.4
Barbiturates	4.7	3.9	4.3	3.2	3.2	2.9	2.6	2.0	2.1	1.7	2.0
Methaqualone	2.1	1.6	2.3	1.9	2.3	3.3	3.1	2.4	1.8	1.1	1.0
Tranquilizers	4.1	4.0	4.6	3.4	3.7	3.1	2.7	2.4	2.5	2.1	2.1
Alcohol	68.2	68.3	71.2	72.1	71.8	72.0	70.7	69.7	69.4	67.2	65.9
Been drunk	—	—	—	—	—	—	—	—	—	—	—
Cigarettes	36.7	38.8	38.4	36.7	34.4	30.5	29.4	30.0	30.3	29.3	30.1
Smokeless tobacco	—	—	—	—	—	—	—	—	—	—	—
Steroids	—	—	—	—	—	—	—	—	—	—	—

SOURCE: Johnston et al., 1995.

TABLE 6.2B. Long-Term Trends in 30-Day Prevalence of Use of Various Types of Drugs for 12th Graders (From the Class of 1986 to the Class of 1995)

					Percentage who used in past 30 days						
	Class of 1986	Class of 1987	Class of 1988	Class of 1989	Class of 1990	Class of 1991	Class of 1992	Class of 1993	Class of 1994	Class of 1995	1994–1995 change
Approximate N =	15,200	16,300	16,300	16,700	15,200	15,000	15,800	16,300	15,400	15,400	
Any illicit drug	27.1	24.7	21.3	19.7	17.2	16.4	14.4	18.3	21.9	23.8	+1.9
Any illicit drug other than marijuana	13.2	11.6	10.0	9.1	8.0	7.1	6.3	7.9	8.8	10.0	+1.2*
Marijuana/hashish	23.4	21.0	18.0	16.7	14.0	13.8	11.9	15.5	19.0	21.2	+2.2*
Inhalants	2.5	2.8	2.6	2.3	2.7	2.4	2.3	2.5	2.7	3.2	+0.5
Inhalants, adjusted	3.2	3.5	3.0	2.7	2.9	2.6	2.5	2.8	2.9	3.5	+0.6
Amyl/butyl nitrites	1.3	1.3	0.6	0.6	0.6	0.4	0.3	0.6	0.4	0.4	0.0
Hallucinogens	2.5	2.5	2.3	2.2	2.2	2.2	2.1	2.7	3.1	4.4	+1.3***
Hallucinogens, adjusted	3.5	2.8	2.3	2.9	2.3	2.4	2.3	3.3	3.2	4.6	+1.4***
LSD	1.7	1.8	1.8	1.8	1.9	1.9	2.0	2.4	2.6	4.0	+1.4***
PCP	1.3	0.6	0.3	1.4	0.4	0.5	0.6	1.0	0.7	0.6	-0.1
Cocaine	6.2	4.3	3.4	2.8	1.9	1.4	1.3	1.3	1.5	1.8	+0.3
Crack	–	1.3	1.6	12.4	0.7	0.7	0.6	0.7	0.8	1.0	+0.2
Other cocaine	–	4.1	3.2	1.9	1.7	1.2	1.0	1.2	1.3	1.3	0.0
Heroin	0.2	0.2	0.2	0.3	0.2	0.2	0.3	0.2	0.3	0.6	+0.3***
Other opiates	2.0	1.8	1.6	1.6	1.5	1.1	1.2	1.3	1.5	1.8	+0.3
Stimulants	5.5	5.2	4.6	4.2	3.7	3.2	2.8	3.7	4.0	4.0	0.0
Crystal meth. (ice)	–	–	–	–	0.6	0.6	0.5	0.6	0.7	1.1	+0.4
Sedatives	2.2	1.7	1.4	1.6	1.4	1.5	1.2	1.3	1.8	2.3	+0.5*
Barbiturates	1.8	1.4	1.2	1.4	1.3	1.4	1.1	1.3	1.7	2.2	+0.5**
Methaqualone	0.8	0.6	0.5	0.6	0.2	0.2	0.4	0.1	0.4	0.4	0.0
Tranquilizers	2.1	2.1	2.1	2.0	1.5	1.3	1.2	1.4	1.0	11.2	1.4*
Alcohol	65.3	66.4	63.9	60.0	57.1	54.0	51.3	51.0 / 48.6	50.1	51.3	+1.2
Been drunk	–	–	–	–	–	31.6	29.9	28.9	30.8	33.2	+2.4
Cigarettes	29.6	29.4	28.7	28.6	29.4	28.3	27.8	29.9	31.2	33.5	+2.3*
Smokeless tobacco	11.5	11.3	10.3	8.4	–	–	11.4	10.7	11.1	12.2	+1.1
Steroids	–	–	–	0.8	1.0	0.8	0.6	0.7	0.9	0.7	-0.2

SOURCE: Johnston et al., 1995.
Level of significance of difference between the two most recent classes: * = .05, ** = .01, *** = .001.

TABLE 6.3. 30-Day Prevalence of Drug Use Among High School Seniors by Race/Ethnicity and Gender (percentage)

Race/Ethnicity	Alcohol			Cigarettes			Marijuana		
	Female	Male	Total	Female	Male	Total	Female	Male	Total
White	49	51	50	35	32	34	15	20	17
Black	37	48	43	14	16	15	13	24	19
Hispanic	47	55	51	27	30	29	16	23	19

SOURCE: CDC, 1993.

lated to tobacco, alcohol, and other drugs. Table 6.4 summarizes the baseline data used to formulate the objective, the target objective for the year 2000, and the progress made to date (U.S. Department of Health and Human Services, 1990, 1995). At least minimal progress was made for each objective, with the exception of the objectives related to perceived harmfulness of marijuana and drug-related deaths, for which negative progress was made.

Reasons for Lack of National Success

This national effort, despite all the financial support it has provided, has led to little success in preventing adolescent drug use (Austin, 1988; Klitzner, 1987; Moore & Saunders, 1991; U.S. General Accounting Office, 1990). There are several reasons for this lack of success, including the use of inappropriate theoretical models, unclear and unrealistic goals for programs, use of programs proven ineffective, and lack of a comprehensive approach.

Lack of Appropriate Theoretical Models

Since 1987, the field of drug prevention among adolescents has been driven predominately by the risk factor model, which defines an adolescent subpopulation more susceptible than normal to the use of alcohol and other drugs. These adolescents are defined as having

one or more risk factors, which include early antisocial behavior, friends who use drugs, parent as substance abuser, pregnancy, economic deprivation, and school transition, among many others (Hawkins, Lishner, Jenson, & Catalano, 1987). This model is so pervasive that many state and federal agencies require applicants for grant money to use it as a basis for their application. However, there are three serious flaws with this model that make it an inappropriate one on which to design adolescent drug prevention programs:

1. The model is based on correlation, not causation, making the model unpredictive.
2. The model results in identifying the majority of students as at-risk, which is not borne out by the statistics on drug use among adolescents (Brown & Horowitz, 1993).
3. It suggests that adolescents are both the problem and the cause, absolving institutions such as schools of responsibility expected "only to do its best with limited resources" (Baizerman & Compton, 1992).

For the field of drug prevention to move forward, theoretical models that are grounded in appropriate, effective, and rigorous research need to be used as the basis for programming.

Unclear, Unrealistic Goals

One of the problems of past and current efforts is a lack of consensus about the goal of drug prevention programs. Some programs

TABLE 6.4. Healthy People 2000: Objectives Related to Alcohol, Tobacco, and Other Drugs Among Adolescents

Baseline 1988	Target 2000	Progress to Date
30% of youth had become regular cigarette smokers by ages 20 through 24	3.5 Reduce the initiation of cigarette smoking by children and youth so that no more than 15% have become regular cigarette smokers by age 20	About 20% of target achieved. In 1993, 27% of youth had become regular cigarette smokers by ages 20 through 24
6.6% of males ages 12 through 17 used smokeless tobacco	3.9 Reduce smokeless tobacco use by males ages 12 through 24 to a prevalence of no more than 4%	About 65% of target achieved
Drug-related deaths were 4 per 100,000 people	4.3 Reduce drug-related deaths to no more than 3 per 100,000 people	About 65% of target achieved
The average age of first use was 12 years for cigarettes, 13 years for alcohol, and 13 years for marijuana	4.5 Increase by at least 1 year the average age of first use of cigarettes, alcohol, and marijuana by adolescents ages 12 through 17	About 10% of target achieved. In 1993, the average first age of use of cigarettes was 11.7; alcohol was 12.9; and marijuana was 13.9
25% of youth ages 12 to 17 used alcohol in the past month; 6% used marijuana; 1% used cocaine	4.6 Reduce the proportion of young people ages 12 to 17 who have used alcohol, marijuana, and cocaine in the past month as follows: alcohol:12.6%; marijuana: 3.2%; cocaine: 0.6%	Approximate percentage of target achieved: alcohol: 55%; marijuana: 45%; cocaine: 140%
33% of high school seniors engaged in recent occasions of heavy drinking of alcoholic beverages	4.7 Reduce the proportion of high school seniors engaging in recent occasions of heavy drinking of alcoholic beverages to no more than 28%	Approximately 95% of target achieved
Youth ages 14 and older consumed 2.54 gallons of ethanol per person	4.8 Reduce alcohol consumption by people ages 14 and older to an annual average of no more than 2 gallons of ethanol per person	About 40% of target achieved
The proportion of high school seniors who perceive social disapproval of drug use was as follows: heavy use of alcohol: 56%; occasional use of marijuana: 71%; trying cocaine once or twice: 89%	4.9 Increase the proportion of high school seniors who perceive social disapproval of drug use as follows: heavy use of alcohol: 70%; occasional use of marijuana: 85%; trying cocaine once or twice: 95%	Approximate percentage of target achieved: alcohol: 15%; marijuana: 20%; cocaine: 35%
The proportion of high school seniors who associate risk of physical or psychological harm with heavy use of drugs was as follows: heavy use of alcohol: 44%; regular use of marijuana: 78%; trying cocaine once or twice: 55%	4.10 Increase the proportion of high school seniors who associate risk of physical or psychological harm with heavy use of drugs as follows: heavy use of alcohol: 70%; regular use of marijuana: 90%; trying cocaine once or twice: 80%	Approximate percentage of target achieved: alcohol: 5%; marijuana: 100%; cocaine: 5%
5% of male high school seniors used anabolic steroids	4.11 Reduce to no more than 3% the proportion of male high school seniors who use anabolic steroids	About 70% of target achieved

SOURCE: U.S. Department of Health and Human Services, 1990, 1995.

have the goal of responsible use, whereas others seek to eliminate any form of experimentation with drugs. The goal of prevention programs is often unstated or so ambiguous that the desired outcome is unclear. This lack of a clear goal for programs has hampered program development, as well as evaluation.

There are many people within organizations with differing views. Some want to delay the onset of use, whereas others may want to focus specifically on illicit drugs. Some are comfortable with adolescent use of alcohol and want efforts focused on drinking and driving. This ambiguity creates problems for prevention programmers and evaluators. Without clear and realistic goals, it is difficult to determine if a program is effective. In addition, it is difficult to plan programs that are consistent with those goals. This mixed message provided to adolescents is exemplified in school-based programs with educational components espousing a no-use message while promoting a responsible use organization such as Students Against Drunk Driving. In class, the message is don't use alcohol. Outside class, the message is that it is acceptable to use as long as one doesn't drive while intoxicated. Other programs or individuals within programs may want to prevent any use of any drug, implying that any drug use is deviant adolescent behavior. For these programs, "no effort has been made to establish the concept of limits. In the minds of many, there are only two choices: abstention or abuse" (Brown & Horowitz, 1993, p. 542). The goal of complete abstention not only is unrealistic, but it sets programs up for failure from the outset and falsely assumes that drug use is equivalent to drug abuse. A good example of the implementation of this goal is the U.S. Department of Education's Drug-Free Schools and Communities Recognition Program. Early on, schools were ineligible for receiving an award for an exemplary program if they had any intervention program, because it indicated that there were students on the campus who were using drugs. This requirement has since been eliminated.

One of the factors contributing to the perception that use equals abuse is the lack of clarification about the prevalence period when reporting drug use statistics. For example, reports will often give a percentage of students who use drugs, but the prevalence period may be lifetime, within the past year, or within the past month. If the statistic used is lifetime prevalence, the perception is given that the extent of the problem is greater than it is because more students will report lifetime use than regular use, such as 30-day prevalence. The reporting of lifetime use supports the assumption that use is equivalent to abuse, when, in fact, most of those students will not go on to be regular users.

Continued Use of Programs and Methods Proven Ineffective

The lack of rigorous program evaluation in the field of drug prevention has left many practitioners frustrated when designing programs. This leaves practitioners with the overwhelming task of designing a program based on what little is known, and transferring findings to uncharted territories. When left with little on which to base a decision, it is understandable that practitioners are implementing programs that may or may not be effective. One would hope that the programs were at least based on strong theories and findings from other effective programs. However, the implementation of programs known to be ineffective is unacceptable. This may sound remarkably uncommon; however, it is occurring daily throughout the nation. The prime example is the wide implementation of the DARE (Drug Abuse Resistance Education) program despite the results of numerous evaluations demonstrating its ineffectiveness (Ennett, Tobler, Ringwalt, & Flewelling, 1994).

DARE is a school-based program in which a trained police officer implements a core cur-

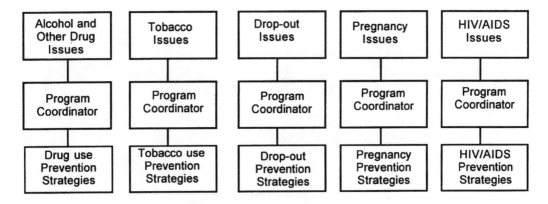

Figure 6.1. Categorical Approach to Adolescent Health Issues

riculum consisting of 17 lessons in the last grades of elementary school, usually offered once a week for 45 to 60 minutes. Since its beginning in 1983, about half of school districts throughout the nation have adopted DARE, and the number continues to rise (Ennett et al., 1994). U.S. Departments of Justice and Education have both supported the implementation of DARE throughout the nation.

Given the widespread use of DARE and the considerable investment of money, it is surprising that implementation continues despite its ineffectiveness. Political pressure, ability of schools to defer implementation to another agency, and community and parental support for the program are all factors that contribute to its continuation. This is an example of institutional enabling, giving the illusion that something is being done to prevent substance use among adolescents when, in fact, nothing is really being accomplished (English, Champlin, & Bickel, 1996).

Categorically, Crisis-Driven Response

The national "war on drugs" continues to demonstrate our historical approach to responding to health-related issues only when a crisis is perceived. When HIV/AIDS became a national issue, funding was provided to prevent further spread of the disease. When re-

search began identifying the relationship of chronic health problems to cigarette smoking, many states passed laws to increase the tax on tobacco, using the revenues for tobacco-specific prevention programs.

Yet rarely, if ever, does an adolescent have a drug problem without other precipitating problems such as depression, abuse, or neglect. This interrelationship of health issues creates a web that needs to be treated as a whole, not as individual strands (Gibbs & Bennett, 1990). The treatment of one will not be effective without addressing the others. Schools, community agencies, and health care providers do not address this web of problem behaviors in an integrated manner. In fact, the families with the most severe problems and the most limited resources are likely to experience the most disorganized social service delivery (Thomas, English, & Bickel, 1993). In any school or community, there are usually several different planning groups with the same goal but separate programs, curricula, and activities. This results in duplication, inefficient use of limited resources, and a system that allows adolescents to fall through the cracks. Their problems tend to be treated categorically, with separate programs having separate coordinators addressing individual problems. Figure 6.1 demonstrates the typical categorical approach to adolescent problems.

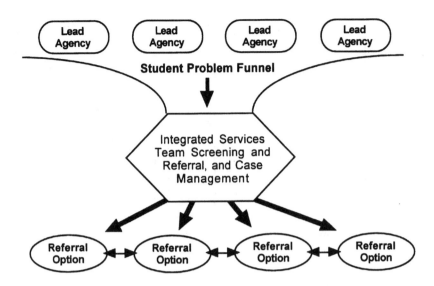

Figure 6.2. Comprehensive Coordinated Approach to Adolescent Health Issues

Categorical, single-issue, crisis-oriented approaches to adolescent health issues, including alcohol and other drug use, are neither successful nor cost-effective in helping the whole being of the adolescent who presents interrelated problems. Sometimes, due to eligibility criteria imposed by separate funding streams, staff can even be prohibited from helping students who do not fit the criteria (Melaville & Blank, 1991; Thomas et al., 1993). Tobacco education funds frequently cannot be used for education about any other drug. Funding for HIV/AIDS may not be available for drug prevention, even though the two are often related. Drop-out prevention programs may not be allowed to use staff to assist with drug prevention efforts despite the fact that both programs would benefit from such a joint effort.

Staff get discouraged trying to work within these artificial frameworks because the problems of adolescent health are so interrelated. What is needed is a comprehensive, coordinated system for early identification, referral, and treatment of adolescents, not their presenting problems. Figure 6.2 demonstrates an approach to working with the whole adolescent and a package of interrelated problems, allowing agencies to treat the adolescent, not the problem (Thomas et al., 1993).

Components of a Comprehensive Drug Prevention Program

Much of the literature discusses a framework for a comprehensive drug prevention program, which includes the following components (Allensworth, Symons, & Olds, 1994; CDC, 1994):

- Needs assessment
- Planning
- Policy
- Staff development
- Education
- Intervention
- Aftercare
- Parent and community involvement
- Evaluation

However, categorical programs work best within a comprehensive framework that promotes adolescent health, rather than separate frameworks for each categorical program. The National Commission on the Role of the School and Community in Promoting Adolescent Health (n.d.) outlines a full range of activities supporting adolescent health in a comprehensive framework that includes activities supporting health promotion through institutionalization. This framework, with activities specific to the prevention of alcohol and other drug use, is provided in Table 6.5.

Despite the numerous recommendations about components or activities that are needed to address drug use prevention, little is known about the effectiveness of each component with the exception of education.

Drug Education: What Works and What Doesn't

Throughout the past several decades, numerous approaches have been tried to prevent drug use among adolescents. However, with years of research on drug education programs, we are beginning to find out which strategies are effective and which are not.

Drug Education: What Doesn't Work

Historically, drug education approaches were ineffective (Austin, 1988; U.S. General Accounting Office, 1990). These include the use of scare tactics, relying heavily on information about the effects of drug use, testimonies of ex-addicts, alternative programs such as weekend risk-taking excursions, and affective approaches. A description and limitations of these programs are provided in Table 6.6. Their effectiveness, if any, was limited to increasing knowledge and changing attitudes, not reducing drug use.

The effort put into these programs, however, is not lost. Over the years, much has been learned about what doesn't work in health education. To avoid mistakes of the past, it is equally valuable to learn both what does and what does not work.

Drug Education: What Does Work

Of all the components recommended for inclusion in a comprehensive drug prevention program, the only one whose effectiveness we know much about is education. Years of research on drug education programs have shown that reductions in drug use can be produced if the curricula contain several key elements (Dusenbury & Falco, 1995; Hansen, 1992). These elements, based on the results of educational programs that have been shown to reduce drug use, are outlined in Table 6.7 and discussed below.

Based on Research and Theory

Criteria for drug education need to be based on educational theory and previous research on effective education programs. Too often, curricula are developed based on what educators believe should be included, rather than building on what is already known. When a curriculum is selected, it is rarely a systematic process (English, Lloyd-Kolkin, & Hunter, 1991). Individual bias toward a particular approach often arises. One person may recommend a particular curriculum because it focuses on self-esteem. Another curriculum may be recommended because it contains good graphics. When curriculum selection is not done systematically, all components of a program do not get examined and, consequently, curricula get selected or written based on a few personal agendas. This process poses a danger of purchasing or developing a cur-

TABLE 6.5. A Full Range of Activities Supporting Adolescent Health Related to Alcohol and Other Drug Use

Type	Description	Examples
Health promotion	Activities that promote positive health behaviors and provide knowledge that increases health-enhancing activities	• Public service announcements • School health education • After-school programs • Programs that build decision making and social skills
Primary prevention	Activities that seek to prevent or stop young people from ever engaging in specific health-endangering behaviors or from experiencing certain health problems	• Specific drug-prevention education programs • Clear policies and procedures surrounding drug use
Early problem identification	Activities that systematically examine most young people in order to uncover physical, educational, emotional, and social problems as early as possible so that effective interventions can be recommended and implemented	• Screening • Drug testing • Regular surveys of drug use and attitudes among adolescents
Assessment	Activities and procedures used to more clearly delineate the severity and nature of any problems so that an effective program can be developed for an individual adolescent and family	ù Drug testing programs
Secondary prevention	Activities that seek to limit or eliminate the negative consequences of current behaviors and health problems by encouraging responsible or changed behaviors or preventing further manifestations of the problem	• Designated driver programs • Adolescent support groups • Mentioning programs • Counseling
Referral	Activities that connect a young person to physical, educational, emotional, and social services in a collaborative fashion	• Referral to a hot-line • Referral to health or social service agencies • Collaboration among service providers • Case management
Treatment	Services that treat young people for particular problems or health conditions but allow them to remain in their normal family, school, and community environment	• Outpatient treatment • Support groups • Counseling • After-care programs
Institutionalization	Programs that seek to treat a young person and his or her problem by placing the adolescent in a new environment. This allows for more optimal monitoring, modification, or control of behaviors or disorders and preparation for reintegration into the community with appropriate support services	• Residential drug treatment programs

Adapted from the National Commission on the Role of the School and the Community in Improving Adolescent Health, n.d.

TABLE 6.6. Ineffective Drug Education Strategies

Approach	Description/Problem
Information-based	
Adolescents were presented with information about the effects of drugs	• Increases knowledge, but doesn't change behavior
	• May encourage experimentation because curiosity is increased
	• Students believe in personal immunity, "it won't happen to me"
Affective education	
Self-esteem, decision-making, goal-setting approaches	• Little connection was made to content and use of drugs
	• Changed attitudes, but not behavior
Alternative programs	
Excursions or other activities that provided adolescents opportunities to learn activities to do other than use drugs	• Activities were not viable alternatives to drug use
	• Adolescents often found that activities were enhanced when under the influence of drugs
Testimonies of ex-addicts	
Ex-addicts, often celebrities, presented their life history to the adolescents	• Teacher had little control over what was said
	• Adolescents rationalized by thinking that it won't happen to them
	• Impression was often left that you can use drugs, go through recovery, and continue life as usual
Scare tactics	
Exaggerated, inaccurate information about drug use was presented	• Adolescents knew it isn't always true
	• Teacher credibility was lost

riculum that will not be as effective as it could be at reducing substance use among youth.

Provides Developmentally Appropriate Content

Content of effective programs provided information about short-term social conse-quences of drug use. The information provided was accurate and relevant, not exaggerated to scare students into not using drugs. Long-term health consequences of drug use are not rele-vant to adolescents. They believe in the con-cept of personal immunity—"it won't happen to me." When told they may get cancer at the age of 50 because they smoke cigarettes now,

TABLE 6.7. Key Components of Effective Drug Prevention Curricula

- Curricula are based on current knowledge of theory and research
- Content is developmentally appropriate, including normative education and short-term social consequences of drug use
- Training is given in social resistance skills, often in the context of comprehensive health education and broader-based skills training, which requires interactive teaching techniques
- Teachers are trained and receive ongoing support
- Adequate time is allocated to the educational program
- Strategies are sensitive to the ethnic and cultural backgrounds of youth
- Program is stringently evaluated by independent investigators
- Full implementation of the program is ensured

they believe it won't happen to them, often because they know people who smoked and lived well past 50 years. The short-term social consequences of drug use are much more relevant to adolescents. These include bad breath, having a driving license suspended, vomiting at a party, or having others not want to kiss them.

In addition to short-term consequences of drug use, education programs most effective at reducing drug use among adolescents contained content about normative education, which teaches that the adolescent norm is not to use or approve of drug use. Most adolescents believe that everyone has tried or uses drugs. In fact, most adolescents have not used drugs and find it unacceptable. Helping adolescents come to believe this information has proven beneficial to educators, allowing them to build on the positive norm.

Provides Skills Training Using Interactive Teaching Techniques and Providing Adequate Time

Effective education programs go far beyond the provision of information to increase knowledge. They provide adolescents with social skills to help them communicate their decision to abstain from drug use, set goals for themselves that the use of drugs would prohibit them from attaining, deal with stress in a healthy manner, and make healthy decisions.

To teach these skills, two things are needed: adequate instructional time and interactive teaching techniques. When students are taught math skills, time is allocated on a daily basis year after year. If adolescents are expected to master the art of communication and other health-related skills, a considerable amount of time needs to be devoted to health education. Allocating small amounts of time in selected grades will not produce adequate results.

In addition, when students are taught skills such as jump shots in basketball, they are provided opportunities to hear about how to make the shot, watch a skilled person make it,

practice, receive feedback, and practice some more. The same approach must be used for social skills. Students need to be taught using interactive instructional methodologies such as role playing and small-group work. Without these types of strategies, mastery of the skills necessary to effectively handle pressure to use drugs will not take place.

Provides Training and Ongoing Support

Many educators are not comfortable or familiar with the instructional methodologies, such as role playing, needed to teach adolescents social skills. Intensive training needs to be provided that goes far beyond the typical staff development days where teachers chose from a menu of presentations. Too often, programs are disseminated to educators with the assumption that staff are qualified enough to implement the program without training. There is an assumption that by recommending training, it is implied that the teachers or other staff are not competent. However, no matter what the skill level of the implementers is, adequate training results in greater commitment to the program, increased implementation and fidelity, and increased effectiveness. Inadequate training may lead to implementation failure and, consequently, program failure. Teachers who are not adequately trained may not understand the program's philosophy, be able to perform, or be motivated to perform what is asked of them by the program.

Educators, like students, also need continued opportunities for learning and skill development. Simply training educators is not enough. They also must be provided with ongoing support, feedback, technical assistance, and opportunities to be observed by educators with more experience who can provide feedback on lesson implementation (Showers & Joyce, 1996).

Ensures Full Implementation

One of the common complaints heard from schools is that there is no time to teach one more thing, even something as important as drug education. Competing demands on teachers' time generally mean that the implementation of prevention programs is far less than optimal. If programs are only partially implemented, or implemented without fidelity, they are unlikely to be effective. Yet, coordinators of drug prevention programs rarely have an accurate account of how much or how well a program is being implemented. The perception is that if a program was purchased and disseminated, it is being used.

Monitoring fidelity of implementation—the degree to which a program is implemented as designed—is critical to program success. Changing a prevention program known to be effective by modifying program components or adding new ones that have not yet been tested can render the program ineffective (Anderson et al., 1987). When a program has been evaluated and proven to be effective, one rarely knows which of the program's components are responsible for the success. Therefore, eliminating components or making major adaptations is likely to result in reduced program effectiveness.

Monitoring implementation can provide prevention specialists with data on level of implementation as well as fidelity of implementation. Monitoring can take the form of interviews, surveys, observations, or forms that teachers complete and submit upon completion of each lesson. Although time-consuming, monitoring is essential to the success of programs. Without it, programs may be deemed failures when, in fact, they may not have been implemented well enough to determine success or failure.

Education Needs to Be Supported With Other Components

Due to the complexity of drug abuse problems, it is clear that a comprehensive approach is needed that does not rely solely on education. Education is a viable strategy for primary prevention activities, but it will do little for the adolescent who is addicted. Therefore, education provided within the context of a comprehensive framework for all adolescent health issues is most promising. An example of such an effective collaboration between schools, community agencies, and health care providers is a student assistance program (SAP).

Student Assistance Programs

All schools have some process for helping students with problems. Most have a team that accepts referrals from teachers, gathers data on the student, and makes recommendations to provide assistance. The types of teams frequently in place in most schools, often called student study teams or child study teams, have as their main focus the provision of school-based solutions to problems that interfere with the adolescent's ability to succeed in school. These solutions may include testing for special education eligibility, recommendations for changing instructional processes, referral to a student attendance review board, or other school-based service. Most often, students are referred to these teams because of behavioral or academic problems (English & Horowitz, 1995). Once again, a crisis-oriented system responds when an adolescent is showing signs of academic failure or problem behavior.

Many students in need of support to help them achieve their academic and human potential are rarely identified through a student study team approach. For example, a child of an alcoholic who is experiencing tremendous pressure to excel may never show signs of academic failure, but is still in need of support to improve his or her health status. An adolescent whose parents are going through a divorce may not yet be showing a decline in grades or behavioral problems, but participating in a support group with other adolescents experiencing the same problems may help prevent such a decline.

On the other hand, SAPs provide a comprehensive, integrated, school-community program for providing early identification, intervention, and aftercare services to adolescents who are experiencing a variety of health problems, including alcohol and other drug use, all of which interfere with the school's foremost function—ensuring academic success for every adolescent.

There are several key elements to a successful SAP, including staff training on behaviors that may indicate a potential health problem, referral of an adolescent to a team, data gathering, team meeting, recommendations, and case management (Anderson, 1993). These elements are similar to student study teams with the following notable exceptions:

1. SAPs offer both academic and nonacademic solutions to student problems.
2. Anyone involved with the youth may make the referral, including self-referrals.
3. The number and type of referral options increased dramatically from only those the school can provide to include referrals to community-based agencies, health care providers, recreational programs, mentoring programs, and others.
4. Collaboration and team participation are increased to include not only school personnel, but possibly representatives from social services, health care, and mental health.
5. The data gathered are not limited to that information provided by the referring teacher. Anyone involved with the adolescent may be called on to provide information, including the parents, coach, bus driver, or librarian.
6. The data gathered do not just supply the negative behaviors of the adolescent but also provide information about other behavioral indicators that a potential problem may be present. The adolescent's strengths are also noted to help the team get a more complete picture of the adolescent.

This view of a school-based program as comprehensive and integrated is a promising one for addressing the interrelated health needs of adolescents that hinder their ability to succeed in school and other areas of life.

The National Commission on the Role of the School and the Community in Improving Adolescent Health (n.d.) provides recommendations for a comprehensive coordinated system that provides services to adolescents, such as those provided through a students' assistance program. Their report (National Commission on the Role of the School and the Community in Improving Adolescent Health, n.d.) notes that in order for any service to be used by adolescents, it must be

Convenient: Services must be physically convenient and offered at times designated by the adolescents as convenient.

Confidential: Parent involvement should be sought, but requiring it may prevent adolescents from obtaining services.

Comprehensive: Although adolescents may seek help for a drug problem, they most likely have multiple problems that require a comprehensive set of services.

Age appropriate: Adolescents desire to be treated as adults, yet still need assistance in becoming fully responsible for their own health.

SAPs can meet all these requirements. An evaluation of such programs in secondary schools throughout the state of California found that 6-month prevalence of alcohol and other drug use in schools with programs remained stable from pre- to posttest whereas students in comparison schools reported increased use of all substances across time (Pollard & House, 1993). The effect was strongest for alcohol and marijuana. Also, students in schools with student assistance programs significantly improved on the Piers-Harris Children's Self-Concept Scale (PH) from pretest to posttest whereas the comparison site students did not show improvement.

SAPs are not easy to create. As was found in an evaluation of a 5-year drug prevention

TABLE 6.8. Common Denominators of Successful Prevention Programs

1. Programs are targeted and focused by a reasonable understanding of the risks and problems encountered by the target group
2. Programs are aimed at long-term change by setting individuals on a new developmental course
3. Successful programs give people new skills to cope more effectively and provide social support in the face of life transitions
4. Successful programs strengthen the natural support from family, community, or school settings
5. Successful programs collect rigorous research evidence to document their success

project that included an SAP as a key element (English & Horowitz, 1995), several major problems may prohibit a school from effectively implementing an SAP:

1. Staff who use the SAP only as a means of getting on-site services for youth.
2. Lack of access to staff development time to train staff on key behavioral indicators of potential health problems.
3. Unwillingness on the part of staff to make the paradigm shift from a student study team to a SAP.

However, with a strong willingness on the part of schools, community agencies, and health care organizations to collaborate, SAPs can be a successful mechanism for providing comprehensive support for the prevention of the use of alcohol and other drugs, among other health problems of adolescents.

Conclusion

With little research available on effective strategies for drug prevention programs, practitioners can look to commonalities across effective prevention programs in a variety of arenas. A review of successful prevention programs identified several commonalities among the 14 programs reviewed (Price, Cowen, Lorion, & Ramos-McKay, 1988). These are described in Table 6.8.

The big question now is "Where do we go from here?" Two major approaches are given serious consideration by practitioners, the *protective factor* model and a *harm minimization* model.

Recently, more and more drug prevention practitioners are discussing the concepts of protective factors and resiliency. Research on individuals identified as being at high risk for developing certain disorders found that although a certain percentage of these children developed various problems at rates higher than the normal population, a greater percentage of the children became healthy and competent young adults (Garmezy, 1991; Werner & Smith, 1992). A typical profile of these resilient children included the following characteristics (Benard, 1991):

- Social competence
- Problem-solving skills
- Autonomy
- Sense of purpose and future

Predictors of resiliency for high-risk youth include protective factors within the family, school, and community. These protective factors include the following (Benard, 1991):

- Caring and support
- High expectations
- Opportunities for meaningful participation

When work within families, schools, and community environments provides adolescents with caring and support, creates high expectations, and provides opportunities to be active participants in their family, school, and community life, adolescents may become resilent and avoid the dangers of alcohol and other drug abuse.

The harm minimization approach includes the following components (O'Hare, Clements, & Cohen, 1988):

1. Providing young people with factual information about drugs
2. Helping them to examine their own attitudes about drugs and drug users
3. Helping them to understand people who experience drug problems and foster a caring attitude
4. Helping them to avoid the harmful consequences of drug use by explaining secondary prevention strategies
5. Raising awareness of the legal, health, and social implications of their own drug use
6. Helping them to understand the role of drug use in past and present societies and cultures

This approach is a viable alternative, particularly if most school-based drug education approaches have been exhausted, because it "offers the opportunity to provide this information without judgment . . . [and] represents a substance use/abuse education process of inclusion and not exclusion" (Horowitz & Brown, 1993, pp. 5-6).

Practitioners need to reexamine their assumptions about adolescent drug use and drug prevention programs, creating an opportunity to refocus their efforts on new theoretical models that support the interrelatedness of drug abuse to other health problems.

References

Allensworth, D., Symons, C., & Olds, S. (1994). *Healthy students 2000: An agenda for continuous improvement in America's schools.* Kent, OH: American School Health Association.

Anderson, B., Odden, A., Farrar, E., Fuhrman, S., Davis, A., Huddle, E., Armstrong, J., & Flakus-Mosqueda, P. (1987). State strategies to support local school improvement. *Knowledge: Creation, Diffusion, Utilization, 9*(1), 42-86.

Anderson, G. (1993). *When chemicals come to school: The core team model of student assistance programs.* Greenfield, WI: Community Recovery Press.

Austin, G. (1988). *Prevention research update number one: Prevention goals, methods, and outcomes.* Portland, OR: Northwest Regional Educational Laboratory.

Austin, G., & Pollard, J. (1993). *Prevention research update number ten: Substance abuse and ethnicity: Recent research findings.* Los Alamitos, CA: Southwest Regional Laboratory.

Bachman, J. G., Wallace, J. M., O'Malley, P. M., Johnston, L. D., Kurth, C. L., & Neighbors, H. W. (1991). Racial/ethnic differences in smoking, drinking, and illicit drug use among American high school seniors, 1976-89. *American Journal of Public Health, 81*(3), 372-377.

Baizerman, M., & Compton, D. (1992). From respondent and informant to consultant and participant: The evolution of a state agency policy evaluation. In A. M. Madison (Ed.), *Minority issues in program evaluation* (New Directions in Program Evaluation No. 53, pp. 5-16). San Francisco: Jossey-Bass.

Benard, B. (1991). *Fostering resiliency in kids: Protective factors in family, school, and community.* San Francisco: Far West Regional Laboratory.

Brown, J., & Horowitz, J. (1993). Deviance and deviants: Why adolescent substance use prevention programs do not work. *Evaluation Review, 17*(5), 529-555.

Centers for Disease Control. (1993, March 24). Youth risk behavior surveillance—United States. *Morbidity and Mortality Weekly Report, 44*(SS-1), 1-57.

Centers for Disease Control. (1994, February 25). Guidelines for school health programs to prevent tobacco use and addiction. *Morbidity and Mortality Weekly Report, 43*(RR-2), 1-18.

Dusenbury, L., & Falco, M. (1995). Eleven components of effective drug abuse prevention curricula. *Journal of School Health, 65*(10), 420-425.

English, J., Champlin, S., & Bickel, A. (1996). *How schools support substance abuse by youth: Enabling in schools.* Redondo Beach, CA: South Bay Youth Project.

English, J., & Horowitz, J. (1995). *Growing up well: Final report.* Los Alamitos, CA: Southwest Regional Laboratory.

English, J., Lloyd-Kolkin, D., & Hunter, L. (1991). *Criteria for comprehensive school health education curricula.* Kent, OH: American School Health Association.

Ennett, S., Tobler, N., Ringwalt, C., & Flewelling, R. (1994). How effective is drug abuse resistance education? A meta-analysis of Project DARE outcome evaluations. *American Journal of Public Health, 84*(9), 1394-1401.

Garmezy, N. (1991). Resiliency and vulnerability to adverse developmental outcomes associated with poverty. *American Behavioral Scientist, 34*(4), 416-430.

Gibbs, J., & Bennett, S. (1990). *Together we can: A framework for community prevention planning.* Seattle, WA: Comprehensive Health Education Foundation.

Hansen, W. B. (1992). School-based substance abuse prevention: A review of the state of the art in curriculum, 1980-1990. *Health Education Research, 7*(3), 403-430.

Hawkins, J. D., Lishner, D. M., Jenson, J. M., & Catalano, R. F. (1987). Delinquents and drugs: What the evidence suggests about prevention and treatment programming. In B. S. Brown & A. R. Mills (Eds.), *Youth at high risk for substance abuse* (DHHS Publication no. ADM 87-1537. Reprinted 1990 as ADM 90-1537, pp. 81-131). Washington, DC: Government Printing Office.

Horowitz, J. (1993). Results from the 1991 California out-of-school youth alcohol and other drug survey. In *Evaluating school-linked prevention strategies.* Los Alamitos, CA: Southwest Regional Laboratory.

Horowitz, J., & Brown, J. (1993, November). *The end of risk and reduction of vulnerability: Viable school-based prevention programs.* Paper presented at the Seventh International Conference on Drug Policy Reform, Drug Policy Foundation, Washington, DC.

Johnston, L., O'Malley, P., & Bachman, J. (1995). *National survey results on drug use from the Monitoring the Future study, 1975-1995.* Washington, DC: Government Printing Office.

Klitzner, M. D. (1987). *Report to Congress and the White House on the nature and effectiveness of federal, state, and local drug prevention/education programs.* Washington, DC: U.S. Department of Education.

Melaville, A. I., & Blank, M. J. (1991). *What it takes: Structuring interagency partnerships to connect children and families with comprehensive services.* Washington, DC: Education and Human Services Consortium.

Moore, D., & Saunders, B. (1991). Youth drug use and the prevention of problems: Why we've got it all wrong. *International Journal on Drug Policy, 2,* 29-33.

National Commission on the Role of the School and the Community in Improving Adolescent Health. (n.d.). *Code blue.* Alexandria, VA: National Association of State Boards of Education.

O'Hare, P. A., Clements, I., & Cohen, J. (1988). *Drug education: A basis for reform.* Paper presented at the International Conference on Drug Policy Reform, Bethesda, MD.

Pollard, J., & House, D. (1993). *Student assistance program demonstration project evaluation: Final report* (ADP Publication No. ADP 93-2, Contract #A-0366-8). Sacramento: California Department of Alcohol and Drug Programs.

Price, R. H., Cowen, E. L., Lorion, R. P., & Ramos-McKay, J. R. (1988). *Fourteen ounces of prevention: A casebook for practitioners.* Washington, DC: American Psychological Association.

Showers, B., & Joyce, B. (1996). The evolution of peer coaching. *Educational Leadership, 53*(6), 12-16.

Thomas, C., English, J., & Bickel, S. (1993). *Moving toward integrated services: A literature review for prevention specialists.* Los Alamitos, CA: Southwest Regional Laboratory.

U.S. Department of Health and Human Services. (1990). *Healthy people 2000: National health promotion and disease prevention objectives.* Washington, DC: Author.

U.S. Department of Health and Human Services. (1995). *Healthy people 2000: Midcourse review and 1995 revisions.* Washington, DC: Author.

U.S. General Accounting Office. (1990). *Drug education: School-based programs seen as useful but impact unknown* (GAO/HRD-91-27). Washington, DC: Author.

Werner E., & Smith, R. (1992). *Overcoming the odds: High-risk children from birth to adulthood.* Ithaca, NY: Cornell University Press.

7

Adolescents and Alcohol Use

Marjorie E. Scaffa

Blasted, blitzed, bombed, buzzed, catatonic, ripped, trashed, wasted. However, you say it, America's youth are drinking alcohol.

- A 16-year-old dies after drinking 26 shots of
alcohol in 90 minutes on a dare at a party.
- A 17-year-old who has been drinking hits his
girlfriend in the face for trying to take the
keys to his car.
- A talented, popular youth lies comatose in a
hospital bed after an alcohol-related automobile crash on the evening before high
school graduation.
- A young woman discovers she is pregnant as
a result of a sexual encounter at an all-you-
can-drink keg party.

Unfortunately, the newspapers recount examples like these in every community across the
country on a far too regular basis.

In April 1992, at a press conference, then
U.S. Surgeon General Antonia Novello stated,

[The unrecognized] consequences of alcohol
rarely have captured the headlines, rarely war-
ranted more than a passing nod of acknowledgment, followed by a shrug of the shoulders.
But many of these consequences are serious,
particularly when underage drinkers binge. . . .

Alcohol consumption frequently leads to crime,
sexual misconduct, personal injuries, higher
school dropout rates, and other consequences
that hamper the ability of adolescents and children to stay healthy, to stay in school, and to
take charge of their futures.

Alcohol is the primary drug of choice in
American society for adolescents and adults
alike. It is readily available. Its use is pervasive.
It holds a unique place in our collective histo-
ries. It provokes feelings of ambivalence in individuals and in society as a whole. For these
reasons, alcohol is one of the most dangerous
drugs in our society and is the most difficult
to deal with effectively.

Alcohol Use in the United States

Alcohol, the Drug

Ethyl alcohol, or ethanol, is produced by a
process of fermentation. Alcoholic beverages
contain various amounts of ethanol. Beer contains about 4% to 5% pure alcohol, whereas
wine has about 12% alcohol. The distillation
process produces alcoholic beverages such as
whiskey, rum, gin, vodka, and tequila. These

drinks are 80 to 100 proof, containing 40% to 50% pure alcohol. Therefore, the alcohol content of one 12 oz. beer is equivalent to a 4 oz. glass of wine or 1 oz. of liquor in a mixed drink.

Alcohol is readily absorbed throughout the gastrointestinal tract and is metabolized by the liver. Regardless of the amount a person consumes or his or her body weight, alcohol is metabolized at a relatively steady rate, about one drink (12 oz. beer, 4 oz. wine, or 1 oz. liquor) per hour.

The acute physiological effects of alcohol include cell dehydration, irritation of the gastrointestinal tract, dilation of the blood vessels causing a flushed appearance, and depression of the central nervous system. Depression of brain functions causes impaired judgment, decreased hearing and visual acuity, release of inhibitions, a mild euphoria, slurred speech, and motor incoordination. Long-term, heavy consumption of alcohol increases the risk of many types of cancer, pancreatitis, cirrhosis of the liver, hepatitis, ulcers, and a number of cardiac conditions.

Historical Context

Drinking habits and customs are a reflection of society at large. Beer, wine, and distilled spirits have been used for centuries to alter mood and enhance sociability. The use of alcoholic beverages has been an established practice in America for over 300 years. The United States ranks 15th in per capita consumption of alcohol when compared to other countries.

Both intentionally and by accident, alcohol has played an important role in American history. The early settlers brought their drinking practices and attitudes with them to their new home. During this time, alcohol was considered a blessing from God and was included as a normal part of family life and special occasions. Early on, farmers recognized the financial profitability of producing alcohol from their grain harvests.

In the early 1800s, alcohol consumption reached a peak, with the average drinker consuming more than six servings of alcohol each day. The temperance movement emerged at this time and advocated controlled, moderate use of alcohol. Around 1900, the temperance movement had evolved into the prohibitionist movement, which culminated in 1917 with the ratification of the 18th Amendment to the Constitution, which made the sale and transportation of alcoholic beverages illegal. By 1933, Prohibition was recognized as a failure. The 18th Amendment was repealed with the passage of the 21st Amendment, which restored alcohol as a legal substance for adults.

During the 1960s and the Vietnam War, many states lowered the drinking age from 21 to 18 or 19. This was due in part to an outcry by military inductees and other young people that they could be drafted to fight and die for their country but could not obtain or drink alcohol legally. Not all states lowered the minimum drinking age, and this created "blood borders" where young people would cross state lines to obtain alcohol.

As alcohol-related motor vehicle crashes increased in the young adult population, the U.S. Congress passed the National Minimum Drinking Age Act of 1984. This legislation required states to increase their legal purchase and public possession age to 21 or risk the loss of significant federal funding for highway safety. Although the minimum drinking age in all 50 states and the District of Columbia has been 21 years for some time now, adolescents continue to obtain access to alcohol and to exhibit high levels of alcohol consumption.

Current Data

Statistics gathered from a variety of sources give credence to the concern of many that alcohol use by youth is a serious problem in

America. The following are but a few of the indications of the magnitude of the problem.

- The average age of first use of alcohol is 12.3 years.
- Half of high school students can be classified as regular drinkers.
- About 3.3 million youth under the age of 17 are diagnosable as alcoholic.
- Teenage drinkers are involved in at least 50% of all fatal automobile crashes.
- Alcohol-related problems are disproportionately found among juvenile offenders as compared to the general adolescent population.

In 1991, the U.S. Surgeon General commissioned the Office of the Inspector General to survey youth in the 7th through 12th grades to determine their attitudes and behaviors related to alcohol use. This survey revealed the following:

- Junior and senior high school students drink 35% of all wine coolers sold in the United States and 1.1 billion cans of beer each year.
- Of the 10.6 million students who drink, 31% drink alone; 41% drink when they are upset because it makes them feel better; 25% drink because they are bored; and 25% drink to feel high.
- Despite the minimum age laws, almost two thirds of students who drink are able to buy their own alcohol.
- Older adolescents (88% of 12th graders) frequently obtain alcohol from their friends, whereas younger adolescents (75% of 7th graders) obtain alcohol from their parents, with or without their parents' knowledge. (U.S. Department of Health and Human Services, 1991)

According to the *Monitoring the Future Study* in 1994 of high school seniors conducted by the University of Michigan for the U.S. Alcohol, Drug Abuse and Mental Health Administration (ADAMHA):

- 2.9% were daily alcohol users
- 28.2% had consumed alcohol six or more times in the past 2 weeks
- 51.7% had been drunk in the past year
- 30.8% had been drunk in the past month (U.S. Department of Health and Human Services, 1994)

Several gender and racial/ethnic differences are evident in alcohol consumption. Boys are more likely than girls to (a) drink alcohol, (b) consume greater quantities, (c) start drinking at a younger age, and (d) become problem drinkers. In general, black or African American adolescents, both male and female, are less likely to use or abuse alcohol than either their white or Hispanic peers.

Impact of Adolescent Alcohol Use

Why do adolescents drink? For many of the same reasons adults drink. Adolescents drink out of habit, to facilitate social interaction, to reduce shyness, to minimize painful emotions such as feelings of inadequacy, to achieve an altered mood state, and to relieve boredom.

Several factors appear to be related to the initiation of alcohol use. These include but are not limited to association with alcohol-using peers, family environment and drinking practices, level of school performance, strength of religious convictions, and personality factors. Some personality characteristics associated with adolescents who abuse alcohol include

- Hostility, aggression, impulsivity, unpredictability
- Depression, dependency, low self-esteem
- Immaturity, anxiety, instability
- A lower value placed on achievement and low expectations for achievement

Depression, when combined with aggression and impulsivity, makes adolescents who use alcohol more at risk for suicide. In fact, suicide is the second leading cause of death for adolescents, and many of these deaths are alcohol-related. Adolescents frequently use alcohol to self-medicate feelings of depression, anxiety, guilt, and fear.

When compared with adolescents who use alcohol, nonusers or abstainers report:

- Better physical and mental health
- Higher academic achievement
- Less preoccupation with money
- Greater ability to get along with others
- Higher levels of overall happiness
- Less incidence of parental problem drinking
- Happier childhoods
- Higher levels of daydreaming
- Higher levels of concern about the future

The impact of alcohol use on the life span and quality of life of adolescents is significant. Motor vehicle crashes and violence are the two leading causes of death and disability among adolescents. Alcohol is a major contributor to these problems. More than 50% of fatal automobile crashes in the 15- to 24-year age group involve alcohol. In addition, about 60% of 8th and 10th graders reported not using seat belts on their most recent ride in a car. Adolescents and young adults are disproportionately represented in driving under the influence (DUI) and driving while intoxicated (DWI) arrests. About 40% of those arrested for drinking and driving offenses are under 25 years of age. About 50% of all homicides in this age group are associated with alcohol use, and over half of the perpetrators of this kind of violence are relatives or acquaintances of the victims.

According to the U.S. Surgeon General's report on adolescents and alcohol (U.S. Department of Health and Human Services, 1991), about one third of all students in the 7th through 12th grades have accepted a ride from a driver who had been drinking. Among students who drink, almost half have been a passenger in a car with a driver who had been drinking. The *Monitoring the Future* study (U.S. Department of Health and Human Serv-

ices, 1994) of high school seniors conducted by the University of Michigan in 1994 included these findings. During the preceding 12 months:

- 9% had received a ticket or warning for moving violations after drinking alcoholic beverages
- 5.4% had been involved as a driver in a motor vehicle collision that had resulted in property damage or personal injury after drinking alcoholic beverages

During the preceding 2 weeks,

- 15.7% had driven a car, truck, or motorcycle after drinking alcohol
- 8.1% had driven a car, truck, or motorcycle after having five or more drinks in a row
- 25.1% had been a passenger in a car where the driver had been drinking

In addition, alcohol has been determined to be a "gateway" drug, in that its use often precedes the use of other drugs. The use of alcohol impairs coordination and cognitive functioning, diminishes problem-solving and decision-making ability, and can lead to unwanted sexual encounters. Alcohol use may also increase the likelihood of contracting AIDS. It appears that alcohol can impair the immune system, thereby increasing the vulnerability to HIV infection, and it may speed the onset of HIV-related symptoms in those already infected with the virus. In addition, the use of alcohol increases the probability of teens engaging in high-risk or unsafe sexual behavior due to a decrease in sexual inhibition and impaired judgment. Studies have shown that men and women who frequently drink alcohol and subsequently engage in sexual intercourse are generally less likely to use condoms.

Long-term, excessive use of alcohol in adolescence can develop into alcoholism. The earlier the drinking begins, the more likely an adolescent is to experience negative consequences. The U.S. Department of Health and Human Services (1997) estimates that about 1 out of every 15 adolescents will eventually develop alcohol abuse and/or dependence.

Influences on Adolescent Alcohol Use

Developmental Issues

Adolescence is a dynamic state of transition from childhood to adulthood. Effective programs for adolescents need to acknowledge and support the dramatic changes that occur during this developmental stage. In general, society views adolescence as a tumultuous time and the use of alcohol by teenagers as a normal part of adolescent risk-taking and rebellion. In reality, adolescents use alcohol for a wide variety of reasons, and most adolescents negotiate the transition from childhood to adulthood without serious difficulties.

Developmentally, adolescents are not a homogeneous group. Different time periods during adolescence require different skills and pose different challenges. The needs of an early adolescent (ages 10-13) are significantly different from those of middle (ages 14-16) or late adolescents (ages 17-19). Prevention strategies need to address both the transition from childhood to adolescence and from adolescence to adulthood.

The use of alcohol during early adolescence (ages 10-13) should not be considered a normal part of growing up, but rather a symptom of impaired psychosocial development, inadequate coping mechanisms, or problems in the adolescent's social/family environment. Alcohol experimentation begun in late adolescence (ages 17-19) is typically a result of permissive societal attitudes toward alcohol use and the contemporary social structure during adolescence. It is also important to recognize that adolescents who have similar alcohol use patterns may have initiated and maintained alcohol use for very different reasons.

During adolescence a variety of developmental issues emerge that may have an impact on the initiation and maintenance of alcohol use, including

- The need to establish a separate identity and emotional/psychological independence
- Increasing importance of relationships with peers
- The emergence of sexual awareness
- Increased cognitive capacity and the development of abstract thinking
- The need to become productive and self-sufficient

These developmental issues can sometimes predispose adolescents to alcohol use and abuse. For example, adolescents frequently view the use of alcohol as a statement of independence and a means to defy or rebel against authority. Use of alcohol becomes the means, although unhealthy, of establishing a separate identity.

In addition, acceptance by peers is of paramount importance to adolescents, and alcohol use provides an easy mechanism for socialization and the development of peer relationships, as it decreases inhibition. A fear of rejection is a significant motivating factor in adolescent alcohol use. Alcohol is also used by adolescents as a stress reliever to mitigate the extreme self-consciousness that accompanies the physical and sexual changes of adolescence.

Increasing productivity is also a developmental task of adolescence. This is often accomplished through participation in extracurricular activities, taking on a part-time job, and involvement in sports. Time and energy spent obtaining and using alcohol detracts from other more useful activities.

Adolescents use alcohol to satisfy a variety of needs, including acceptance, intimacy, acknowledgment, independence, and self-esteem. Unfortunately, alcohol use has the potential to delay adolescent growth and development in numerous areas, most notably in intellectual, social, and emotional maturation. Therefore, it is extremely important that prevention programs facilitate other, more healthy, means for adolescents to fulfill these needs.

Family/Parental Issues

Although society has a stereotypic perspective that family stress, adolescent-parent conflict, and a deterioration in family relationships are inevitable and to be expected during adolescence, research indicates that family upheaval is not the norm. It appears, from several large-scale surveys of adolescents and their parents, that about 75% of families experience warm, caring, and pleasant relationships during the adolescent transition. Of the 25% of families who report family discord, most indicate that the problems were evident prior to adolescence.

Several research studies have indicated that parents are the single strongest influence on adolescent use of alcohol, followed closely by peers (Goplerud, 1991). However, it is important to recognize that parental effects on adolescent drinking are complex and dynamic, changing over time.

Often, parents are less concerned if their adolescent drinks alcohol than if they use other drugs. This results in part from the fact that alcohol is a familiar drug, legal for people over 21 years of age, and used by a majority of parents. Some studies suggest a relationship between adolescent alcohol use and parental control. Adolescents whose parents exert a moderate degree of control in the relationship tend to have lower rates of alcohol abuse than those whose parents exert either high or low levels of control. Parental monitoring of adolescents appears to be the most significant deterrent to adolescent alcohol abuse and other problem behaviors.

Habits and attitudes related to alcohol develop within the family context. The way adults relate to alcohol within the family environment can have a significant and enduring impact on the children. A number of studies have shown a positive correlation between parental and adolescent use of alcohol. Adolescents often model or imitate their parents' use of alcohol. In addition, a permissive attitude toward drinking by parents is correlated with higher levels of alcohol use by adolescents. In general, parental modeling appears to have a greater influence on boys, whereas parental norms appear to have a greater influence on girls.

According to the U.S. Surgeon General's report on adolescent drinking (U.S. Department of Health and Human Services, 1991), almost two thirds of all students say that their parents disapprove of underage drinking. However, 35% of the students who drink say their parents tolerate their use of alcohol under certain conditions, which limit the quantity, frequency, or location of their drinking. Almost 15% of students who drink reported that their parents do not say or do anything about their drinking.

At least one out of every six adolescents, or 6.6 million children under the age of 18, live in a household with at least one alcoholic parent. Children of alcoholics are at significantly higher risk than their peers for developing alcoholism themselves. In general, it can be anticipated that if one parent is alcoholic, then about 50% of the children will develop substance abuse problems. If both parents are alcoholic, this percentage rises to 80%. The increased risk to children of alcoholics appears to be due to an interaction of genetic and environmental factors. In addition, adolescent children of alcoholics tend to have higher rates of depression and lower self-esteem than the general high school population. Children of alcoholics may develop a distorted perception of "normal" drinking as a result of parental modeling at home.

In families in which adolescents feel rejected, lack supervision, perceive emotional tension, and are deprived of affection, it is more likely that the adolescent will develop excessive drinking habits. Other family characteristics that appear to be related to adolescent substance abuse include inconsistent or inadequate limit setting, lack of emotional closeness between family members, poor communication, lack of parental involvement in their children's activities, and high levels of disagreement between parents. Adolescents who abstain from alcohol typically have outlooks similar to their parents and are more involved in family activities. An emotionally healthy attachment to the parents is associated with low alcohol consumption. Several guidelines for parents are suggested. These include

- Acting as positive role models in both attitude and behavior
- Setting realistic expectations and limits and enforcing them fairly and consistently
- Being moderately involved in adolescent activities
- Avoiding the involvement of teenage children in marital issues

Peer Issues

Parents typically believe that the primary cause of adolescent alcohol use is peer pressure. Although peer influence during adolescence is stronger than at any other time of life, attributing alcohol use solely to this factor is an oversimplification. Peer influence is a short-lived phenomenon, and long-range goals, values, decisions, and attitudes are more determined by family and parental influences.

Research indicates that adolescent alcohol use is influenced by both peers and the family, but the balance of influence shifts depending upon the circumstances. When there are problems or stressors in the home, peers will tend to be more influential. Evidence suggests that when the motivation for alcohol use is curios-

ity and experimentation, peers are more likely to be influential. When the motivation for alcohol use is to cope with psychosocial and emotional problems, family factors are more likely to be involved.

Adolescents typically choose their friends in a way that maximizes compatibility of values, attitudes, and behaviors. Teens are influenced by their friends' attitudes and behaviors and also choose friends who reinforce their own norms. This suggests that adolescents who have had positive relationships with family members, teachers, and peers during childhood tend to choose friends who also accept traditional values and social norms. On the other hand, teens who have not been able to get their needs met through social relationships and feel alienated from society tend to choose friends who have also been rejected or have rebelled against society.

Peer groups or "crowds" take on a variety of forms and, in adolescence, begin to exert some influence in defining one's identity. An adolescent may belong to one or more crowds, for example, an academic crowd (the brains), an athletic crowd (the jocks), a social crowd (the popular teens), and/or an alcohol/drug-oriented crowd. Identifying with a particular group provides a rudimentary foundation for the development of an individual identity. If an adolescent chooses to associate with an alcohol/drug oriented crowd, then his or her risk of developing alcohol/drug-related problems increases greatly.

The benefits of belonging to a peer group and the consequences of deviating from the crowd are typically strongest during early adolescence. Therefore, the demand to conform and the likelihood of submitting to peer pressure are greatest during early adolescence. Susceptibility to peer pressure appears to increase from the 3rd through the 8th grades, hit a peak, and then diminish during high school. It is critical to acknowledge that not all peer pressure is negative. Peers can influence positive, health-enhancing behaviors as well as antisocial, destructive behaviors.

Due to the importance of peer relationships in adolescent development, many prevention and treatment programs use a strong peer education or peer counseling component. Many programs attempt to enhance adolescents' ability to resist peer pressure but do little to attenuate the values and norms in the adolescents' social system that perpetuate this pressure. Programs can and should capitalize on the phenomenon of positive peer pressure, as well as attempt to defuse the effects of negative peer pressure.

Risk and Protective Factors

Lately, much attention has been focused on the role of risk factors in the development of alcohol and other drug problems. Risk factors are considered to be those precursors that increase an individual's vulnerability to developing alcohol-related problems. A variety of risk factors have emerged in the alcohol and drug abuse research. However, many of the risk factors for alcohol abuse are also risk factors for other types of problem behaviors, including youth suicide, teenage pregnancy, juvenile delinquency, and conduct disorders.

The risk factors for alcohol use are different from those for alcohol abuse. In addition, risk factors vary for the initiation, maintenance, and escalation of alcohol use. Different groups of youth will have different constellations of risk factors.

Protective factors, also sometimes called resiliency factors, are those that appear to increase an individual's resistance to developing alcohol-related problems. More research needs to be conducted on these factors, as they may be useful in the development of more effective prevention strategies. The major protective factors that contribute to resiliency in youth include

- Flexibility, adaptability, autonomy
- Empathy, caring
- Good communication and problem-solving skills
- A sense of humor
- Social competence
- A sense of purpose
- Opportunities for participation
- High expectations for achievement

Risk and protective factors may be organized into levels. These levels are individual, interpersonal, institutional, and societal (see Table 7.1). Individual risk/protective factors have to do with an individual's genetic composition, personality, school performance, and behavior patterns. Interpersonal risk/protective factors are related to a person's family and peer relationships. Institutional risk/protective factors include the variety of established organizations that people encounter throughout their lifetime including school, work, and the health care and legal systems. Societal risk/protective factors include general societal attitudes and media coverage of alcohol.

Psychosocial risk factors that have an individual and/or interpersonal component associated with alcohol abuse include

- Problems with identity formation
- Persistent academic underachievement
- Emotional detachment/rejection of parents
- Difficulties in developing responsible autonomy
- Persistent isolation/rejection from peers
- Involvement in delinquent activity, truancy, and/or precocious sexuality

Some risk factors are considered causal, as the behavior cannot occur in the absence of the risk factor; for example, alcohol use cannot occur in the absence of access to alcohol. Other risk factors are considered contributory, as they interact with causal risk factors to develop combinations that lead to the onset, ex-

TABLE 7.1. The Most Important Factors in Predicting Adolescent Alcohol Use

---

Risk Factors

Individual
- A prior history of personality problems, especially those related to anger, aggression, impulsivity, or depression
- School failure and academic difficulties, especially if they have resulted in grade retention
- Involvement in other problem behaviors, including precocious sexual activity, truancy, or drug, criminal, or delinquent behavior

Interpersonal
- Distant or hostile relations with parents or guardians
- Familial disruption, reconstitution, and marital conflict
- Membership in a peer group or friendship group that encourages or tolerates use of alcohol or other drugs

Institutional
- School transitions that involve movement into a more impersonal, more anonymous, and less protected environment
- Involvement in the part-time labor force in excess of 20 hours per week
- Lack of access to meaningful roles in the community
- Growing up in poverty

Protective Factors

Individual
- Academic success
- A sense of self-efficacy and personal responsibility
- Well-developed social and interpersonal skills
- Adequate decision-making skills and intellectual abilities

Interpersonal
- Having at least one close relationship with a parent, teacher, relative, or mentor who can provide both guidance and emotional support
- Membership in a peer group that actively discourages use of alcohol or other drugs and encourages academic, athletic, or artistic accomplishment as routes to popularity and status

Institutional
- A sense of bonding to school and other societal institutions
- An acceptance of societally approved values and expectations for behavior

---

SOURCE: Goplerud, 1991.

acerbation, and maintenance of alcohol use. As with many psychiatric illnesses, positive family history appears to be the single most predictive risk factor for adolescent alcohol abuse.

Adolescents identified as "at risk" are those who exhibit multiple risk factors. In 1986, the importance of risk factors was recognized by public policymakers through the passage of the Comprehensive Drug Abuse Rehabilitation and Treatment Act. This legislation mandated schools, communities, and agencies to develop programs for youth at risk. Nine categories of high risk youth were developed:

- Children of alcoholics and other drug abusers
- Victims of physical, sexual, or psychological abuse
- School dropouts
- Pregnant teenagers
- Economically disadvantaged youth
- Delinquent youth
- Youth with mental health problems
- Suicidal youth
- Youth with disabilities

The Public Health Model of Prevention (see Figure 7.1), with its triad of host, agent, and environment variables, can provide a framework for conceptualizing the interaction of risk factors. It is this interaction of risk factors that is responsible for the development of alcohol abuse.

The host refers to the individual and his/her associated risk factors, the agent is alcohol, and

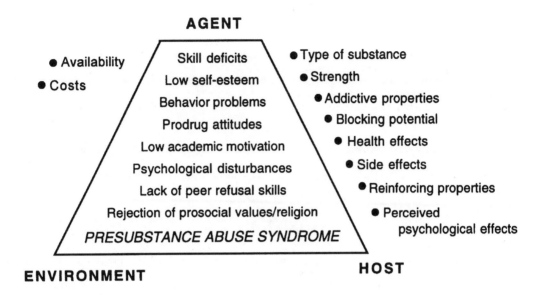

AGENT

- Availability
- Costs

Skill deficits
Low self-esteem
Behavior problems
Prodrug attitudes
Low academic motivation
Psychological disturbances
Lack of peer refusal skills
Rejection of prosocial values/religion
PRESUBSTANCE ABUSE SYNDROME

- Type of substance
- Strength
- Addictive properties
- Blocking potential
- Health effects
- Side effects
- Reinforcing properties
- Perceived psychological effects

ENVIRONMENT

HOST

Figure 7.1. Public Health Model
SOURCE: Kumpfer, 1990.

the environment encompasses the interpersonal, institutional, and societal risk factors. Interactions can occur between the host and the agent, between the agent and the environment, and between the environment and the host. The cumulative effect of all these factors may predispose a youth to use alcohol or other drugs. A vulnerable adolescent may, as a result, manifest the *presubstance abuse syndrome* (depicted in the triangle in Figure 7.1). The environment and host interactions can be quite complex and actually include a variety of interrelated contexts that affect the individual, including the immediate family environment, the social/peer environment, school environment, and the community environment.

Prevention and Health Promotion Goals

Healthy People 2000 is a statement of National Health Promotion and Disease Prevention Objectives (U.S. Department of Health and Human Services, 1990). Its development was facilitated by the U.S. Public Health Service, with input from over 300 national organizations, all of the state health departments, and the Institute of Medicine. This document can serve as a guideline for the development and evaluation of prevention programs.

The objectives in *Healthy People 2000* related to adolescents and alcohol cover a wide range of alcohol-related behaviors and are summarized in Table 7.2. Specific national outcome criteria for evaluation purposes are included in the original document.

Adolescent alcohol and drug use and abuse is a complex, multidimensional dynamic phenomenon with a multiplicity of risk factors. It is for this reason that unidimensional interventions are likely to be ineffective. It is critically important that adolescents have access to a continuum of alcohol-related services including prevention/education, early intervention, treatment, and aftercare.

Prevention/Education

For prevention/education to be successful, it needs to be broad-based and multifocused.

TABLE 7.2. Healthy People 2000, Adolescents and Alcohol Objectives

Alcohol consumption
- Increase by at least 1 year the average age of first use of alcohol by adolescents ages 12 through 17
- Reduce the proportion of young people who have used alcohol in the past month
- Reduce the proportion of high school seniors and college students engaging in recent occasions of heavy drinking of alcoholic beverages (five or more drinks in a row)
- Reduce alcohol consumption by people ages 14 and older to an annual average of no more than 2 gallons of ethanol per person

Alcohol attitudes
- Increase the proportion of high school seniors who perceive social disapproval associated with the heavy use of alcohol
- Increase the proportion of high school seniors who associate risk of physical or psychological harm with the heavy use of alcohol

Education
- Provide to children in all school districts and private schools primary and secondary school educational programs on alcohol and other drugs, preferably as part of quality school health education

Legislation/regulation
- Extend to 50 states administrative driver's license suspension/revocation laws or programs of equal effectiveness for people determined to have been driving under the influence of intoxicants
- Increase to 50 the number of states that have enacted and enforced policies to reduce access to alcoholic beverages by minors
- Increase to at least 20 the number of states that have enacted statutes to restrict promotion of alcoholic beverages that is focused principally on young audiences
- Extend to 50 states legal blood alcohol concentration tolerance levels of .04% for motor vehicle drivers age 21 and older and .00% for those younger than age 21

Morbidity/mortality
- Increase to at least 75% the proportion of primary care providers who screen for alcohol and other drug use problems and provide counseling and referral as needed

Comprehensive programs must include both micro and macro strategies. Micro strategies are aimed at individuals in specific settings, for example, individual counseling in the school. Macro strategies are aimed at communities and the nation as a whole, for example, mass media campaigns against alcohol and legislative approaches such as the minimum drinking age.

Providing accurate information to adolescents regarding the consequences of alcohol use is a prerequisite, but in and of itself is insufficient. The messages that are conveyed to young people must be reinforced in a variety of settings including the school, home, and community. Programs must start early in the child's developmental process, preferably as early as preschool and kindergarten, but certainly no later than pre-adolescence, because by age 15 many adolescents are drinking heavily.

Traditional public health categories of prevention are related to alcohol use and its risk factors. These categories are primary, secondary, and tertiary prevention. Primary prevention is focused on the general population, which includes individuals and groups who may be at risk but who have not yet developed any symptoms of misuse or abuse of alcohol. For adolescents, primary prevention is directed at nonusers and abstainers for the purpose of reducing the expected incidence rates of alcohol consumption.

Secondary prevention is targeted at individuals and groups who demonstrate the precursors or symptoms of abuse. It is directed at users who are in the early stages of abuse and who have experienced some negative consequences. Early intervention strategies fall into the category of secondary prevention. Tertiary prevention is targeted at individuals who are addicted or dependent on alcohol. Following treatment for alcoholism, tertiary prevention has as its goal the prevention of

TABLE 7.3. Prevention Principles

Prevention researchers and practitioners encourage planners to incorporate the following considerations in developing prevention programs (Goplerud, 1991):

- Build on previous prevention successes and failures in the literature
- Clearly understand the target population and its needs
- Give adequate attention to strategic planning, structure, and management issues
- Concentrate resources; do not overextend the program beyond its means
- Respond to needs of individual participants, both explicit and unarticulated
- Appreciate complexity; build in a variety of approaches and coordinate with other agencies and programs
- Be flexible; address risk factors at several levels
- Reduce barriers to program participation
- Reach out and be accessible; aggressively recruit program participants
- Be culturally sensitive in planning, implementation, and evaluation
- Provide services throughout the age spectrum
- Use appropriate, positive adult role models
- Involve parents
- Involve the school system
- Expect differential effects, as not all adolescents will respond to the program in exactly the same way

relapse. Aftercare services can be included in this category.

Prevention strategies that have demonstrated some promise with adolescents include:

- Peer pressure resistance training
- Normative education to counteract false perceptions of prevalence of alcohol use among teenage peers
- Inoculation against mass media messages
- Peer leadership skills development and peer education
- Reasonable policies and consequences consistently applied
- Recreational and alternative activities

Students' decision making about alcohol use is affected by a combination of factors including alcohol-related information, self-confidence, acceptance by friends, ability to cope with school and family pressures, availability and involvement in recreational alternatives, presence of adult role models, and fair, strict, and consistent policies at school, at home, and in the community.

The most effective alcohol prevention programs for adolescents incorporate strategies that address adolescents' internal states (self-esteem, stress and coping skills, depression), interpersonal skills (communication, refusal skills, and ability to develop friendships), and environmental forces (media influences, adult role models, policies and consequences at a variety of levels). Table 7.3 lists some principles of good prevention programs.

In addition, prevention programs should target youth with multiple risk factors and foster healthy adolescent development rather than focusing solely on deterring problem behavior. Programs that focus more systematically on institutional and interpersonal risk factors and less on individual risk factors have the potential for affecting larger numbers of adolescents.

Early Intervention Strategies

Although many adolescents who use alcohol moderate their use as they age, a significant minority do not and progress to more serious involvement with alcohol and its consequences. Due to high relapse rates associated with substance abuse treatment programs, many in the field have advocated the need for early intervention programs. Early intervention programs, those that intervene before alcohol use-related problems become serious, may offer better outcomes at a lower cost to both the individual and society.

Early intervention is sometimes referred to as secondary prevention because it identifies individuals in the early stages of problem drinking and attempts to reduce both the use of alcohol and its related consequences. Early intervention services are designed to

- Screen, assess, and refer individuals in the early stages of problem drinking
- Provide low-intensity, short-term services including counseling and support and self-help groups
- Provide services that address the problem behaviors associated with alcohol use, including behavior modification strategies, remedial education, recreation programs, and enhanced supervision (Klitzner, Fisher, Stewart, & Gilbert, 1992)

Early intervention services may be provided in a variety of settings, including schools, juvenile justice agencies, health care facilities, and community organizations.

Early Intervention in the Schools

Early intervention programs in the schools typically include school policies regarding alcohol and drug use, staff training, and direct services to students.

The U.S. Department of Education (USDE) advocates that a strong school policy be the cornerstone upon which all substance abuse programs are built. The policy should be broadly disseminated, clearly stated, and consistently and fairly implemented and enforced. The USDE supports school policies that prohibit the use of alcohol on school grounds, at school-sponsored functions, and at any time students are representing the school. As an early intervention strategy, school policies are most effective when they include a specific mechanism to refer students to appropriate services.

Staff training is an essential element in school-based programs. Appropriately, teachers view their role solely as educators, not counselors. However, teachers and other school personnel need to be trained to identify the signs and symptoms of alcohol use and abuse in order to be more effective in appropriately referring students for early intervention services.

Direct early intervention services for students frequently include Student Assistance Programs (SAPs). SAPs are the most rapidly growing form of early intervention and are modeled after Employee Assistance Programs (EAPs) frequently found in the business world. Students referred to SAPs are identified as "at risk" by peers, family members, or school personnel. SAPs may be coordinated by in-house school staff or by contracting with outside agencies. SAPs typically serve several functions, including

- Educating school staff about substance abuse issues
- Assessing students who have been referred for services
- Developing relationships with treatment and counseling resources in the community
- Implementing counseling and support groups in the school itself

Early Intervention and the Juvenile Justice System

Early intervention in the juvenile justice system is different from other types of early intervention programs due to more limited contact with adolescents. Only if alcohol use, possession, or intoxication is observed by a law enforcement officer will an adolescent be brought into the juvenile justice system. Two basic types of early intervention exist in this setting: preadjudication and postadjudication programs.

Preadjudication interventions typically include lecture and release strategies; diversion to educational, mental health, or social service agencies; and/or informal probation or supervision for 3 to 6 months by the probation department. Postadjudication interventions occur after an adolescent has been found guilty of committing an illegal act.

The most rapidly growing type of postadjudication intervention in the juvenile justice system is restitution and/or community service. This strategy may include monetary restitution to the victim, for example, paying for car repairs after an alcohol-related traffic crash; service to the victim, for example, repairing property after an alcohol-related incidence of vandalism; and/or service to the community in which the offense occurred. In addition, the judge may choose to refer the adolescent to specialized programs for substance abuse.

Early Intervention in Health Care Settings

The National Center for Health Statistics (1983) reports that 73% of all American youth ages 5 to 24 years old see a physician at least annually, and 50% have seen a doctor in the past 6 months. Health care utilization rates are typically higher for substance users than for nonusers. In spite of this, early intervention in health care settings is seriously lacking.

Health care professionals need increased education about screening, assessment, and intervention with children and adolescent substance users. Early intervention in health care settings can be provided in private practices, clinics, and hospitals. Health care professionals can provide identification, screening, assessment, and referral services, as well as brief office interventions.

Assessments for adolescent alcohol abuse usually take the form of pencil and paper questionnaires, face-to-face interviews, laboratory tests, and a physical examination. Brief office interventions are also valuable. Typically, they involve a minimal amount of time and minimal cost. These interventions have

the potential to reach large numbers of patients because they can be administered by health care professionals who are not substance abuse specialists.

Brief office interventions can be as simple as a direct suggestion by a physician or as complex as behavioral contracting. Other strategies may include referral to self-help programs, relevant reading material, counseling, and instruction in self-monitoring techniques.

Treatment Approaches

Unfortunately, adolescent alcohol abuse is probably the most frequently missed pediatric diagnosis in primary care. In detecting adolescent alcohol abuse, professionals should be aware that adolescents usually do not have the same physical signs of alcohol dependence as adults. For example, rarely will an adolescent have cirrhosis of the liver or demonstrate serious symptoms of alcohol withdrawal. In addition, lower expectations for role performance in work, self-care, and family relationships make detection of adolescent alcohol abusers more difficult. For example, a teen who is tardy to class or who has a disheveled appearance may be dismissed as a "typical" adolescent, whereas an adult demonstrating the same behaviors may provoke suspicion of alcohol abuse.

The symptoms of alcohol abuse among adolescents are basically the same as among adults. Preoccupation with alcohol, including how one is going to acquire it, when and where one will be able to consume it, and how one will cover up its use, is an early symptom of alcohol abuse. Other symptoms include increased tolerance, or the need to use more and more of the substance to achieve the desired effect; blackouts, an inability to recall events that occurred while one was under the influence; loss of control; denial; increased quantity and frequency of use; and problems related to alcohol consumption, such as decreased academic performance and arrest for driving while intoxicated.

In reviewing the literature on adolescent substance abuse treatment, three major conclusions emerge.

- Treatment is better than no treatment.
- The relapse rate among adolescents is high, ranging anywhere from 35% to 85% in various studies.
- No particular treatment approach has proven to be more effective than others.

Experts speculate that better matching of clients to particular treatment regimens will improve outcomes. Adolescent treatment programs need to take into account and address the following issues:

- Severity of substance involvement
- Substance abuse patterns and history
- Concurrent psychiatric problems
- Criminality and other deviant behavior
- Educational problems and dropping out of school
- Family dysfunction, including abuse
- Lack of involvement in productive roles

Currently, the resources in most communities for adolescent treatment are inadequate. It cannot be assumed that treatment programs for adults can effectively intervene with adolescent substance use problems. Adolescent treatment programs need to acknowledge the multiple problems associated with alcohol use and use a multimodality approach.

Adolescent alcohol abusers, like their adult counterparts, require a variety of treatment options. According to recent research, inpatient and outpatient treatment programs appear to be equally effective when used appropriately. The key issue is to match the unique characteristics and needs of the client with the unique characteristics and strengths of the programs.

Outpatient programs may focus on the individual adolescent or the family as the unit of care. Outpatient family therapy programs are useful when the adolescent alcohol abuse is a symptom of dysfunction within a family. The goal of this type of intervention is to resolve dysfunctional patterns in the family and thereby reduce adolescent alcohol use.

Outpatient treatment directed at the individual adolescent typically includes group, individual, and family therapy as well as substance abuse education. These programs allow adolescents to continue living at home and attending school. They are particularly beneficial for adolescents who are motivated to stop using alcohol and who have a healthy support system.

Inpatient treatment programs remove clients from dysfunctional environments that are counterproductive to their treatment. Short-term treatment may last 2 to 8 weeks, typically in hospital or residential settings. Characteristically these programs are more intense than outpatient treatment and provide external controls for adolescents with little internal control.

Long-term treatment provides ongoing structure and support for adolescents with poor home environments. These programs may last for 3 to 6 months or longer. The primary goals are the development of age-appropriate skills and the enhancement of the capacity for abstinence.

The most effective treatment programs, whether inpatient or outpatient, employ multiple modalities. The most common modalities used are individual, group, and family therapy; self-help groups; alcohol education; and activity/leisure programs.

Individual therapy allows adolescents to focus on their unique personal issues and circumstances in a one-to-one relationship. Group therapy encourages the expression of feelings and provides an opportunity for feedback from peers. The goals of group therapy are to provide support and encouragement and to reinforce constructive self-enhancing thinking and behavior. There are many different types of family therapy, but the strategic and structural approaches, based on general systems theory, are most often used in alcohol and drug treatment settings.

Self-help groups are a core component of most treatment programs. These often take the form of Twelve-Step programs, such as Alcoholics Anonymous, Alateen, and Adult Children of Alcoholics. Teenagers in treatment often need to attend multiple self-help groups to deal with their own alcohol issues and to cope with a substance-abusing parent.

Education, as part of a treatment protocol, involves both academic and substance abuse components. The academic component attempts to prevent the adolescent from falling further behind in school through tutoring and academic counseling. The substance abuse education component provides information about the effects of alcohol and its consequences for the adolescent's life and health.

Adolescents with alcohol problems spend a great deal of their leisure time "partying" and need to develop alternative recreational pursuits. Occupational therapy and therapeutic recreation services can provide activities that build life skills and increase self-esteem. These may involve both work and leisure activities, for example, games/sports, arts and crafts, hiking/camping, volunteer work, and part-time employment. Activity-based interventions are particularly important for adolescents because they encourage the integration of thought and behavior and give clients the opportunity to practice new skills in a nonthreatening environment. Newly achieved success in these activities may translate into better coping strategies when the adolescent returns to life in the community.

School-Based Programs and Curriculum Guidelines

For the majority of children and adolescents, school is the environment in which they spend most of their waking hours when they are not at home. As a result, the school can have a profound influence on child development, including health-related behaviors.

Schools are one of the primary vehicles for the socialization of children and adolescents and therefore are an important component of any alcohol prevention effort. Socialization is a developmental process through which individuals internalize cultural values and assimilate social norms. Schools are a place where children can acquire the knowledge and skills necessary to become responsible, productive members of society. In addition to helping students acquire academic abilities, the school is also a vehicle for the development of personal and social skills and habits. Adaptation to the school environment, with its associated values and norms, is a critical developmental milestone. If a child is unable to successfully adapt to the school environment, the consequence is often poor academic performance, troubled relationships with peers and teachers, anxiety/depression/alienation, and/or possible alcohol/drug use.

Although the field of substance abuse prevention is still in its infancy, it has made significant progress since the first prevention strategies were implemented in the late 1960s. Much has been learned from prevention failures as well as successes. Programs designed to increase knowledge are often quite successful, but it has become blatantly obvious that knowledge alone is insufficient to prevent alcohol abuse. Programs designed to change attitudes and behaviors are more difficult to develop but appear to hold promise for the future.

Unfortunately, many school-based prevention programs are based on the premise that characteristics of the individual are the primary cause of alcohol use and abuse. These programs typically ignore the influence of school environmental factors including school policies, organizational structure, classroom practices, and social climate. Environmental factors are critical as the use of alcohol, both by adolescents and adults, is contextual and results from the complex interplay of individual, social, and environmental variables. Recent successes by smoking prevention programs have demonstrated the power that changes in the social milieu can have on health behavior.

For a school-based alcohol prevention program to be effective, it must include a variety of strategies as opposed to making sole use of the traditional informational, in-class teaching approach. Schools can provide alcohol education, SAPs, appropriate alcohol-related policies and norms, and alternative health-enhancing activities. Regardless of the specific components of the program, alcohol prevention should be an important part of school life that is reflected in the curriculum, organization, policies, and social environment of the school.

The Seattle Social Development Program, a cooperative effort between the Seattle Public Schools and the Center for Social Welfare Research at the University of Washington, was developed to prevent alcohol and other drug use and delinquency among adolescents. The program is designed to facilitate the formation of social bonds among elementary and middle school children and their families, the school, and nondelinquent peers.

Parent involvement is crucial to the success of the program. Parents of 1st- and 2nd-grade students receive positive parenting skills training with an emphasis on recognizing and reinforcing children's positive behaviors. Parents of 2nd- and 3rd-grade children are trained to facilitate the development of basic reading and math skills in a home environment that is conducive to learning. Parents of middle school students receive information about alcohol and other drug use and training in family management techniques.

In an effort to provide a positive learning environment and promote bonding between students and their teachers, as well as students

and their peers, classroom teachers are trained in proactive classroom management, interactive teaching, and cooperative learning techniques. Proactive classroom management attempts to prepare students to monitor their own behavior and that of their peers, become independent learners, and develop prosocial behaviors. Interactive teaching emphasizes the collaboration between student and teacher in determining learning objectives and strategies for each individual child. This increases student commitment to educational goals and the likelihood of academic success. Cooperative learning techniques encourage students to work together toward a common goal and develop positive peer pressure and prosocial relationships.

Evaluation of the Seattle Social Development Program has demonstrated improved attitudes toward school, increased positive attachment to family members and teachers, improved scholastic performance on standardized math tests, increased time spent doing homework, and increased academic aspirations. The findings also suggest a decrease in aggressiveness among boys and self-destructive behaviors among girls, as well as reductions in suspensions, expulsions, and self-reported alcohol and other drug use at school.

Curriculum Guidelines

Alcohol education is best incorporated within a comprehensive school health education program. A high-quality school health education program is a planned, sequential, and developmentally appropriate series of health-related instruction modules taught by trained health education specialists. The goal of comprehensive school health education is not only to enhance knowledge, but also to develop positive health-related attitudes and behaviors. School health education programs are most successful when a sufficient amount of in-class time is devoted to the subject, when teachers are trained and motivated to present the content, and where there is strong administrative support.

Many school health education curricula already exist, and a number of these have a significant emphasis on alcohol and other drug abuse. Curricula that are approved by the Center for Substance Abuse Prevention (CSAP, 1992) for use in kindergarten through 12th grade must conform to the following criteria. The curricular materials must:

- Contain a strong no-use message
- Consist of at least 25% or more alcohol and other drug use prevention material
- Make clear that the use of illicit drugs is wrong and harmful
- Make clear that young people are responsible for their own decisions and not provide them with excuses for their behavior
- Use no illustrations or dramatizations that could teach people how to obtain, prepare, or ingest illegal drugs
- Be scientifically accurate and up-to-date
- Be appropriate for the developmental age, interests, and needs of the students
- Reflect an understanding of the target group's cultural systems and assumptions
- Not use recovering addicts or alcoholics as role models
- Be school-based
- Be available to the general public

A comprehensive school health curriculum is an important component of an alcohol prevention program, but a curriculum in isolation will probably have minimal long-term effect. Schools need to enhance the development of the whole child, not simply promote academic competencies. Strategies to enhance cognitive, psychological, and social development are integral components of progressive educational practice. A child's needs for autonomy, belongingness, and competence must be addressed in the school environment if he or she is expected to grow into a caring, responsible, and productive member of society. To achieve this broader goal, changes in classroom management, instructional practices, curriculum, and social organization and climate will be essential. Experts in the field recommend certain fundamental principles to enhance the effectiveness of school-based programs.

- Alcohol prevention should be infused within a comprehensive program of promoting the healthy development of children.
- Efforts to promote healthy cognitive, psychological, and social development need to begin early with preschool and elementary students.
- The school environment should provide positive social influences that enhance the socialization process and encourage the adoption of positive social norms.

Linking Strategies and Model Programs

There is no one answer, no matter how comprehensive, to the problem of alcohol use and abuse among adolescents. Each community in the nation is unique, and for a prevention program to be effective, it must take into account the specific characteristics, structure, and cultural diversity inherent in the target community.

Collaborative efforts across various sectors of the community that are well planned, well coordinated, and ongoing are likely to have the strongest impact on adolescent alcohol use and abuse. Characteristically, these programs incorporate multiple interventions that are directed at multiple levels. For example, some interventions may be directed at individuals, some at families, others at small groups and organizations, and still others at the community at large.

Prevention programs need to acknowledge and address the interrelationships between alcohol use behavior and the social and physical environment. Alcohol use and abuse occurs in a context and, therefore, the social environment is also a target for intervention.

One of the objectives in *Healthy People 2000* is to "establish community health promotion programs that separately or together address at least three of the Healthy People 2000 priorities and reach at least 40% of each state's population" (U.S. Department of Health and Human Services, 1990). The concept or philosophy behind this objective is that effective prevention programs must be designed to address multiple health problems and include not only strategies that influence individual behavior, but also social norms and attitudes. Because social norms are influenced by a variety of institutions, educational, political, religious, legal, and media, the active involvement and commitment of a broad cross section of the community is critical. Effective strategies are designed to influence the social norms that operate in communities where people live and work. The commitment and active participation of many sectors of a community—schools, churches, businesses, government agencies, health care providers, and community organizations—enhances the potential for long-lasting changes in attitudes, social norms, and behavior.

A comprehensive community health promotion program, as outlined in *Healthy People 2000*, should include

- Participation from at least three of the following community groups: government, education, business, religion, health care, media, voluntary agencies, and the public
- A community needs assessment to ascertain specific problems and resources
- Measurable objectives that address at least one of the following: health outcomes, risk factors, public awareness, or services
- A monitoring and evaluation process
- Multifaceted, culturally relevant interventions that have multiple targets for change and multiple approaches to change

A project that was specifically designed to address the issues related to underage drinking and that attempted to follow the recommen-

dations offered in *Healthy People 2000* is described next.

Society's Dilemma: Youth and Alcohol

In January 1992, a project funded by the National Highway Traffic Safety Administration, entitled "Society's Dilemma: Youth and Alcohol," got under way in the Washington, D.C., metropolitan area. The project was designed to examine the problem of underage drinking in the Washington, D.C., metropolitan area and was conducted by the Washington Regional Alcohol Program (WRAP), the Metropolitan Washington Council of Governments (COG), and the University of Maryland Alcohol and Drug Abuse Prevention Resource Center (see Figure 7.2). These three agencies, one located in Virginia, one in Washington, D.C., and the third in Maryland, collaborated to

- Create a broad-based coalition that included representatives from businesses, schools, the alcohol industry, government at the state and local levels, and key community groups
- Conduct a comprehensive needs assessment that included the identification of problems and resources, as well as the collection of baseline data for evaluation purposes
- Develop a strategic plan of action that had the buy-in and support of the key groups in the community coalition

The comprehensive needs assessment included input from a variety of sources and used a number of strategies for data collection. The key components of the needs assessment process consisted of

- A survey of current laws and pending legislation related to underage drinking in each of the political jurisdictions in the region
- A report from each jurisdiction regarding its specific demographics, indicators of underage drinking, available resources to address the problem, and activities currently under way

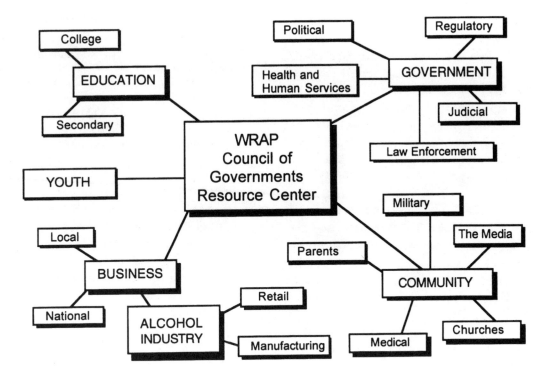

Figure 7.2.　Coalition Target Groups

- A market survey designed to elicit the opinions and attitudes of the general public regarding adolescent alcohol use
- A household telephone survey of adults and a street (or key location intercept) survey of adolescents to assess attitudes, perceptions, and behaviors related to underage drinking
- Focus group interviews with all coalition target groups
- A compilation of all existing youth and alcohol data from local and state police departments, alcohol beverage control agencies, and campus police departments
- A community forum with adolescents from across the region to debate and discuss issues related to underage drinking
- A review of print and broadcast reports to monitor the involvement of local and regional media with respect to the issues of interest

As a result of the needs assessment activities, it became clear that action was needed in four major areas: law enforcement, prevention/education, public policy, and community coordination and communication. Coalition representatives from both the public and the private sectors developed 20 objectives and over 150 action steps in those four major areas to include in a strategic planning document. In addition to action steps, each objective was supported by specific data from the needs assessment, and outcome measures were developed for evaluation purposes.

The strategic plan was designed as a guide for use by communities, regional groups, or states to facilitate the development of their own individualized strategic plans based on their real and perceived needs and resources. The next steps in the process include implementation of the strategic plan across the Washington, D.C., metropolitan area and monitoring/evaluation to determine whether the objectives have been met and if the program has successfully achieved its ultimate goal of reducing underage drinking.

Due to the diverse racial/ethnic population and the urban, suburban, and rural communities located in the metropolitan Washington, D.C., area, this project can serve as a model for other regions across the country in attempting to address adolescent alcohol use.

Two other exemplary programs identified by the Alcohol, Drug Abuse and Mental Health Administration (ADAMHA) are briefly described below.

Community Organizing for Prevention in Lincoln, Nebraska. This comprehensive prevention program was designed to change alcohol use norms in rural Nebraska by organizing training retreats and seminars for community leaders, teachers and other school personnel, parents, and youth.

Teams from various communities came together for a 4-day training to prepare them to implement the following activities:

- "Proud to be Drug Free" Summer Youth Retreats
- "Setting the Limits" parent training program
- "Decisions About Alcohol and Other Drugs" training for teachers to enable them to effectively implement a revised school curriculum

A Train the Trainer methodology was employed to reach large numbers of participants.

"Solid Ground" in Carson City, Nevada. This program, created by the Young Volunteers of Nevada, encouraged juveniles on probation to get involved in community service experiences that would expand their skills and enhance their sense of self-worth. The volunteer experiences attempted to expose the probationers to new activities and new peers while enhancing their personal and vocational aspirations and skills.

Participants were referred to the program by juvenile probation officers and were involved in the following activities:

- Completion of an interest and aptitude inventory and counseling
- Completion of a resume, job application form, videotaped role play of a job interview, and a seminar in stress management and impulse control
- 25 hours of volunteer work in a setting that complemented their interests and aptitudes as identified through the assessment

Over 100 organizations or agencies were involved in the volunteer experiences including nonprofit businesses, local and state government agencies, and volunteer organizations. In addition, local high schools offer school credit if participants continue their volunteer work after completion of the Solid Ground program.

Summary

Clearly, the use of alcohol by adolescents can have serious implications for their health and well-being and for their futures as productive members of society. Each individual, family, school, church, community organization, and government agency has an obligation and responsibility to address the concerns related to underage drinking and to protect our young people.

Opportunities to make a difference occur daily if we are only open to doing our part. In our roles as parents, friends, teachers, employers, scout leaders, health care professionals, community leaders, and concerned citizens, we can make a difference in the lives of adolescents.

We must act individually and collectively to ensure not only the health and safety of our children, adolescents, and young adults, but also the future of our country, as our young people are our greatest American resource.

References

Center for Substance Abuse Prevention. (1992). *Alcohol and other drugs resource guide: Curriculum* (MS445). Washington, DC: U.S. Department of Health and Human Services.

Goplerud, E. N. (1991). *Preventing adolescent drug use: From theory to practice* (CSAP Prevention Monograph-8). Washington, DC: Alcohol, Drug Abuse, and Mental Health Administration.

Klitzner, M., Fisher, D., Stewart, K., & Gilbert, S. (1992). *Early intervention for adolescents.* Princeton, NJ: Robert Wood Johnson Foundation.

Kumpfer, K. I. (1990). Prevention of alcohol and drug abuse: A critical review of risk factors and prevention strategies. In D. Shaffer, I. Philips, & N. B. Enzer (Eds.), *Prevention of mental disorders, alcohol and other drug use in children and adolescents.* Rockville, MD: U.S. Department of Health and Human Services.

National Center for Health Statistics. (1983). *Physician visits: Volume and interval since last visit* (Series 10, No. 144). Washington, DC: U.S. Department of Health and Human Services.

U.S. Department of Health and Human Services. (1990). *Healthy people 2000: National health promotion and disease prevention objectives.* Washington, DC: Author.

U.S. Department of Health and Human Services (1991). *Youth and alcohol: A national survey* (RPO799). Washington, DC: Author.

U.S. Department of Health and Human Services. (1994). *Monitoring the future study (high school senior survey).* Washington, DC: Author.

U.S. Department of Health and Human Services. (1997). *Ninth special report to the U.S. Congress on alcohol and health.* Washington, DC: Author.

8

—— ❧ ——

Recognizing and Preventing Sexually Transmitted Diseases Among Adolescents

Sarath Gunatilake

A wide variety of diseases can be transmitted through sexual intimacy. Chlamydia, trichomoniasis, gonorrhea, syphilis, human papilloma virus (HPV), genital herpes, hepatitis B, and human immunodeficiency virus (HIV) are the most widely known, but there are more than 15 other identified sexually transmitted diseases (STDs). Every year, there are about 250 million new cases of STDs reported worldwide (Khanna, Van Look, & Griffin, 1992). In the United States, an estimated 12 million cases of new sexually transmitted infections occur every year, two thirds of them among men and women under age 25. Every year 3.8 million teenagers acquire an STD. Adolescents thus account for nearly a third of the 12 million new cases of STDs that occur annually in the United States (Irwin, Brindis, Holt, & Langlykke, 1994). At the current rates, as many as 56 million individuals—

more than one American in five–may be infected with an incurable STD other than HIV (Alan Guttmacher Institute, 1993).

The Extent of Some STDs

Gonorrhea

Gonorrhea is the United States' most frequently reported communicable disease, with 620,478 cases reported in 1991. The actual incidence of the disease may be three times higher. An estimated 2 million people acquire gonococcal infection each year in the United States (Cates, 1987). This disease is associated with considerable morbidity, producing inflammation of the urethra, epididymis, and the rectum in men and painful pelvic inflammatory disease (PID) in women (Hook & Holmes, 1985). The latter is an important risk factor for ectopic pregnancy and infertility; about 25% of women who have had PID are unable to conceive (Westrom, 1975). Pregnant women with active gonococcal infection are at increased risk for obstetrical complications and can give birth to infants with gonococcal eye infections. People with gonorrhea are also at risk for a disseminated form of the disease, in which skin, joints, and other sites may become involved. Sexual contacts of people with active disease are at risk for acquiring gonorrhea; a large proportion of carriers of gonorrhea are asymptomatic. The incidence of gonorrhea is highest in young adults under age 25, unmarried people, people of low socioeconomic status, and people with multiple sexual contacts, such as prostitutes (Washington & Arno, 1986).

Syphilis

Annually, over 16,000 cases of primary and secondary syphilis are reported among adolescents in the United States (Irwin et al., 1994). Primary syphilis produces ulcers of the genitalia, pharynx, or rectum, and secondary syphilis produces complications such as contagious skin lesions, lymphadenopathy, and condylomalata. The disease then progresses into a latent phase in which syphilis may be clinically inapparent. If left untreated, one third of cases progress to the potentially severe cardiovascular and neurologic complications of tertiary syphilis (Clark & Danbolt, 1964). Victims of tertiary syphilis have decreased life expectancy, and they often experience significant disability and diminished productivity as a result of their disease. Long-term hospitalizations are often necessary for patients with severe neurologic deficits or psychiatric illness. Syphilis may also be associated epidemiologically with acquired immunodeficiency syndrome (AIDS); a possible relationship between diseases that cause genital ulcers, such as syphilis, and infection with HIV is being investigated (Holmberg et al.,

1988). The incidence of syphilis has increased in recent years and is currently at its highest rate since 1950 (CDC, 1988). A growing proportion of cases is also reported among prostitutes and people who use illicit drugs.

The incidence of syphilis in pregnant women is also increasing. Transmission of the disease to the fetus results in congenital syphilis, a condition resulting in fetal or perinatal death in 40% of affected pregnancies, as well as increased risk of medical complications in newborns who survive.

Chlamydia

An estimated 940,000 adolescents acquire chlamydia infections each year in the United States (Irwin et al., 1994). This organism is responsible for about half of all cases of nongonococcal urethritis and acute epididymitis in men and about half of the cases of mucopurulent cervicitis in women (McMillan & Weiner, 1985). It has been estimated that chlamydia infections are responsible for about 25% to 50% of the 1 million cases of PID that are reported annually in the United States. PID is an important cause of infertility and ectopic pregnancy in American women (CDC, 1985). About half of the sexual partners of people with chlamydia infection are also infected with this organism. The economic costs of chlamydia infection are estimated to be over $1 billion per year. Chlamydia infection is more common in people under age 25, especially adolescents (CDC, 1985). Other risk factors for chlamydia infection in asymptomatic people include having multiple sexual partners, a new sexual partner in the preceding 2 months, and a sexual partner with a chlamydia infection.

About 8% to 12% of pregnant women have cervical chlamydia infections. Infection during pregnancy can produce postpartum endometritis, and the organism is transmitted to the fetus in over half of deliveries. Each year, more than 155,000 infants are born to chlamydia-infected mothers (CDC, 1985).

Genital Herpes Simplex

Primary episodes of genital herpes occur each year in about 200,000 to 500,000 Americans (Chuang, Su, Perry, et al. 1983), and as many as 20 million people are already infected (Guinan, Wolinsky, & Reichman, 1985). An estimated 1,270,000 adolescents have genital herpes simplex virus infection (Irwin et al., 1994). The chief morbidity associated with infection with herpes simplex virus (HSV-1 or HSV-2) are painful vesicular and ulcerative lesions that erupt in the anal, genital, and oral areas. About 4% of symptomatic primary episodes require hospitalization (Corey et al., 1983). Sexual contacts of people with active and inactive disease are at risk of becoming infected. Pregnant women with genital herpes infection can transmit the infection to the newborn during vaginal delivery. An estimated 400 to 1,000 cases of neonatal herpes occur each year in the United States (Nahmias, Keyserling, & Kerrick, 1983). If the infection is untreated, death occurs in 65% of infants; less than 10% of survivors with central nervous system infection have normal development. Genital herpes costs the United States an estimated $500 million per year (Cates, 1988).

Hepatitis B

Each year in the United States, over 300,000 people become infected with hepatitis B virus (HBV), and more than 10,000 require hospitalization (Immunization Practices Advisory Committee, 1987). Although most infections resolve with time, 6% to 10% of patients develop an asymptomatic chronic carrier state that places them at risk for developing chronic active hepatitis, cirrhosis, and primary hepatocellular carcinoma. The United States has an estimated pool of 1 million to 1.5 million chronic carriers of HBV (Alan Guttmacher Institute, 1993). About 4,000 hepatitis B-related deaths occur each year as a result of liver cancer (Immunization Practices Advisory Committee, 1985). An estimated 16,500 births occur to HBV-infected women each year in the United States. Infants whose mothers are positive for hepatitis B "e" antigen have a 70% to 90% chance of becoming infected perinatally, and virtually all (85%-90%) infants who do become infected develop chronic HBV carrier status (Stevens et al., 1985). The principal risk factors for HBV infection in the United States are intravenous drug abuse; heterosexual contact with HBV-infected persons, HBV chronic carriers, or multiple partners; and male homosexual activity. Certain population groups, such as immigrants from Asia and Africa, may also be at increased risk. In recent years, a growing number of intravenous drug abusers have become infected; currently, between 60% and 80% of people who use illicit parenteral drugs have serologic evidence of HBV infection. This population now accounts for the largest proportion of HBV cases in the United States (Immunization Practices Advisory Committee, 1985).

Risk Factors for STD Among Adolescents

Type of STD and Ethnicity

As mentioned, 3.8 million teenagers—roughly one person in seven ages 13 to 19—acquire an STD every year. Considering the fact that 63% of the females and 86% of the males have had sexual intercourse by age 19, roughly one in four adolescents who are sexually active are at risk for developing a STD. Some STDs are more easily transmissible than others: For example, in a single act of unprotected intercourse with an infected partner, a woman has a 1% risk of acquiring HIV, a 30%

risk of getting genital herpes, and a 50% chance of contracting gonorrhea; a man's risk of infection ranges from 1% for HIV and 30% for genital herpes. Chlamydia is more common among adolescents than among older men and women. Some studies have reported chlamydia prevalence rates of 10% to 29% among sexually active adolescents and a rate of up to 10% among teenage boys who have already had sex. Because chlamydia may be responsible for up to 50% of the cases of PID, it also explains why women ages 15 to 19 have the highest rate of hospitalization for acute PID. Hospitalization for chronic PID is twice as common among non-white females.

Adolescents ages 15 to 19 also have higher rates of gonorrhea than sexually active men and women in any 5-year age group between the ages of 20 and 44. Adolescents of color are at a much higher risk of developing gonorrhea than their white counterparts. The reported rate of gonorrhea in 1991 was 40 times higher among African Americans and more than two times higher among Hispanics than among whites (Alan Guttmacher Institute, 1993). The risk for adolescents of color is even greater for infectious syphilis. In 1991, the reported rate of infectious syphilis among African Americans was 62 times higher than among whites; the rate for Hispanics was 6 times higher. It is also alarming to note that the infectious syphilis rates more than doubled between 1986 and 1990 among females ages 15 to 19. Adolescents are also at high risk for developing human papilloma virus (HPV). It is estimated that up to 15% of sexually active women ages 13 to 19 are infected with HPV. Cervical cancer, which kills more than 4,500 American women each year, is strongly associated with several strains of HPV.

Gender

Female adolescents are at disproportionately increased risk of developing STDs due to physiological factors, such as an immature cervix that is more vulnerable to infection, and social factors, such as lack of assertiveness and pressure to agree to sex (Woolf, Jones, & Lawrence, 1996). A woman is twice as likely as a man to contract gonorrhea, chlamydia, chancroid, or hepatitis-B during a single act of unprotected intercourse with an infected partner. Although they are at a higher risk for developing STDs, women are less likely to experience symptoms of the infections they develop; that is, they are more likely to have asymptomatic infections. Therefore, it is more difficult to diagnose these STDs in women until serious problems and consequences ensue. For example, it is known that up to 75% of the chlamydia infections in women are asymptomatic compared to 25% in men.

Every year, more than 2 million women suffer an episode of PID, the most common complication of STDs. About one woman in nine between the ages of 15 and 44 are treated for PID during their reproductive years. Adolescent females account for at least 200,000 cases of PID every year (Irwin et al., 1994). The most frequent complication of PID is infertility. An estimated 100,000 to 150,000 women become infertile each year as a result of PID secondary to STDs. One woman in seven may become infertile after a single episode of PID. It is estimated that up to 30% of the U.S. couples who are infertile may have acquired the condition due to STDs that result in the development of PID.

Women who have had PID are also 10 times more likely than other women to have an ectopic pregnancy. About half of more than 88,000 ectopic pregnancies that occur each year are the result of a previous attack of an STD (Alan Guttmacher Institute, 1993). Ectopic pregnancy is also the leading cause of maternal mortality among African American women.

Adolescent Sexual Behavior

Because adolescence is a time of sexual curiosity, experimentation, and risk taking, adolescents have the highest risk of exposure to STDs. Many adolescents mistakenly believe that it is not possible for them to come into contact with anyone who is infected. They view multiple sex partners as an achievement rather than a health risk. Adolescents also tend to have spontaneous rather than premeditated sex, which hinders use of preventive measures (Woolf et al., 1996). Because of the influence of physiological, individual, family, community, and social factors, early initiation of sexual intercourse among adolescents is on the rise (Miller & Moore, 1990). The percentage of women ages 15 to 19 who reported having sexual intercourse rose from 36% in 1971 to 47% in 1982 and 53% in 1988. The percentage of never-married males ages 17 to 19 living in metropolitan areas who reported having sexual intercourse increased from 66% in 1979 to 76% in 1988. Currently, it is estimated that, by the age of 19, more than 63% of females and 86% of males have become sexually active. It is estimated that there is about a 15% incremental increase per year in the number of adolescents who are sexually active (Irwin et al., 1994). The number of adolescents who report having sex with multiple sexual partners is also on the increase. Between 1971 and 1988, the percentage of sexually experienced women ages 15 to 19 living in urban areas who claimed to have had sex with four or more partners increased from 14% to 31%. In another study of the general population of adolescents, 4% of white females, 6% of African American females, 11% of white males, and 23% of African American males reported having six or more sexual partners (Moore & Peterson, 1989). Early initiation of sexual intercourse may lead to a higher number of sexual partners over one's lifetime. Having more than one partner over a given period of time or over one's lifetime increases the risk of exposure to STDs. An estimated number of 12 million to 17 million women ages 15 to 44 may be at increased risk for acquiring STD because of exposure to multiple sex partners.

A full discussion of the factors contributing to the recent trends in sexual behavior among adolescents is beyond the scope of this chapter. However, in order to plan strategies for the prevention and treatment of STDs, one must understand the research findings on why and how adolescents tend to initiate sexual intercourse early and have sex with multiple partners. Summarizing the research through the 1980s, Miller and Moore (1990) provide a comprehensive discussion on the subject, delineating biological, psychosocial, family, and sociocultural antecedents and peer influences on adolescent sexual behavior patterns. For example, there appears to be a strong relationship between hormone levels, pubertal development, and sexual activity. However, hormone levels cannot account for all of the societal increases in early sexual intercourse (Miller & Moore, 1990). At the same time, adolescents' cognitive and emotional development often lags behind their biological development. Adolescents who are physically capable of sexual and reproductive behavior may lack cognitive and behavioral skills necessary to choose a responsible course of action and understand its long-term consequences and implications. There is also a correlation between sexual activity and academic achievement. In one 10-year longitudinal study, it was found that adolescents who experienced sexual intercourse sooner placed a higher value on and expectation for independence and a lower value and expectation on academic achievement (Donovan & Jessor, 1985).

Many aspects of the family also affect sexual behavior. For example, several studies have shown that adolescents—daughters, in particular—from single-parent families are more likely to begin sexual intercourse at younger ages than their peers from two-parent families (Miller & Moore, 1990). There is less parental supervision in single-parent homes, both because there are fewer parents and because single mothers are more likely to work full-time than are mothers in two-parent households. Also, among single parents who are dating, their own sexual behavior may have a role model effect. Adolescent girls whose parents exert greater supervision over their dating also report less sexual activity (Miller, McCoy, & Olson, 1986). The more years of education completed by parents, the less likely their teens are to be sexually active (Forste & Heaton, 1988); and low educational goals and poor educational achievement are associated with greater sexual activity among both adolescent boys and girls (Miller & Sneesby, 1988).

Sociocultural antecedents including race, religion, and social class also have a strong influence on adolescent sexual behavior. Young women ages 15 to 19 who said religion was important to them and attended church more frequently were less likely to report having had sexual intercourse (Forste & Heaton, 1988). Also, the highest level of premarital intercourse occurred among those with no religious affiliation. The effects of religion and sexual behavior operate in both directions; adolescents who are more religious are less likely to engage in sexual intercourse, and adolescents who become sexually active at young ages have a tendency to become less religious (Thornton & Camburn, 1989).

Race is one of the most powerful factors differentiating early from late initiators of sexual activity. There are large black-white differences in sexual activity in the raw data, and these differences do not disappear when controls for other factors including poverty are introduced. The gap between first intercourse and marriage is especially long for black adolescents, about 12 years for women and 19 years for men, because they usually initiate sex relatively early and marry late (Alan Guttmacher Institute, 1994). Living in poverty is also associated with both early sexual activity and pregnancy. As socioeconomic status decreases, rates of sexual activity and early pregnancy rise (Miller & Moore, 1990). The influence of poverty may operate through other factors such as lack of options and desirable alternatives for the future, community norms, supervision practices, and social and economic variations among neighborhoods.

Peer group influences also affect sexual behaviors strongly. In a Harris (1988) poll, social pressure was identified by 73% of the girls and 50% of boys as a reason why adolescents do not wait until they are older to have sexual intercourse. One longitudinal peer network study reported that sexual behavior of white girls was influenced by their best male and female friends: That is, girls who were virgins when the study began were more likely to have intercourse between the waves of the survey if they had sexually experienced friends. In contrast, white males appeared to pick their friends on the basis of prior sexual activity rather than being influenced by friends' behavior. Blacks appeared neither to be influenced by friends' sexual behavior nor to pick their friends on that basis (Billy & Udry, 1985). Other studies also suggest both best friends' and siblings' sexual behavior predict the same behaviors among young adolescents (Miller & Moore, 1990).

Peers are a major source of health information for adolescents, with their importance increasing as adolescents enter the mid-adolescent years. Although adolescents view health care providers as providing the most reliable information, they often find it difficult to spontaneously disclose sensitive information to providers. In one study, 44% of the adolescents said if they thought they had a STD, they would be too embarrassed to ask a physician about it (Irwin et al., 1994). Adolescents therefore look to their peers as the primary source of information about STDs and other health issues (Opinion Research Corporation, 1993).

Available Services and Recommendations to Prevent the Spread of STDs

The available strategies to prevent the spread of STDs can be classified by the stage of illness they target. Primary prevention strategies are intended to prevent infection. They are implemented before any disease occurs and involve reducing or eliminating the risk factors for STDs. As currently practiced, the main site of primary prevention activities is the school. Secondary prevention strategies are implemented to prevent adverse health outcomes once an infection has occurred and involve early detection and treatment of patients with STDs. Because treating an infected person breaks the chain of transmission, many STD prevention strategies directed toward the infected individual serve both primary and secondary prevention functions. The sites of secondary prevention activities are the clinical settings that include school-based and community clinics, physicians' offices, and other health care institutions.

STD Prevention Programs in School Settings

Schools have played a major role in helping adolescents take more responsibility for their sexual behavior and health. Some form of health education and health promotion activities in relation to STDs and sexual behavior is present in almost all schools. Driven by the concern about HIV infection, many schools expanded their health education programs to address sexuality education more specifically. The Sex Information and Education Council of the United States found that as of 1992, 47 states and the District of Columbia recommended or required education on HIV, AIDS, and sexuality. Adolescents are generally receptive to school settings as a source of health information, often find health classes to be more interesting than other classes, and report

that they find the material taught in these classes to be useful (Harris & Associates, 1988). The U.S. Public Health Service (1993) prepared a report entitled *School Health: Findings from Evaluated Programs* to provide information on school health programs throughout the nation. Table 8.1 provides a summary of some examples included in this report on school health programs intended to provide sexuality education and change behaviors of adolescents toward engaging in safer sexual practices.

In spite of continued efforts, school health programs have not been able to achieve their intended outcomes. For example, three recent commissioned reports by the National Commission on the Role of School and the Community in Improving Adolescent Health (1990) concluded that for the first time in U.S. history, adolescents are regressing in health and social well-being. Drug abuse, suicide, STDs, pregnancy, homelessness, delinquency, crime, and unintentional violent deaths have increased. Healthy dietary and exercise habits, routine health care, and education have decreased. Furthermore, there is grudging recognition that these social and health problems are significantly interrelated and that their associated diseases are co-morbid (Hechinger, 1992; U.S. Office of Technology Assessment, 1991).

An analysis of the examples cited in Table 8.1 demonstrates some major gaps in the current practice of school health education and related programs. First, a large number of programs existing today focus on providing health information to increase knowledge. The most common content of the prevention messages included in most sexuality education programs are shown in Figure 8.1. Enhanced knowledge does not necessarily lead to desired behaviors. Although traditional sex education has been successful in achieving the limited goal of increasing knowledge, students do not appear to change their sexual behavior unless the program provides specific information on how to resist sexual pressures and how to prevent pregnancy and disease (Kirby, 1984). Ad-

TABLE 8.1. School-Based Programs for STD Prevention and Sexuality Education

Program	Objectives	Population Studied	Program Setting and Components	Findings
Postponing Sexual Involvement, Atlanta, Georgia (Howard & McCabe, 1990)	To help young people postpone sexual involvement	7th- and 8th-grade low-income minority teens in 19 schools	Five classroom-period educational series	Participants were five times less likely to have begun having sex. Participants experienced fewer pregnancies
Project Accept, San Diego, CA (Shulkin et al., 1991)	To increase knowledge of HIV transmission; to change behavioral intentions to correspond with safer sexual practices	Young adults in four classes, San Diego State University	Didactic presentations; group discussion by peer educators	Program improved knowledge, attitudes, and behavioral intentions to practice safer sex
Reducing the Risk, California (Kirby, Waszak, & Ziegler, 1991)	To reduce unprotected intercourse among students	10th graders in 13 high schools from 10 school districts	15-session sexuality education curriculum; building cognitive and behavioral skills	Program had the greatest impact on sexual initiation. After 18 months, 29% of intervention students had had sex compared with 38% of nonparticipants
Self Center Program, Baltimore, Maryland (Zabin et al., 1988)	To increase knowledge, postpone intercourse, increase clinic attendance, reduce the risk of pregnancy	7th- to 12th-grade African American students living in public housing in the inner city; 667 males, 1,033 females studied for 3 years	Classroom presentations, educational and counseling services, medical services at a nearby storefront clinic	37% fewer pregnancies among program participant females; 24% to 29% fewer females participated in unprotected intercourse; male participants showed significant increases in knowledge
Reproductive Health Programs of six school-based clinics, multiple sites (Kirby et al., 1991)	To influence sexual behavior and contraceptive usage among teenagers	9th- to 12th-grade students from low-income families with large proportion of African American and other minorities with limited access to health care in California, Michigan, Florida, Texas, and Indiana	School-based clinic; comprehensive health program with emphasis on reproductive health, sexuality education, and family planning, provided at the school clinic	One clinic school with a strong AIDS education program showed sharp increases in condom use; pregnancy rates were equal to the nonclinic schools

SOURCE: U.S. Public Health Service

The prevention messages may include:

1. Abstaining from sex and from injecting drugs is the surest way to prevent STDs, including HIV infection.
2. A mutually monogamous relationship in which neither partner is infected with an STD nor uses injected drugs is the safest sexual relationship.
3. If abstinence or monogamy is not possible, always use condoms during sexual intercourse. Avoid sexual practices involving the exchange of body fluids, such as vaginal, anal, or oral sex without a condom.
4. Limit the number of sex partners.
5. Know the symptoms of STDs and seek care as soon as symptoms are suspected.
6. When infection is detected, take all medications as directed, and ensure that all sex partners are also examined and/or treated before resuming sexual intercourse.

Figure 8.1. Prevention Messages

SOURCE: Woolf, Jones, and Lawrence, 1996.

ditional efforts to enhance skills and competencies to deal with undesirable peer pressure, reinforcements in terms of changes in school environment and societal norms, and other policy changes are necessary to bring about meaningful changes in health behaviors. Very few school health programs in existence today address all these components of health behavior change.

Second, greater efforts are associated with the use of didactic instructional methods rather than including other methods that use modeling, role playing, and Socratic discussion with feedback (Botvin, 1986; Flay et al., 1985; Perry, 1987). Adolescents' suggestions for how to improve health education in the schools point to a number of areas where attention should be focused. These include the use of smaller groups for open discussion of health-related topics, the use of question-and-answer periods in which all questions would be answered completely and honestly, and health teachers who can listen and who are not ashamed to talk about certain topics. Adolescents also note the importance of up-to-date information, support media, the use of outside specialists, and the value of nonbook "real life" learning (Byler, Lewis, & Tofman, 1969). There is enough evidence from available literature that the use of adolescent peers as role models and facilitators appears to contribute to program effectiveness (Perry, 1987). Curricula have been designed that combine sexuality education with interactive instruction

emphasizing values and norms for responsible behavior and decision making so that students learn the communication skills needed to say "no" or "not yet" to sexual intercourse or unprotected sex (Barth et al., 1992).

Third, it is known that programs that focus on changing social influences yield the largest effect on health behaviors (Flay et al., 1985). Social influences targeted in these programs include media influences, peer pressure, modeling by adults, and perceived social norms. There is a striking similarity of social influences that affect the incidence of STDs and those that contribute to other high-risk behaviors that lead to adolescent drug abuse, teen pregnancy, and so on. Therefore, it makes a lot of sense to design programs that affect the multitude of social influences that contribute to a number of co-morbid diseases or adolescent health problems at the same time. However, very few of the available school health programs attempt to deal with the whole social environment that contributes significantly to a complex of multiple and often co-morbid health problems.

Fourth, health promotion and disease prevention strategies must be developed at multiple levels: the individual, the schools, the community, the family, and other places that are frequented by adolescents. The more points of leverage, the larger the extent of health behavior change and duration. Unfortunately, because of logistical difficulties and the limitation of resources, many programs limit their focus to the classroom or the school-based clinic. Comprehensive communitywide approaches that encourage abstinence by teaching communication and life skills, provide accurate information on contraceptive methods and STD prevention, and facilitate access to contraceptives have been implemented in a limited number of places (Alan Guttmacher Institute, 1994). In some cases, such programs have been successful in reducing the birth rate among adolescents (Vincent, Clearie, & Schluchter, 1987).

Fifth, the cultural sensitivity of some of the school-based programs is also in question (Elster, Pranzarine, & Holt, 1993). Most health professionals are middle class and white. Therefore, the issues, approaches, and strategies that are critical for health promotion are already incongruent with the lives and experiences of many of America's adolescents of color. In terms of the prevalence of risk factors for the development of STDs, there is little doubt that this is the group that is most in need of health promotion programs that take into account their values, attitudes, traditions, and customs. Health promotion and prevention strategies must engage in better "social marketing" of their programs and products. Such marketing requires paying attention to socioeconomic and cultural factors as well as messages that are targeted to reach a specific population.

Sixth, most school health programs described in the U.S. Public Health Service Study (1993), as well as many others, lack rigorous evaluation designs. The majority of the programs described compare pre- and postintervention knowledge, attitudes, and beliefs. Only a small number reported data on behavior, health status, and educational performance. Also of note is the lack of long-term evaluations that document the persistence of the beneficial effects of the interventions demonstrated in the short term. A few programs that did report long-term follow-up tended to show a diminution of the program effects over time.

In summary, successful school-based programs and interventions share a number of characteristics, including the following: (a) theoretical grounding in social learning or social influence theories, (b) a focus on reducing specific sexual risk-taking behaviors, (c) experiential activities to convey the information on the risks of unprotected sex and how to avoid those risks and to personalize the information, (d) instruction and discussion on social influences and pressures, (e) reinforcement of individual values and group norms against unprotected sex that are age and experience appropriate, and (f) activities to increase relevant skills and confidence in those skills (Kirby et al., 1994).

Clinical Services for the Prevention of STDs

The clinical services for the prevention of STDs include screening STDs for early diagnosis and treatment, counseling, partner notification, and follow-up. A full discussion of STD diagnosis and treatment is beyond the scope of this chapter. However, certain aspects of STD screening, counseling, and partner notification, which should be included in a comprehensive STD education program, are discussed below. There appears to be a fair amount of consensus on procedures to be followed on screening, counseling, and treating STDs. The U.S. Preventive Services Task Force (1989) is a panel of 20 experts from medicine and related fields who conducted a 4-year comprehensive review of 169 interventions to prevent 60 different illnesses. The following is a list of recommendations by the U.S. Preventive Services Task Force on screening and counseling for STDs, adapted for the use of adolescent population.

Screening for STDs

1. *Screening for Hepatitis B:* Pregnant adolescents and all pregnant women should be

tested for the hepatitis-B surface antigen (HBsAg) at their first prenatal visit. The test may be repeated in the third trimester if the mother engages in high-risk behavior such as intravenous drug abuse or if exposure to hepatitis B during pregnancy is suspected. Hepatitis-B vaccine should be offered to susceptible individuals in high-risk groups, including homosexually active men, intravenous drug users, recipients of certain blood products, and people in health-related jobs with frequent exposure to blood and blood-related products.

2. *Syphilis:* Routine serologic testing is recommended for people at increased risk for syphilis, such as prostitutes, people who engage in sex with multiple partners in areas in which syphilis is prevalent, and sexual contacts of people with active syphilis. The optimal frequency of tests has not been determined and is left to clinical discretion. All pregnant women should be tested at their first prenatal visit and at delivery; and additional testing at 28 weeks of gestation is recommended for women at increased risk of acquiring syphilis during pregnancy.

3. *Gonorrhea:* Routine cultures for gonorrhea should be obtained in high-risk groups such as prostitutes, people with multiple sexual partners or a sexual partner with multiple sexual contacts, sexual contacts of people with culture-proven gonorrhea, and people with a history of repeated episodes of gonorrhea. The optimal frequency of such testing has not been determined. Pregnant women should receive endocervical cultures for gonorrhea at their first prenatal visit. An additional test later in pregnancy is recommended for those at increased risk for acquiring gonorrhea during pregnancy. Erythromycin 0.5% ophthalmic ointment or tetracycline 1% ophthalmic ointment should be applied topically to the eyes of all newborns as soon as possible after birth and no later than 1 hour of age.

4. *Chlamydia:* Routine testing for *Chlamydia trachomatis* is recommended for asymptomatic persons who attend clinics for STDs, attend other high-risk health care facilities (e.g., adolescent and family planning clinics), or have other risk factors for chlamydial infection (e.g., age less than 20, multiple sexual partners, or a sexual partner with multiple sexual contacts). The optimal frequency of such testing has not been determined and is left to clinical discretion. Recent sexual partners of people with positive cultures also require testing and treatment. Pregnant women in the high-risk categories listed above should be tested for chlamydia at the first prenatal visit. Erythromycin 0.5% ophthalmic ointment or tetracycline 1% ophthalmic ointment should be applied topically to the eyes of all newborns as soon as possible after birth and no later than 1 hour of age.

5. *Herpes simplex:* All pregnant women during their first prenatal visit and adolescents attending STD clinics should be asked whether they or their sexual contacts have had genital herpetic lesions. Those with active lesions should be cultured, but cultures are not necessary in the absence of active disease.

U.S. Preventive Services Task Force (1989) Recommendations on Counseling

1. *Clinicians should take a complete sexual and drug use history on all adolescent and adult patients.* Sexually active patients should receive complete information on their risk for acquiring STDs. They should be advised that abstaining from sex or maintaining a mutually faithful monogamous sexual relationship with a partner known to be uninfected are the most effective strategies to prevent infection with HIV or other STDs. Patients should be advised against sexual activity with individuals whose infection status is uncertain. A nonreactive HIV test does not rule out infection if the sexual partner has not been monogamous for at least 6 months before the test. Patients who

choose to engage in sexual activity with multiple partners or with people who may be infected should be advised to use a condom at each encounter and to avoid anal intercourse. Women should be informed of the potential risks of HIV infection during pregnancy. People who use intravenous drugs should be encouraged to enroll in a drug treatment program, warned against sharing drug equipment and using unsterilized syringes and needles, and given sources for uncontaminated injection equipment or referred to community programs with this information. Patients should be offered testing in accordance with recommendations on screening for syphilis, gonorrhea, chlamydia, genital herpes, hepatitis B, and infection with HIV.

2. *Condoms need not be recommended to prevent infection in long-standing mutually monogamous relationships in which neither partner uses IV drugs or is infected with HIV.* Those patients who need to use condoms should be informed that they do not provide complete protection against infection and must be used in accordance with the following guidelines to be effective:

- Latex condoms, rather than natural membrane condoms, should be used. Torn condoms, those in damaged packages, or those with signs of age (brittle, sticky, discolored) should not be used.
- The condom should be put on an erect penis, before any intimate contact, and should be unrolled completely to the base.
- A space should be left at the tip of the condom to collect semen; air pockets in the space should be removed by pressing the air out toward the base.
- Water-based lubricants should be used. Those made with petroleum jelly, mineral oil, cold cream, and other oil-based lubricants should not be applied because they may damage the condom.
- Insertion of nonoxynol 9 in the condom increases protection, but vaginal application in addition to condom use is likely to provide greater protection.

- If a condom breaks, it should be replaced immediately.
- After ejaculation and while the penis is still erect, the penis should be withdrawn while carefully holding the condom against the base of the penis so that the condom remains in place.
- Condoms should not be reused.

Partner Notification and Dealing With Sex Partners

Breaking the chain of transmission is central to the prevention of STDs both from an individual and a public health (community) point of view. Therefore, sex partners of patients diagnosed with STDs should be evaluated, examined, and, in circumstances in which infection is considered likely, treated in spite of the absence of clinical signs of infection or before a confirmatory laboratory diagnosis is made. Informing their sexual partners may be a specially difficult and sensitive topic for adolescents. Frank face-to-face discussion with adolescents, role playing, rehearsals involving questions such as "How will you tell your partner(s) about this?" "What if he (she) gets angry and starts crying?" "What will you say?" have been found to be useful (Coates & Lo, 1990). Sex partners of patients diagnosed with specific STDs require different management strategies. Table 8.2 provides a useful set of guidelines in partner notification for STDs.

Health Service Delivery Needs of Adolescents

The existing health care delivery system for adolescents focuses primarily on illness rather than health promotion and disease prevention. This perspective is particularly problematic in the case of adolescents who engage in a multitude of risk-taking behaviors, which often result in socially caused morbidity and mortality. Financial barriers to care are also significant; more than 15% of adolescents lack either pub-

TABLE 8.2. Management of Sex Partners

Disease	Intervention
Gonorrhea	Partners should be referred for evaluation and treatment according to the following schedule: If the index patient is symptomatic, partners should be evaluated and treated for gonorrhea and chlamydia if their last sexual contact with the patient was within 30 days of onset of the patient's symptoms. If the index patient is asymptomatic, partners should be evaluated and treated for gonorrhea and chlamydia if their last sexual contact with the patient was within 60 days of diagnosis. Patients must be instructed to avoid sexual intercourse until patient and partner(s) are cured (when therapy is completed and patient and partner are without symptoms). The mothers of infants with gonococcal infection and their sex partners should be evaluated and treated.
Nongonococcal urethritis	If the index patient is symptomatic, partners should be evaluated and treated for gonorrhea and chlamydia if their last sexual contact with the patient was within 30 days of onset of the patient's symptoms. If the index patient is asymptomatic, partners should be evaluated and treated for gonorrhea and chlamydia if their last sexual contact with the patient was within 60 days of diagnosis. Patients must be instructed to avoid sexual intercourse until patient and partner(s) are cured (when therapy is completed and patient and partner are without symptoms).
Mucopurulent cervicitis	Partners should be managed appropriately for the specific STD (chlamydia or gonorrhea) identified in the index patient. Partners of patients treated presumptively should receive the same treatment as the patient.
Chlamydia	If the index patient is symptomatic, partners should be evaluated and treated for gonorrhea and chlamydia if their last sexual contact with the patient was within 30 days of onset of the patient's symptoms. If the index patient is asymptomatic, partners should be evaluated and treated for gonorrhea and chlamydia if their last sexual contact with the patient was within 60 days of diagnosis. Patients must be instructed to avoid sexual intercourse until patient and partner(s) are cured (when therapy is completed and patient and partner are without symptoms). The mothers of infants with chlamydia infection and their sex partners should be evaluated and treated.
Trichomoniasis	Partners should be treated. Patients should be instructed to avoid sex until therapy is completed and patient and partner are without symptoms.
Bacterial vaginosis	Routine treatment of partners is not recommended.
Syphilis	Sexual transmission occurs only when mucocutaneous syphilitic lesions are present; such manifestations are uncommon after the first year of infection. All partners exposed to a patient with early syphilis (primary, secondary, or latent with duration < 1 year) should be evaluated clinically and serologically. Partners exposed to a patient with early syphilis within the preceding 90 days might be infected yet seronegative; they should be treated presumptively. It may be advisable to presumptively treat people exposed more than 90 days ago if serologic test results are not immediately available and follow-up is uncertain. Long-term sex partners of patients with late syphilis should be evaluated clinically and serologically for syphilis. The time periods usually used for identifying at-risk partners are 3 months plus duration of symptoms for primary syphilis, 6 months plus duration of symptoms for secondary syphilis, and 1 year for early latent syphilis.
Chancroid	Partners exposed to chancroid within 10 days before onset of the patient's symptoms should be examined and treated, whether symptomatic or not.
HIV infection	Sexual and needle-sharing partner of HIV-infected persons must receive HIV prevention counseling (see text) and must be offered HIV testing.
Genital herpes	Symptomatic partners should be managed as would any patient with genital lesions. Asymptomatic individuals may benefit from evaluation and counseling.
Genital warts	Examination of sex partners is not necessary for management of genital warts, because the role of reinfection is probably minimal. Sex partners may have warts and desire treatment, and they also may benefit from counseling.

TABLE 8.2. *Continued*

Disease	Intervention
Hepatitis B	Susceptible partners should receive postexposure hepatitis B immunoglobulin prophylaxis within 14 days of their last exposure. This should be followed by the standard three-dose immunization series with hepatitis-B vaccine beginning at the time of hepatitis-B immunoglobulin administration. (See Chapter 18 for more details.)
Ectoparasites	Partners of patients with lice or scabies within the past 30 days should be examined and treated.
Pelvic inflammatory disease	Treatment of partners of women with pelvic inflammatory disease is imperative, because of the risk of reinfection. Because diagnostic testing for *Chlamidia trachomatis* and *Neisseria gonorrhoeae* is thought to be insensitive in asymptomatic males, all sex partners should be treated empirically with regimens effective against these infections. In clinical settings in which only women are seen, special arrangements should be made to provide care for male sex partners of women with pelvic inflammatory disease. When this is not feasible, clinicians should ensure that partners are referred for treatment.

SOURCE: Centers for Disease Control, 1993.

lic or private health insurance coverage. In addition to access and availability of curative, preventive, and health promotion services, the other important criteria for an adolescent health care facility include quality, confidentiality, flexibility, and coordination of services.

Confidentiality of health services is of highest importance for adolescents. Fear of disclosure can lead to serious delays in the diagnosis and treatment of STDs. In a recent survey, 58% of high school students had health concerns they wanted to keep private from their parents, and 68% had concerns about the confidentiality of the services they receive from school-based clinics (Irwin et al., 1994).

School-Based and School-Linked Health Services

In recent years, schools have expanded their role in the delivery of some health services. School-based and school-linked health centers have the potential of not only linking adolescents to needed health services, but also creating linkages between health promotion in the school and health promotion in the health setting. Although studies specifically comparing adolescents' willingness to use different sites for health-related services have not been done, there appear to be fairly high levels of willingness to use school-based clinics among youth, especially when sensitive health problems such as STDs are involved (Elster et al., 1993). This is not surprising, because school-based services eliminate many of the barriers that adolescents identify in relation to obtaining health care.

A focus on school-based health programs is appropriate for several reasons: There is optimism about new funding for school-based primary care; school-based clinics fulfill many access criteria; and the over 600 clinics currently believed to exist do improve care delivery for many adolescents. School-based and school-linked programs serve a large proportion of in-school adolescents, many of whom have no other regular source of care. The number of states with programs or demonstration projects has grown from 9 in 1991 to 32 in 1993. The Robert Wood Johnson Foundation (1993) has funded a $23.2 million state-community partnership grant program to increase availability of school-based health services for children and youth with unmet health needs.

Recommendations for STD Programs for Adolescents

The American Medical Association (Elster et al., 1993) and the U.S. Public Health Service

(Irwin et al., 1994) have many suggestions and recommendations for reorganizing the programs for preventing STDs among adolescents. The following discussion attempts to summarize some of these recommendations.

• Prevention efforts for adolescents should be broadly based and include both health-promoting activities and activities directed at disease prevention. Strategies should be based on scientific principles and should build on strengths of the adolescent and positive outcomes rather than focusing on weaknesses and negative outcomes.

• Prevention programming should be relevant for the targeted audience. This necessitates involving adolescents and parents in the planning process and ensuring that material is appropriate for targeted age, gender, developmental level, and cultural group.

• Prevention efforts should be coordinated among various settings and various professional disciplines. Adolescents need to hear consistent health messages reinforced by different social settings.

• Health promotion must become a societal priority to ensure the allocation of proper financial and human resources. This requires leadership by physicians, educators, community leaders, and adolescent advocates.

• Health promotion and prevention strategists must engage in better "social marketing" of their products. Such marketing requires attention to socioeconomic and cultural variations as well as messages that are tailored for and targeted to reach a specific population. Differences in language and communication styles of the particular groups must be taken into account. For instance, radio may be a more effective medium for reaching Hispanic populations than television or print medium.

• To be more effective in communities of color, health professionals must expand those organizations and agencies where adolescents receive health education. Many adolescents of color who have left the educational system are at even greater health risk than those in schools. Health promotion and prevention strategies must be developed and incorporated into other organizations where many adolescents of color are found—namely, institutional settings such as detention centers, training centers, residential programs, and homeless and runaway shelters.

• In intervening in communities of color, health prevention strategists cannot afford to be myopic and focus only on the specific disease of interest. Rather, they must also view themselves as advocates and recognize that the lives of individuals living in high-risk communities cannot be changed without addressing the concomitant issues of poverty, homelessness, and racism.

• Greater emphasis should be given to evaluation research. Although research is difficult to fund with scarce financial resources, evaluating the effectiveness of the preventive intervention is necessary to ensure that funds are being used efficiently and that the benefits outweigh the deficits. Therefore, it is necessary to ensure that surveillance and monitoring of health services utilization and outcomes specific to adolescent health are an integral part of any reinvigorated public health system, and that they are explicitly linked to any new governance structures (e.g., an alliance of health plans).

• School-based health centers should be allowed to qualify as "essential community providers," whether or not they are federally funded, as long as they meet standards of quality adopted by the Secretary of Health and Human Services.

• Strong mechanisms and incentives must be created to ensure that mainstream providers (i.e., health plans) contract with community-based providers and school-based health centers that serve adolescents.

- Estimates are needed of the number, type (e.g., physician, nurse, physician assistant, social worker, psychologist and other mental health professional, nutritionist, etc.), and distribution of adolescent health care providers needed currently and projected for the next 50 years, based on demographic changes expected and the target of a 55:45 ratio of primary care providers to subspecialists.

- The case for adolescent health care must be established as a primary care component of all disciplines (e.g., pediatrics, general internal medicine, family practice, nursing, etc.).

- Institutions must consider ways in which training of primary care practitioners can occur in outpatient and community-based settings for adolescents. Build a case for the benefits of academic health centers improving their integrated networks by affiliating with sites that care for adolescents. Consider essential community providers and school-related services as sites for training.

- A model adolescent health curriculum for undergraduate and postgraduate trainees in all relevant disciplines can be designed to be incorporated into expanded primary care training sites around the country. Consider ways to integrate the curriculum into sites that currently do not have adolescent health training programs. Work with agencies now setting workforce priorities (e.g., American Association of Medical Colleges, Health Resources and Services Administration) to ensure that adolescent health training components are included.

References

Alan Guttmacher Institute. (1993). *Facts in brief: Sexually transmitted diseases (STDs) in the United States–1993.* New York: Author.

Alan Guttmacher Institute. (1994). *Sex and America's teenagers.* New York: Author.

Barth, R. P., et al. (1992). Enhancing social and cognitive skills. In B. C. Miller et al. (Eds.), *Preventing adolescent pregnancy* (pp. 53-82). Newbury Park, CA: Sage.

Billy, J. O. G., & Udry, J. F. (1985). The influence of the male and female best friends on adolescent sexual behavior. *Adolescence, 20,* 21-32.

Botvin, G. J. (1986). Subsance abuse prevention research: Recent developments and future directions. *Journal of School Health, 56*(9), 369-374.

Byler, R. V., Lewis, G. M., & Tofman, R. J. (1969). *Teach us what we want to know.* New York: Mental Health Material Center.

Cates, W., Jr. (1987). Epidemiology and control of sexually transmitted diseases: Strategic evolution. *Infectious Disease Clinics of North America, 1,* 1-23.

Cates, W., Jr. (1988). The "other STDs": Do they really matter? *Journal of the American Medical Association, 259,* 3606-3608.

Centers for Disease Control. (1985). Syphilis and congenital syphilis, 1985-1988. *Morbidity and Mortality Weekly Report, 37,* 486-489.

Centers for Disease Control. (1988). Syphilis and congenital syphilis, United States, 1985-1988. *Morbidity and Mortality Weekly Report, 37,* 486-489.

Centers for Disease Control and Prevention. (1993). Sexually transmitted diseases treatment guidelines. *Morbidity and Mortality Weekly Report, 42*(RR-14), 1-102.

Chuang, T. Y., Su, W. P. D., Perry, H. O., et al. (1983). Incidence and trend of herpes progenitalis: A 15-year population study. *Mayo Clinic Proceedings, 58,* 436-441.

Clark, E. G., & Danbolt, N. (1964). The Oslo study of the natural course of untreated syphilis: An epidemiologic investigation based on a restudy of the Boeck-Bruusgaard material. *Medical Clinics of North America, 48,* 613-623.

Coates, T. J., & Lo, B. (1990). Counseling patients zero-positive for human immunodeficiency virus: An approach to medical practice. *Western Journal of Medicine, 153*(6), 629-634.

Corey, L., Adams, H. G., Brown, Z. A., et al. (1983). Genital herpes simplex virus infections: Clinical manifestations, course, and complications. *Annals of Internal Medicine, 98,* 958-972.

Donovan, J. E., & Jessor, R. (1985). Structure of problem behavior in adolescence and young adulthood. *Journal of Consulting and Clinical Psychology, 53,* 890-904.

Elster, A., Pranzarine, S., & Holt, K. (Eds.). (1993). *American Medical Association state-of-the-art conference on adolescent health promotion proceedings.* Arlington, VA: National Center for Education in Maternal and Child Health.

Flay, B. R., et al. (1985). Are social-psychological smoking prevention programs effective? The Waterloo study. *Journal of Behavioral Medicine, 8*(1), 37-59.

Forste, R., & Heaton, T. B. (1988). Initiation of sexual activity among female adolescents. *Youth and Society, 20,* 250-268.

Guinan, M. E., Wolinsky, S. M., & Reichman, R. C. (1985). Epidemiology of genital herpes simplex virus infection. *Epidemiology Review, 7,* 127-146.

Howard, M., & McCabe, J. B. (1990). Helping teenagers postpone sexual involvement. *Family Planning Perspectives* 22(1), 21-26.

Hook, E. W., & Holmes, K. K. (1985). Gonococcal infections. *Annals of Internal Medicine, 102,* 229-243.

Harris, L., & Associates. (1988). *Health: You got to be taught—An evaluation of comprehensive health education in American public schools* (Study No. 874024). New York: Metropolitan Life Insurance Company.

Hechinger, F. M. (1992). *Fateful choices: Healthy youth for the 21st century.* New York: Carnegie Corporation.

Holmberg, S. D., Stewart, J. A., Gerber, A. R., et al. (1988). Prior herpes simplex virus type 2 infection as a risk factor for HIV infection. *Journal of the American Medical Association, 259,* 1048-1050.

Immunization Practices Advisory Committee. (1985). Recommendations for protection against viral hepatitis. *Morbidity and Mortality Weekly Report, 34,* 313-324, 329-335.

Immunization Practices Advisory Committee. (1987). Update on hepatitis B prevention. *Morbidity and Mortality Weekly Report, 36,* 353-360, 366.

Irwin, C. E, Brindis, C., Holt, K. A., & Langlykke, K. (Eds.). (1994). *Health care reform: Opportunities for improving adolescent health.* Arlington, VA: National Center for Education in Maternal and Child Health.

Khanna, J., Van Look, P. F. A., & Griffin P. D. (1992). *Reproductive health: A key to brighter future: Biennial report 1990-91.* Geneva: World Health Organization.

Kirby, D. (1984). *Sexuality education: An evaluation of programs and their effects.* Santa Cruz, CA: Network.

Kirby, D., Waszak, C., & Ziegler, J. (1991). Six school-based clinics: Their reproductive health services and impact on sexual behavior. *Family Planning Perspectives, 23*(1), 6-16.

Kirby, D., et al. (1994). School-based programs to reduce sexual risk behaviors. *Public Health Reports, 109,* 339-360.

McMillan, J. A., & Weiner, L. B. (1985). Efficacy of maternal screening and therapy in the prevention of chlamydial infection of the newborn. *Infection, 13,* 263.

Miller, B. C., McCoy, J. K., & Olson T. D. (1986). Dating age and stage as correlates of adolescent sexual attitudes and behavior. *Journal of Adolescent Research, 1,* 361-371.

Miller, B. C., & Moore, K. A. (1990). Adolescent sexual behavior, pregnancy, and parenting: Research through the 1980s. *Journal of Marriage and Family, 52.*

Miller, B. C., & Sneesby, K. R. (1988). Educational correlates of adolescents' attitudes and behavior. *Journal of Youth and Adolescence, 17,* 521-530.

Moore, K., & Peterson, J. (1989). *The consequences of teenage pregnancy, final report.* Washington, DC: Child Trends, Inc.

Nahmias, A. J., Keyserling, H. L., & Kerrick, G. M. (1983). Herpes simplex. In J. S. Remington & J. O. Klein (Eds.), *Infectious diseases of the fetus and newborn infant* (pp. 636-678). Philadelphia: W. B. Saunders.

National Commission on the Role of School and the Community in Improving Adolescent Health. (1990). *Code blue: Uniting for healthier youth.* Alexandria, VA: National Association of State Boards of Education.

Opinion Research Corporation. (1993). *Teen sex attitudes* (Prepared for CBS/Good Housekeeping).

Perry, C. L. (1987). Results of prevention programs with adolescents. *Drug and Alcohol Dependency, 20*(1), 13-19.

The Robert Wood Johnson Foundation. (1993). *Making the grade: Call for proposals.* Princeton, NJ: Author.

Shulkin, J. J., Mayer, J. A., Wessel, L. G., de Moor, C., Elder, J. P., & Franzini, L. R. (1991, September). Effects of a peer-led AIDS intervention with university students. *Journal of American College Health, 40,* 75-79.

Stevens, C. E., Toy, P. T., Tong, M. J., et al. (1985). Perinatal hepatitis B virus transmission in the United States: Prevention by passive-active immunization. *Journal of the American Medical Association, 253,* 1740-1745.

Thornton, A. D., & Camburn, D. (1989). The influence of the family on premarital sexual attitudes and behavior. *Demography, 24,* 323-340.

U.S. Office of Technological Assessment. (1991). *Adolescent health: Vol. 1. Summary and policy options* (OTA-H-468). Washington, DC: Author.

U.S. Preventive Services Task Force. (1989). *Guide to clinical preventive services.* Baltimore, MD: Williams and Wilkins.

U.S. Public Health Service. (1993). *School health: Findings from evaluated programs.* Washington, DC: U.S. Department of Health and Human Services.

Vincent, M. L., Clearie, A. F., & Schluchter. (1987). Adolescent pregnancy through school and community-based education. *Journal of the American Medical Association 257,* 3382-3386.

Washington, A. E., & Arno, P. S. (1986). The economic cost of pelvic inflammatory disease. *Journal of the American Medical Association, 255,* 1735-1738.

Westrom, L. (1975). Effect of acute pelvic inflammatory disease on fertility. *American Journal of Obstetrics and Gynecology, 121,* 707-713.

Woolf, S. H., Jones, S., & Lawrence, R. S. (Eds.). (1996). *Health promotion and disease prevention in clinical practice.* Baltimore, MD: Williams and Wilkins.

Zabin, L. S., Hirsch, M. B., Streett, R., Emerson, M. R., Smith, M., Hardy, J. B., & King, T. M. (1988). The Baltimore Pregnancy Prevention Program for Urban Teenagers: I. How did it work? *Family Planning Perspectives, 20*(4), 182-187.

9

HIV/AIDS

Britt Rios-Ellis
Margarita Figueroa

HIV/AIDS infection among adolescents is quickly becoming recognized as one of the leading health problems facing the youth of our nation. AIDS is now the sixth leading cause of death among young people ages 15 to 25 (CDC, 1995). Although HIV and AIDS do appear to be more prevalent among urban populations, about one third of adolescent AIDS cases are found in cities with populations under 500,000 (Lindegren, Hanson, Miller, Byers, & Onorato, 1994). Furthermore, many adolescents infected with HIV are not aware of their seropositive status and therefore do not receive needed medical care (DiLorenzo et al., 1993). This lack of knowledge not only places their sex and needle-sharing partners at risk for HIV infection, but also inhibits the adolescent from receiving appropriate HIV/AIDS-related medical care and counseling. Because the incubation period from HIV infection to the presentation of AIDS-related symptoms can range from 4 to an average of 11 years, one can assume that many young adults ages 20 to 29 became infected in their adolescence (Brookmeyer, 1991; Zimet et al., 1992). The fact that almost 20% of the population with AIDS is between the ages of 13 and

29 points strongly to the growing risk of infection during adolescence (CDC, 1994a).

Definition

The human immunodeficiency virus (HIV) and the resultant acquired immune deficiency syndrome (AIDS) pose critical problems for both the adolescent and health and human service professionals working with the adolescent population.

HIV is an infection that slowly attacks the immune system by depleting the body's CD-4 (T) cells. An average person has 800 to 1,300 CD-4 cells per mm/blood^2. HIV eliminates an average of 80 to 100 CD-4 cells per mm/blood^2 during the first year of infection and about 50 cells per year thereafter (Bartlett, 1993). As the immune system begins to decline, the adolescent is no longer able to fight off infectious diseases and becomes prone to a myriad of illnesses.

Health educators working within the school system are faced with not only the physiological ramifications of the adolescent student with AIDS and/or HIV, but also prevention, education, elimination of risk in case of an emergency, and assuaging parental fear and anxiety. Health educators can play a key role in providing social support, education, and prevention strategies, as well as referrals to appropriate medical personnel for adolescents with HIV/AIDS and those at risk of HIV infection.

The principal routes of HIV transmission for the adolescent include anal, vaginal, and oral sexual intercourse; injecting drug use; and exposure through blood or blood products. Adolescents can also become exposed to the virus through tattoos, piercing with unsterilized needles, and shaving with unsterilized razors that have been exposed to the virus. Additional factors that appear to increase risk behavior include the use of alcohol and noninjecting drugs, homelessness, mental health status, low self-esteem, poverty, sexual molestation and rape, and other variables that contribute to the disenfranchisement of youth in our nation.

Statement of the Problem

Fifteen years into the HIV/AIDS epidemic, health and social service professionals are rapidly identifying the need to specifically target adolescents with tested and effective HIV infection prevention campaigns. For many individuals, the recognition that HIV and AIDS affect all populations has meant that simultaneous work must be done to debunk myths, prejudices, and the denial that surround attitudes toward HIV infection risk behaviors and transmission factors. These variables have played an especially critical role in HIV prevention among adolescents.

Those working with adolescents, whether on a personal or professional level, find it difficult to acknowledge the range of risk-taking behaviors that take place among a population

that many believe has not reached the stage of maturity necessary to deal with the consequences of their actions. Nevertheless, the more that HIV risk behaviors are acknowledged and targeted among adolescents, the greater will be the capacity of health and social service professionals to work appropriately with the adolescent and thus assist in reducing HIV infection among this population. Public health and social service professionals have faced angered and frustrated parents, adolescents who perceive themselves invulnerable to HIV infection, and grave restrictions on the information deemed appropriate for HIV/AIDS-related discussions on the school health front. Meanwhile, HIV and AIDS prevalence among adolescents continues to increase at a dramatically rapid rate. Furthermore, transmission factors among adolescents do not necessarily replicate those of other populations with HIV and AIDS and differ according to geographic location and race/ethnicity (Lindegren et al., 1994).

According to *Healthy People 2000* (U.S. Department of Health and Human Services, 1990), there are a number of objectives that directly mention HIV prevention among adolescent populations. The following objectives have specific ramifications for the adolescents' ability to learn about HIV, prevent HIV infection, and procure the necessary testing and treatment for HIV:

- Reduce the proportion of adolescents who have engaged in sexual intercourse to no more than 15% by age 15 and no more than 40% by age 17. (Baseline 1988: 27% of girls and 33% of boys by age 15; 50% of girls and 66% of boys by age 17)

- Increase to at least 50% the proportion of sexually active, unmarried people who used a condom at last sexual intercourse. (Baseline 1988: 19% of sexually active, unmarried women ages 15 through 44 reported that their partners used a condom at last sexual intercourse)

- Increase to at least 75% the proportion of primary care and mental health care provid-

TABLE 9.1. AIDS Cases by Gender, Age at Diagnosis, and Race/Ethnicity Through June 1997 for Ages 13-29, United States

Age	White, Non-Hispanic	Black Non-Hispanic	Hispanic/ Latino	Asian/Pacific Islander	American Indian/Alaskan Native	Total
Male						
13 to 19	773	653	386	21	17	1,852
20 to 24	6,929	5,746	3,458	131	63	16,350
25 to 29	34,486	21,058	13,613	474	269	69,978
Total	42,188	27,457	17,457	626	349	88,180
Female						
13 to 19	190	725	178	6	1	1,100
20 to 24	1,313	3,153	1,195	29	25	5,715
25 to 29	3,756	8,066	3,303	58	44	15,227
Total	5,259	11,944	4,676	93	70	22,042

SOURCE: CDC, 1997.

ers who provide age-appropriate counseling on the prevention of HIV and other sexually transmitted diseases (STDs). (Baseline 1987: 10% of physicians reported that they regularly assessed the sexual behaviors of their patients)

- Increase to at least 95% the proportion of schools that have age-appropriate HIV education curricula for students in 4th through 12th grades, preferably as part of quality school health education. (Baseline 1989: 66% of school districts required HIV education but only 5% required HIV education in each year for 7th through 12th grade)

- Provide HIV education for students and staff in at least 90% of colleges and universities

- Increase to at least 90% the proportion of family planning clinics, maternal and child health clinics, STD clinics, tuberculosis clinics, drug treatment centers, and primary care clinics that screen, diagnose, treat, counsel, and provide (or refer for) partner notification services for HIV infection and bacterial STDs (gonorrhea, syphilis, and chlamydia). (Baseline 1989: 40% of family planning clinics for bacterial STDs)

Although the *Healthy People 2000* objectives have now been in place for half a decade, HIV infection among adolescents is growing. According to the CDC, although the number of new AIDS cases among individuals born prior to 1960 appears to be declining, new cases among younger people continue to increase. Rising rates of infection among youths of all racial/ethnic groups and both genders have been found in the ages encompassing the late teens and early twenties (CDC, 1994a).

Certain groups of adolescents appear to have particularly high AIDS case rates when compared to the adolescent population at large. Specifically, gay/bisexual youth, African American and Latino adolescents, those who use or are chemically dependent on drugs and alcohol, those who are sexually active, and homeless youth. Table 9.1 shows AIDS cases by gender, age at diagnosis, and race/ethnicity.

According to the CDC exposure categorization procedures, the key risk categories for men and women ages 13 to 29 are those who have sex with men, inject drugs, have hemophilia/coagulation disorder, engage in heterosexual contact, receive transfusions, have mothers with/at risk for HIV infection, and other/risk not reported or identified. This categorization process, although revealing in terms of some risk factors, still neglects to determine the specific sexual behaviors that

TABLE 9.2. Male AIDS Cases by Age at Diagnosis and Exposure Category Through June 1997 for Ages 13 to 24, United States

Age	Have Sex With Men	Inject Drugs	Have Sex With Men and Inject Drugs	Have Hemophilia/ Coagulation Disorder	Engage in Heterosexual Contact	Receive Transfusions	Other/ Risk Not Reported/ Identified	Total
13 to 19	629	114	83	713	62	80	171	1,852
20 to 24	10,259	2,038	1,717	599	655	103	979	16,350
Total	10,888	2,152	1,800	1,312	717	183	1,150	18,202

SOURCE: CDC, 1997.

place adolescents and young adults at risk. Tables 9.2 and 9.3 define AIDS cases by age and risk category by gender.

Significance of HIV/AIDS for the Teacher and the Classroom

The classroom setting provides the student with a unique opportunity to gain useful and accurate knowledge needed to prevent HIV infection. Although many adolescents believe that they already know a great deal about STDs and HIV, the educator is challenged with the task of teaching new materials while simultaneously facilitating the development of positive behavior change and maintenance of healthy behaviors. This requires that the educator, be aware of HIV/AIDS education protocol and HIV/AIDS counseling, understand testing and medical care services, serve as an advocate for HIV/AIDS prevention and education, be comfortable discussing the risks involved with

various sexual behaviors, be able to discuss and instruct role playing regarding safer sex strategies (including the correct demonstration of latex condoms and the use of a water-based lubricant or spermicide), and have an excellent knowledge base regarding the HIV/AIDS-related programs available in the educator's community to enable successful referral to the appropriate resources when needed.

Lenora Johnson (1991), the HIV Prevention Education Project Coordinator for the Association for the Advancement of Health Education, stated,

> The thought of doing something good for someone lies suspended in our own silenced fears and our own hidden perceptions that AIDS is a disease that only happens to "those kinds of people." We teach of the senselessness of fear, yet, even within those of us that are well-informed, fears continue to linger. Each of us has an individual challenge to question our own thoughts, fears, and commitment toward the epidemic. (p. 8)

TABLE 9.3. Female AIDS Cases by Age at Diagnosis and Exposure Category Through June 1997 for Ages 13 to 24, United States

Age	Inject Drugs	Have Hemophilia/ Coagulation Disorder	Engage in Heterosexual Contact	Receive Transfusions	Other/Risk Not Reported/ Identified	Total
13 to 19	164	10	590	76	261	1,101
20 to 24	1,650	14	3,067	112	877	5,720
Total	1,814	24	3,657	188	1,138	6,821

SOURCE: CDC, 1997.

TABLE 9.4. Factors That Place Teens at Risk for HIV Infection

Primary factors
- Unprotected anal, vaginal, and oral sex
- Injecting drug use
- Tattooing and body piercing with unsterilized or shared equipment

Secondary factors
- Use of noninjecting drugs, including alcohol
- Exchange of sex for drugs, food, clothing, and/or shelter
- STD infection
- Sexual abuse, molestation, and rape
- Low educational attainment
- Poverty
- Homeless or runaway status
- Lack of access to health care and health education
- Low socioeconomic status
- Low self-esteem
- Poor mental health status

HIV Risk Factors Among Adolescents

The risk factors presented in Table 9.4 include both those that have been thoroughly established in the medical literature, such as unprotected sexual intercourse and IV drug use, and those that are suspected to play a strong role in the potential for at-risk behavior among the adolescent population. It is imperative that the educator working in HIV/AIDS education recognize that an effective prevention and education program must endeavor to incorporate social, behavioral, psychological, cultural, linguistic, and socioeconomic factors into the prevention and education strategies used.

Condom Use and Sexual Behavior

The CDC reports that every year, 1 million adolescents become pregnant in the United States alone (1993a). According to the 1992 Youth Risk Behavior Survey, 45.1% of adolescents in school have engaged in sexual activity, and 70.1% of out-of-school youth have had intercourse (CDC, 1994b). By the end of ado-

lescence (age 20), 75% of females and 86% of males report being sexually active (CDC, 1991). In addition, rates of STDs among this population are at an all-time high. About 17% of adolescents ages 13 to 19 become infected with an STD annually (Select Committee on Children, Youth & Families, 1992). Infection with an STD has been shown to increase risk of HIV infection, especially if the STD results in genital ulcers or other irritation. From 1981 to 1991, while rates of gonorrhea declined among all other age groups, adolescents ages 10 to 19 represented 24% to 30% of all infected persons. During the aforementioned decade, adolescents also represented 10% to 12% of all cases of syphilis (CDC, 1993a). Other STDs that warrant attention among the U.S. adolescent population include chlamydia, human papilloma virus (HPV), herpes simplex virus type 2 (HSV2), and pelvic inflammatory disease (PID). Of the STDs that can affect both genders, gonorrhea, chlamydia, HPV, and HSV2 are higher in adolescent women than men (Lindegren et al., 1994). It appears that changes in the epithelial tissue of the cervix due to the development of the adolescent female's sexual and reproductive organs may contribute to an increased risk of STD and HIV infection (Cates, 1991).

Although the obvious solution for both of the aforementioned problems appears to be abstinence, an abstinence-alone sexual education program is pernicious in view of the dramatic increase in sexual activity among today's adolescents. Abstinence-based education programs do not take into account the cultural, socioeconomic, historical, social, and psychological factors that preclude sexual activity among teenagers. Achieving an abstinent adolescent population may be the long-term goal among school settings, however, educators need to equip students with an optimal amount of alternatives that facilitate and empower healthy choices. Although parental advocates of abstinence education appear to be receiving a great deal of media coverage, the results of a 1991 Roper poll demonstrated that 64% and 47% of adults favored condom availability in high schools and junior high schools, respectively. In addition, 9 out of 10 parents of adolescent males and 8 out of 10 parents of adolescent females stated that they approved of condom advertisements on television (Buchta, 1989).

Among the most controversial issues facing the educator is that of condom education and distribution within the school setting. Although many schools are initiating condom education and distribution campaigns, many parent groups still believe that these methods of HIV/AIDS prevention convey an attitude that condones sexual activity. Parental attitudes reflected in the moralistic arguments surrounding the definition of what types of sexual education are appropriate in the school setting most often point to the dire need for parental, as well as adolescent, sexual education. The beliefs many parents have regarding their child's sexual behaviors are not only unrealistic, but often harmful. To date, the correct use of latex condoms with a water-based lubricant provides the most effective means of HIV and STD prevention (CDC, 1993b). We also know that for adolescents to use condoms, they must be sexually efficacious enough to trust in their ability to use a condom in a technically correct fashion and also believe that sex with a condom can be enjoyable (Jemmot, Jemmot, & Fong, 1992).

Educators must also recognize that the sexual practices in which adolescents engage are rapidly diversifying. Efforts to determine risk behaviors and their potential for HIV infection must recognize that heterosexual adolescents often engage in unprotected sex. Educators and parents must also be cognizant of the fact that adolescents often engage in a variety of sexual behaviors, which include unprotected anal and oral sex. Among adolescent females attending public health clinics, 10% to 21% report having engaged in anal intercourse (Boyer & Kegeles, 1991; Catania et al.,

1990). In addition, there is a dramatic increase in the number of adolescent females and males who report engaging in oral sex (Wilson & Medora, 1990). Young women often feel pressured and rationalize anal and oral sex as "safe" sexual behaviors that will not place them at risk for pregnancy. In addition, many adolescent females engage in oral sex so as to not be perceived as "teasing" their male sexual partners when they refuse vaginal intercourse. They may also believe that oral sex is safe and will not result in HIV and STD infection.

The majority of the intervention data available demonstrate that the school health setting is often ideal for educating adolescents in HIV prevention. In addition, research by Kirby et al. (1991) has shown that school health interventions not only can reduce short-term risk-taking behavior but can also decrease adolescent sexual activity and increase contraceptive use. School health educators must emphasize that sexual risk behaviors, as opposed to risk groups, are the factors that will determine risk of HIV and STD infection.

Chemical Use and Dependency

Although the focus of school-based HIV/AIDS prevention has consisted in the most part of sexual abstinence and safe sex education, many adolescents are involved in alcohol and illicit drug use. The use of these chemicals often clouds preventive thinking and results in increased risk-taking behaviors, such as unsafe sex and needle sharing. In a study of adolescents in Massachusetts, 16% and 25% of the subjects stated that they were less likely to use condoms after alcohol consumption and illicit drug use, respectively (Hingson, Strunin, Berlin, & Heeren, 1990).

In a study of 100 drug users enrolled in a detoxification program in New York City, 79% of the subjects reported never having used condoms, and 50% stated that they had shared needles during the previous year. The subjects reported engaging in these behaviors despite the fact that 91% reported that condoms are an effective way to prevent HIV transmission and that sharing needles was rated by the subjects as being the HIV/AIDS-related behavior with the highest risk for contagion (Dengeli, Weber, & Torquato, 1990).

Although the aforementioned study found that IV drug users did have a considerable amount of knowledge concerning HIV/AIDS-related behaviors, an educational program in Cleveland, Ohio, was shown to increase HIV/AIDS knowledge considerably (Feucht, Stephens, & Gibbs, 1991). This study suggests that HIV/AIDS-related educational programs can provide an increased awareness for injecting drug users concerning the impact of their behaviors. The high degree of drug use in minority communities is surely a reflection of poverty and despair (Brown, Murphy, & Primm, 1988; De La Cancela, 1989). Sufian et al. (1990) state of their report of injecting drug use,

> This article indicates that not only are cultural differences important, but also that social structures and social relationships affect the epidemic. In particular, ethnicity/race is a social structure of extreme importance in the United States. Ethnic/racial differences may affect life chances, world views, the probability that one will become a drug user, drug use behaviors, the probability of having sex with a drug user, whether a person becomes infected with HIV, and more. (p. 131)

Four factors have been found to predict needle sharing in an investigation of 7,660 IV drug users (Guydish, Abramowitz, Woods, Black, & Sorensen, 1990). Needle sharing was more common among IV drug users entering treatment facilities at a later time span in their drug use and among IV drug users who reported using cocaine; younger IV drug users were more likely to report sharing, and blacks were less likely to share than whites. Whether these factors hold true for other populations is questionable; however, it is clear that the more restrictive state laws are concerning the selling of sterile needles and syringes, the more likely IV drug users are to share or rent "works" with which to inject drugs. When one considers the fact that narcotic addicts inject heroin once every 4 to 6 hours and that cocaine addicts may inject 10 or more times daily, the need for sterile syringes and needles becomes glaringly apparent in the face of the ever changing HIV/AIDS epidemic (Hochhauser & Rothenberger, 1992). This supposition is supported by a recent investigation, which found that 80% of a Philadelphia population that injected daily reported sharing needles, and 66% said that they used shooting galleries (Liebman, McIlvaine, Kotranski, & Lewis, 1990). The fact that younger age has been increasingly associated with needle sharing is of concern to those working with adolescents.

Although school-based HIV/AIDS-related prevention and education can be an effective means by which to educate adolescents, 12.7% of adolescents had dropped out of school in 1993 (CDC, 1994c). Dropout rates are much higher for African American and Hispanic adolescents residing in the inner cities. For chemically dependent adolescents, needle exchange programs and harm reduction methods are the most effective means by which we can help adolescents remain HIV-free and reduce the incidence of infection among those already living with the virus.

Although the HIV-related discussion regarding chemical use and dependency is often centered around the harmful effects of crack cocaine and cocaine, alcohol also plays a detrimental role in both HIV infection and full blown AIDS. Alcohol plays a role in promoting HIV infection in that those who drink alcohol may also engage in a variety of risk-taking activities that include unsafe sexual practices. Furthermore, when an individual engages in a risk-taking activity, he or she will be more likely to "forget" to practice safer sex behaviors such as using condoms and lubricant (Biglan et al., 1990). A study of heterosexual couples found that when they combined drinking with sexual activity, they were much less likely to practice safe sex (Bagnall, Plant, & Warwick, 1990). Alcohol also decreases the body's ability to respond immunologically (MacGregor, 1988). It appears that these immunosuppressive effects increase vulnerability to infection in the non-HIV infected individual exposed to the virus and increase the virus' ability to replicate in the HIV-infected individual. Research has identified three areas in which alcohol and HIV/AIDS are interrelated: alcohol and its debilitating effects on the immune system, alcoholism and sexuality, and alcohol and sexual practices (Molgaard, Nakamura, Hovell, & Elder, 1988).

Adolescents may also be at risk for HIV infection due to the use of other drugs such as cocaine, crack cocaine, methamphetamines, and heroin. For severely chemically dependent populations, rehabilitation is the optimal solution. It is vital that rehabilitation programs offer peer education and are relevant to the adolescent population. Harm reduction techniques, such as needle exchange or cleaning programs, drug substitution, and other methods can also be very effective in reducing the risk of HIV and hepatitis-B infection (Strang, 1992). According to Springer (1991), the connection of sex and drugs must be recognized for its increased effects on the libido (at least initially), the selling of sex for money or drugs, the ability of mood-altering substances to increase poor and inaccurate judgment, the immunosuppressive ability of many drugs, the risk of pediatric infection through the use of unsafe needles, and the increased vulnerability of the drug user through needle routes and adulterated drugs (drugs that have been "cut" with substances that can bring additional harm to the immune system).

As HIV infection and AIDS continue to increase among the adolescent population, the Harm Reduction Model brings forth new perspectives and new weapons with which to fight HIV infection among chemically dependent and drug-using adolescents. The Harm Reduction Model supports condom distribution and education as well as needle exchange programs. Due to the fact that this model views public health costs rather than individual personal expense, the costs of condom and clean needle distribution are offset by the savings in medical and social service costs. Although a model that promotes complete abstinence from chemicals is optimal, it is unrealistic to believe that all adolescent chemical dependents will be able to move as quickly as desired into a state of full abstinence. In the meantime, health professionals need to be able to assist adolescents in practicing safer drug-using behaviors. Use of this model not only will help adolescents at risk in remaining HIV-free but will also facilitate an environment wherein those who are already HIV positive will not infect others through drug-using and unsafe sex behaviors.

As health professionals, we must continue to understand and work toward the elimination of factors that increase an adolescent's proclivity toward drinking and chemical use and dependency. If health and social service professionals do not simultaneously address factors such as parental alcoholism and drug use, abuse, economic hardship, low educational levels, discrimination, and lack of opportunity, efforts to reduce HIV risk behavior will continue to confront what can be insurmountable obstacles to positive behavior change.

Sexual Orientation, Adolescents, and HIV Risk Behavior

Many health education programs do not adequately address the risk of HIV infection for adolescent gays, lesbians, and bisexuals. Although newly identified AIDS cases among adult men who have sex with men have decreased from 64% to 45% from 1981 to 1995, new cases among young men who have sex with men are on the rise. In major urban centers such as San Francisco and New York City, 9% to 12% of young men who have sex with men are infected with HIV (CDC, 1994a).

Bisexual males may be less likely to identify with gay populations and therefore may not believe themselves to be at risk for HIV/AIDS. Because HIV/AIDS education has often been targeted at groups in general and homosexual white males in particular, bisexual males may not receive the education necessary to protect themselves from HIV infection. Women may also become infected with the virus via sexual relations with HIV-positive bisexual males. Hispanic/Latina and African American/black women are three and five times more likely (respectively) to become infected by sleeping with a bisexual male (Chu, Peterman, Doll, Buehler, & Curran, 1992). Because there is a greater degree of homophobia in the Latino and African American communities than among the general population, Latino and African American males are reluctant to identify themselves as homosexuals.

Another possible reason behind the continuation of unsafe sex practices is desirability of high-risk sex. If fear is used as a short-term deterrent, the focus is not on reducing the desirability of high-risk behaviors, which has the potential of producing long-term change. The continuation of an approach that is motivated by fear may in fact have a whiplash effect in terms of actual behavior change, resulting in a type of a "forbidden fruit" paradox that enhances the desirability of the sexual practices that place the individual at risk, whether heterosexual, homosexual, or bisexual (Hook, 1990). The potential is especially marked among adolescents who believe themselves invulnerable to infection and therefore are more likely to take risks.

A study by Roffman, Gillmore, Gilchrist, Mathias, and Krueguer (1990) demonstrates that gay and bisexual males do acknowledge the need for the behavioral changes required for them to begin practicing safer sex. About 73% of homosexuals and 61% of bisexuals interviewed indicated that they needed assistance in changing their high-risk sexual behaviors. Although the desired vehicle for assistance varied from bisexual to gay populations, the fact that these at-risk individuals are admitting the need to change provides hope to health educators working with these populations.

One factor that appears to reduce the levels of risk behaviors in homosexual males is the individual's knowledge of a seropositive HIV test result. Homosexual males tested to be seropositive have been shown to reduce unsafe sex practices. This may result not only from knowledge acquisition, but also from the fact that seropositive individuals are more likely to report the greatest amount of at-risk behaviors and thus have greater capacity for change (McCusker et al., 1988). The fact that HIV-positive males engage in high-risk behavior with a greater number of sexual partners than HIV-negative populations is also supported by additional research (Meyer-Bahlburg et al., 1991).

When sexual behavior was examined in a study of 65,389 HIV/AIDS-positive males, 26% reported bisexual behavior. Non-Hispanic white males were more likely to report homosexual behavior and less likely to report bisexual behavior than were their black and Hispanic counterparts. Respectively, 31% and 41% of the HIV/AIDS-positive Hispanic and black males stated that they had had sex with men. Another important component in this investigation is that males who have experienced bisexual behavior were more than twice as likely to have used IV drugs, when compared to their homosexual counterparts. When examining the effects of bisexual male behavior on the HIV/AIDS-positive female population, 11% stated that their only risk factor was having had sex with a bisexual male.

Adolescence is often a time of sexual inquiry, thus making the ability to negotiate safer sex practices contingent on the ability to feel comfortable with one's own sexuality.

HIV prevention programs must address alternative sexual orientation as well as experimentation in same sex behaviors among adolescents. Often homosexuality and other alternative sexual identities are not adequately discussed in the school health setting (Krieger, 1995). This lack of discussion leaves the adolescent at risk of engaging in risky behaviors without the knowledge and skills necessary to negotiate abstinence from the behavior or safer precautionary measures.

Homophobia among adolescents also leads to the practice of risky behaviors among heterosexual adolescents. Westerman and Davidson (1993) conducted research demonstrating that the more homophobic an adolescent, the more likely the adolescent is to believe that HIV/AIDS is a gay disease and feel invulnerable to infection. The authors also found that the degree to which an adolescent is homophobic positively influences the adolescent's intention to engage in sexual intercourse after knowing his or her partner for only a short time. In addition, the more homophobic adolescents were twice as willing to engage in sexual intercourse without the use of a condom.

Minority Populations

According to the CDC, regardless of route of transmission, gender, or geographic region, Hispanic/Latino and African American individuals are disproportionately affected by HIV/AIDS (CDC, 1994a). Hispanic/Latinos represent 9% of the U.S. population and 17.4% of AIDS cases, and African Americans represent 12% of the U.S. population and 34% of AIDS cases (CDC, 1995). About 50% of all cases of AIDS within the Hispanic/Latino and African American communities are related to injecting drug use (IDU), whereas IDU accounts for only 19.7% of AIDS cases among Anglos (National Council of La Raza, 1995). Among women of color, IDU or sexual intercourse with someone who engages in IDU accounts for 71.9% of cases among His-

panic/Latina and 67.8% of African American women (National Council of La Raza, 1995).

Due to the fact that Latinos and African Americans are more likely to become infected through sexual activity with an IDU or through direct IDU, health education efforts need to include a focus on rehabilitation and chemical dependency treatment, access to clean injection equipment, and harm reduction strategies for IDU. In addition, programs that target Hispanics/Latinos and African Americans must be specific to culture and literacy level. In addition, programs for Hispanics/Latinos must also be linguistically appropriate.

Sex with IDU is also common among African American and Hispanic/Latina women. As of December 1994, 17.3% of African American women and 25.6% of Hispanic/Latina women were infected through sex with an IDU (National Council of La Raza, 1995). For programs to be effective, processes of role playing and sexual negotiation strategies that are culturally and linguistically appropriate must be included. For many women of color, the economic livelihood of themselves and their families often depends on their relationships with men. In addition, due to marginalization resulting from female gender, poverty, lack of education, racism, and ethnocentrism, a relationship with a male may play an even larger role in promoting a woman's self-esteem.

According to the CDC (1994a), HIV risk to women due to unprotected sexual intercourse continues to rise, especially among young women of color. Unfortunately, many women of color have few bases from which to negotiate abstinence or safer sex. One Hispanic/Latina woman who attends a weekly HIV/AIDS discussion group stated,

I saw a condom for the first time here in our discussion group. I had seen them before in the pharmacy, but never outside of the little packets. I—but I don't think I'm going to use them, I like it better without them. You know, naked—I guess I could be at risk but I'm not going to use them anyway—Can you imagine a marriage with a condom? Ay, how can that be? You don't have real intimacy then. There's always distrust. How can you feel free to love each other if you always thinking about using a condom to protect yourself? (Weiss, 1992, pp. 17-18)

Another woman expressed similar views:

I know a woman whose boyfriend was HIV-positive. And even she didn't want to use a condom. I guess we just love so much and give so much of ourselves and we will do anything. All she cared about was that he loved her. (Weiss, 1992, pp. 17-18)

Many women believe that their lives lose value without a male partner and that the demand for safe sex will cause potential male partners to abstain from becoming involved in relationships (Cochran, 1988; Shayne & Kaplan, 1988). This is particularly relevant during adolescence when a young woman's self-esteem is dependent on her relationships with males and her subsequent popularity.

Another investigation suggests that the HIV/AIDS information provided to the general public may have proven to be somewhat counterproductive in some minority cultures. Women who suggest condom use may be considered "loose" and sometimes may even be beaten, especially when the condom is suggested not for use as a means of contraception, but rather as protection from disease infection (Armstrong, 1988).

Although infection patterns in the United States demonstrated high rates of transmission through IV drug use and homosexual/bisexual behavior in males, these patterns are shifting dramatically as HIV/AIDS increasingly is transmitted via heterosexual contact. In 1983, heterosexual HIV/AIDS infection accounted for only 1% of all AIDS cases in the United States (Haverkos & Edelman, 1988). Recent statistics from the CDC conclude that 43% of female AIDS cases and 4% of males AIDS cases are caused by heterosexual contact (CDC, 1994a). This steady rise in the spread of

HIV/AIDS via heterosexual behavior becomes even more alarming when differences in race and gender are examined. The HIV transmission rates of black and Hispanic men via heterosexual contact are 10 and 4 times higher, respectively, when compared to the heterosexual transmission rates of their white counterparts (Holmes, Karon, & Kreiss, 1990). Women infected with HIV via heterosexual contact represent 32% of all HIV/AIDS cases in women, whereas in males, heterosexual transmission accounts for only 2% of all cases in men (Hochhauser & Rothenberger, 1992). When race is combined with gender, the incidence of transmission via heterosexual contact is over 11 times more likely for black and Hispanic women when compared to their white counterparts. Black and Hispanic women were also more likely to have sexual partners who used IV drugs or engaged in bisexual behavior (Holmes et al., 1990).

According to Holmes et al. (1990, p. 862), four factors increase the rate of heterosexually contracted HIV/AIDS in inner-city populations. They are:

1. The pattern of sexual behavior, including early onset of sexual intercourse, prostitution, and sex with prostitutes
2. Epidemic spread in these populations of STDs, including genital ulcer disease, which themselves may promote heterosexual spread of HIV
3. Transmission of HIV by IDU
4. Increasing use of drugs such as crack cocaine, which promotes high-risk sexual behavior, including traditional forms of prostitution and exchange of sex for drugs—a form of prostitution often involving teenagers

Runaway and Homeless Youth

Homeless youth include those who have left their homes without parental consent (runaways), those who have been thrown out of their homes by their parents or guardians (throwaways), and those who do not have access to basic shelter (street youth) (Rotheram-Borus, Koopman, & Ehrhardt, 1991). Due to the fact that homeless youth have little or no social and economic support, they are often in situations that render them susceptible to HIV infection. Homeless youth are more likely to have sex at a younger age (12.5 years); engage in IDU; have STDs; be teen mothers; engage in the trade of sex for food, shelter, money, or drugs; and have been sexually abused (Rotheram-Borus et al., 1991).

Homeless and runaway youth are disproportionately infected with HIV. Of the 1.5 million homeless and runaway youth in the United States, about 60,000 or 4% are infected with HIV (Stricof, Novick, & Kennedy, 1990). The seropositivity rate of these youth is 2 to 10 times higher than that reported for other U.S. adolescents (Rotheram-Borus et al., 1991). Many homeless youth use sex work as a principal means of survival. Meeting immediate needs such as shelter, food, and clothing can influence judgment and override any long-term concerns the adolescent may have about becoming infected with HIV.

In a study of HIV seroprevalence in a facility for runaways and homeless adolescents, it was determined that 80% of the population used alcohol, 68% smoked marijuana, 48% used cocaine, 38% used crack, and 6% percent used IV drugs. About 29% admitted having exchanged sex for food, money, shelter, or drugs, and 91% reported being sexually active with an average of 2.8 sexual partners per week. The average seroprevalence in nine different groups of runaway adolescents was 5.3% from October 1987 to December 1989 (Stricof, Kennedy, Nattell, Weisfuse, & Novick, 1991). In addition, an estimated 25% of homeless youth in New York City and Los Angeles state that they exchange sex for money or drugs (Rotheram-Borus et al., 1992).

In a study of runaway and nonrunaway youth, runaways were found to have a signifi-cantly larger number of illnesses including STDs; they were more likely to have been sexually abused, had experienced sexual activity at a younger age (19% prior to age 10), were more likely to be involved in prostitution, and had used all of the drugs listed on the survey to a much greater degree. The runaways also had higher rates of psychological trauma, including suicide attempts, depression, and other related mental illnesses (Yates, MacKenzie, Pennbridge, & Cohen, 1988).

As a result of the aforementioned factors, homeless youth may not think about the long-term consequences of unprotected sexual activity. They may lack sexual efficacy, need immediate comfort (whether physical, economic, or shelter related), and feel fairly hopeless in their ability to change their long-range outcomes. Peer street outreach, shelter, food, educational and job training programs, chemical dependency rehabilitation programs, and HIV testing and treatment services must be made more readily available to this high-risk population.

Conclusion—What Works?

Considering the information presented here, it may appear that the task of preventing and dealing with HIV and AIDS among the U.S. adolescent population is not achievable. Throughout our country's 18-year history with the epidemic, one fact has become increasingly clear: HIV/AIDS cannot be prevented or treated in and of itself. The impact of the social and economic structure of our society and our educational system must increase its response to the virus. Health educators must work in a dual effort toward the appropriate dissemination of information, in addition to advocating policy that will improve the chances for youth in the United States.

A thorough review of the literature suggests that the following program methodology can be effective in HIV prevention:

- Culturally and linguistically appropriate education and intervention
- Literacy level-specific education and intervention
- Frank and open discussion of the risk of unprotected sexual activity
- Sexual negotiation and role-playing strategies that actively engage the students in discussion, brainstorming, and problem solving
- Accurate and careful instruction regarding the use of condoms and needle cleaning
- Frank and open discussion of the benefits of both sexual and chemical abstinence
- Frank and open discussion and modeling of sexual decision making
- Programs that provide housing, education, and opportunities for underprivileged youth
- Community-based programs that link schools with community-based prevention efforts
- Use of HIV seropositive and seronegative peer educators in the classroom setting
- Chemical dependency and treatment programs designed specifically for adolescent populations
- Needle exchange and sterilization education programs for chemically dependent youth
- Street outreach programs involving peer education and condom use education and distribution
- Readily available HIV testing services designed specifically for adolescent populations
- Frank and open discussion regarding homophobia, sexual orientation, and the increasing risk of heterosexual transmission for women and children
- Social marketing strategies that make safer-sex negotiation and abstinence socially desirable
- Programs that include extensive discussion regarding the difference between contraceptive methods and their ability to prevent pregnancy versus HIV and STDs
- Program development that focuses on adolescent decision making, organization, and empowerment
- Programs that emphasize changing of group social norms
- Programs that increase self- and sexual efficacy among adolescents

Although adult health educators often wish to believe that adolescents will use the information provided in the classroom to completely alter their sexual and chemical use patterns, educators must remain cognizant of the fact that knowledge alone does not change behavior. In addition, knowledge must be taught in a practical setting that emphasizes hands-on learning techniques. Research has shown, for example, that drug users are often very aware of the modes of HIV transmission but are misinformed regarding risk reduction techniques (Des Jarlais & Friedman, 1988).

Theories used to predict behavior must not be used exclusively and must be adapted to meet the needs of the adolescent target population. Theoretical approaches must be combined in HIV prevention programs so that the multidimensionality of HIV risk behavior is not lost to programmatic needs (Ahia, 1991). Skill-based theoretical education, as exemplified by the self-efficacy theory (Bandura, 1992), combined with approaches drawn from the harm reduction model, for example, influence both the individual's behavior and perceptions regarding ability to carry out the behavior, as well as the social and environmental structure within which that behavior takes place. Simultaneous hands-on condom instruction combined with distribution and recognition of the benefits regarding widespread changes in condom-related behavioral norms will promote the long-term behavioral efficacy necessary to prevent HIV infection throughout an individual's sexual life.

Most important, educators must be ready to be open and compassionate in working toward HIV prevention among diverse adolescent populations. We must be ready to listen, involve adolescents in their own solutions, and recognize that the choices and decisions of youth today represent a more complex and difficult paradigm than those of the past.

References

Ahia, R. N. (1991). Compliance with safer-sex guidelines among adolescent males: Application of the Health Belief Model and Protection Motivation Theory. *Journal of Health Education, 22*(1), 49-52.

Armstrong, D. (1988). Management of infectious diseases in patients with the acquired immunodeficiency syndrome. *Kansenshougaku Zasshji, 62*(Suppl.), 247-286.

Bagnall, G., Plant, M., & Warwick, W. (1990). Alcohol, drugs and AIDS-related risks: Results from a prospective study. *AIDS Care, 2*(4), 309-317.

Bandura, A. (1992). A social cognitive approach to the exercise of control over AIDS prevention. In R. DeClemente (Ed.), *Adolescents and AIDS: A generation in jeopardy* (pp. 89-116). Newbury Park, CA: Sage.

Bartlett, J. G. (1993). *The Johns Hopkins University Hospital guide to medical care of patients with HIV infection.* Baltimore, MD: Williams & Wilkins.

Biglan, A., Metzler, C. W., Wirt, R., Ary, D., Noell, J., Ochs, L., French, C., & Hood, D. (1990). Social and behavioral factors associated with high-risk sexual behavior among adolescents. *Journal of Behavioral Medicine, 13*(3), 245-261.

Boyer, C. B., & Kegeles, S. M. (1991). AIDS risk and prevention among adolescents. *Social Science and Medicine, 33*(1), 11-23.

Brookmeyer, R. (1991). Reconstruction and future trends of the AIDS epidemic in the United States. *Science, 253,* 37-42.

Brown, L., Murphy, D., & Primm, B. (1988). The acquired immunodeficiency syndrome: Do drug dependence and ethnicity share a common pathway? *National Institute on Drug Abuse (NIDA) Monograph, 270,* 188-194.

Buchta, R. M. (1989). Attitudes of adolescents and parents of adolescents concerning condom advertisements on television. *Journal of Adolescent Health Care, 10,* 220-223.

Catania, J. A., Coates, T. J., Greenblatt, R. M., Puckett, S., Carman, M., & Miller, J. (1990). Predictors of condom use and multiple partnered sex among sexually active adolescent women: Implications for AIDS-related health interventions. *Journal of Sex Research, 26,* 514-524.

Cates, W. (1991). Teenagers and sexual risk taking: The best of times and the worst of times. *Journal of Adolescent Health, 12,* 84-94.

Centers for Disease Control and Prevention. (1991, January). Premarital sexual experience among adolescent women, United States, 1970-1988. *Morbidity and Mortality Weekly Report, 39,* 929.

Centers for Disease Control and Prevention. (1993a). *CDC surveillance summaries,* Vol. 42(SS-3). Atlanta, GA: Public Health Service.

Centers for Disease Control and Prevention. (1993b). Update: Barrier protection against HIV infection and other sexually transmitted diseases. *Morbidity and Mortality Weekly Report, 42*(30).

Centers for Disease Control and Prevention. (1994a). HIV and AIDS: Trends in the epidemic. *Fact sheet, 1-7.*

Centers for Disease Control and Prevention. (1994b). Health risk behaviors among adolescents who do and do not attend school—United States, 1993. *Morbidity and Mortality Weekly Report, 43*(9), 129-132.

Centers for Disease Control and Prevention. (1994c). Sexual behaviors and drug use among youth in dropout-prevention programs—Miami, 1994. *Morbidity and Mortality Weekly Report, 43,* 873-876.

Centers for Disease Control and Prevention. (1995). First 500,000 AIDS cases—United States, 1995. *Morbidity and Mortality Weekly Report, 44*(46), 849-853.

Centers for Disease Control and Prevention. (1997). *HIV/AIDS Surveillance Report, 9*(1), 12.

Chu, S., Peterman, T., Doll, L., Buehler, J., & Curran, J. (1992). AIDS in bisexual men in the United States: Epidemiology and transmission to women. *American Journal of Public Health, 82*(2), 220-224.

Cochran, S. (1988, August). *Risky behavior and self-disclosure: Is it safe if you ask?* Paper presented at the American Psychological Association, Atlanta, GA.

De La Cancela, V. (1989). Minority AIDS prevention: Moving beyond cultural perspectives toward sociopolitical empowerment. *AIDS Education and Prevention, 1*(2), 141-153.

Dengeli, L., Weber, J., & Torquato, S. (1990). Drug users' AIDS-related knowledge, attitudes, and behaviors before and after AIDS education sessions. *Public Health Reports, 105*(5), 504-510.

Des Jarlais, D. C., & Friedman, S. R. (1988). The psychology of preventing AIDS among intravenous drug users: A social learning conceptualization. *American Psychologist, 43,* 865-870.

DiLorenzo, T. A., Abramo, D. M., Hein, K., Clare, G. S., Dell, R., & Shaffer, N. (1993). The evaluation of targeted outreach in an adolescent HIV/AIDS program. *The Journal of Adolescent Health, 13,* 301-306.

Feucht, T., Stephens, R., & Gibbs, B. (1991). Knowledge about AIDS among intravenous drug users: An evaluation of an education program. *AIDS Education and Prevention, 3*(1), 10-20.

Guydish, J., Abramowitz, A., Woods, W., Black, D., & Sorensen, J. (1990). Changes in needle sharing behavior among intravenous drug users: San Francisco, 1986-88. *American Journal of Public Health, 81*(8), 995-997.

Haverkos, M., & Edelman, R. (1988). The epidemiology of the acquired immunodeficiency syndrome among heterosexuals. *Journal of the American Medical Association, 260,* 1922-1929.

Hingson, R. W., Strunin, L., Berlin, B. M., & Heeren, T. (1990). Beliefs about AIDS, use of alcohol and drugs, and unprotected sex among Massachusetts adolescents. *American Journal of Public Health, 80*(3), 295-299.

Hochhauser, M., & Rothenberger, J. (1992). *AIDS Education.* Dubuque, IA: Wm. Brown.

Holmes, K., Karon, J., & Kreiss, J. (1990). The increasing frequency of heterosexually acquired AIDS in the United States, 1983-88. *American Journal of Public Health, 80*(7), 858-862.

Hook, E. (1990, October-December). Behavioral relapse among homosexually active men: Implications for STD control. *Sexually Transmitted Diseases,* pp. 161-162.

Jemmot, J. B., Jemmot, L. S., & Fong, G. T. (1992). Reductions in HIV risk-associated sexual behaviors among black male adolescents: Effects of an AIDS prevention intervention. *American Journal of Public Health, 82,* 372-377.

Johnson, L. (1991). Beyond knowledge and practice: A challenge in health education. *Journal of Health Education, 22*(1), 8.

Kirby, D., Barth, R. P., Leland, N., et al. (1991). Reducing the risk: Impact of a new curriculum on sexual risk-taking. *Family Planning Perspectives, 23,* 253-263.

Krieger, L. (1995). *What are adolescents' HIV prevention needs?* San Francisco: UCSF Center for AIDS Prevention Studies.

Liebman, J., McIlvaine, D., Kotranski, L., & Lewis, R. (1990). AIDS prevention for IV drug users and their sexual partners in Philadelphia. *American Journal of Public Health, 80*(5), 615-616.

Lindegren, M. L., Hanson, C., Miller, K., Byers, R. H., & Onorato, I. (1994). Epidemiology of human immunodeficiency virus infection in adolescents, United States. *Pediatric Infectious Disease Journal, 13*(6), 525-535.

MacGregor, R. R. (1988). Alcohol and drugs as co-factors for AIDS. *Advances in Alcohol and Substance Abuse, 7*(2), 47-71.

McCusker, J., Stoddard, A., Mayer, K., Zapka, J., Morrison, C., & Saltzman, S. (1988). Effects of HIV antibody test knowledge on subsequent sexual behaviors in a cohort of homosexually active men. *American Journal of Public Health, 78*(4), 462-467.

Meyer-Bahlburg, H., Exner, T., Lorenz, G., Gruen, R., Gorman, J., & Ehrhardt, A. (1991). Sexual risk behavior, sexual functioning, and HIV-disease progression in gay men. *The Journal of Sex Research, 28*(1), 3-27.

Molgaard, C., Nakamura, C., Hovell, M., & Elder, J. (1988). Assessing alcoholism as a risk factor for acquired immunodeficiency syndrome (AIDS). *Social Science and Medicine, 27*(11), 1147-1152.

National Council of La Raza. (1995). *Injecting drug use and HIV/AIDS in the Hispanic community.* Washington, DC: NCLR Center for Health Promotion.

Roffman, R., Gillmore, M., Gilchrist, L., Mathias, S., & Krueguer, L. (1990). Continuing unsafe sex: Assessing the need for AIDS prevention counseling. *Public Health Reports, 105*(2), 202-208.

Roper Organization, Inc. (1991). *AIDS: Public attitudes and education needs.* New York: Gay Men's Health Crisis.

Rotheram-Borus, M. J., Koopman, C., & Ehrhardt, A. A. (1991). Homeless youths and HIV infection. *American Psychologist, 46*(11), 1188-1197.

Rotheram-Borus, M. J., Meyer-Bahlburg, H., Koopman, C., Rosario, M., Exmer, T., Henderson, R., Matthiew, M., & Gruen, R. (1992). Lifetime sexual behaviors among runaway males and females. *The Journal of Sex Research, 29,* 15-29.

Select Committee on Children, Youth, and Families (1992). *Report to House of Representatives, 102nd Congress* (ISBN 0-16-039006-0). Washington, DC: Government Printing Office.

Shayne, V., & Kaplan, B. (1988). AIDS education for adolescents. *Youth and Society, 20*(2), 180-208.

Springer, E. (1991). Effective AIDS prevention with active drug users: The harm reduction model. In M. Shernoff (Ed.), *Counseling chemically dependent people with HIV illness.* New York: Haworth.

Strang, J. (1992). Harm reduction for drug users: Exploring the dimensions of harm, their measurement, and strategies for reductions. *AIDS & Public Policy Journal, 7*(3), 145-152.

Stricof, R., Kennedy, J., Nattell, T., Weisfuse, I., & Novick, L. (1991). HIV-seroprevalence in a facility for runaway and homeless adolescents. *American Journal of Public Health, 81*(Suppl.), 50-53.

Stricof, R., Novick, L. F., & Kennedy, J. (1990). AIDS and IV drug use: Prevention strategies for youth. In M. Quackenbush & M. Nelson, with K. Clark (Eds.), *The AIDS challenge* (pp. 273-295). Santa Cruz, CA: Network Publications.

Sufian, M., Friedman, S., Neaigus, A., Stepherson, B., Rivera-Beckman, J., & Des Jarlais, D. (1990). Impact of AIDS on Puerto Rican intravenous drug users. *Hispanic Journal of Behavioral Sciences, 12*(2), 122-134.

U.S. Department of Health and Human Services. (1990). *Healthy People 2000: National health promotion and disease prevention objectives* (DHHS Publication No. PHS 91-50213). Washington, DC: Author.

Weiss, E. (Producer). (1992). All things considered: AIDS & Hispanics series (Broadcast Transcripts-February 25 to March 1). Washington, DC: National Public Radio.

Westerman, P. L., & Davidson, P. M. (1993). Homophobic attitudes and AIDS risk behavior of adolescents. *Journal of Adolescent Health, 14,* 208-213.

Wilson, S. M., & Medora, N. P. (1990). Gender comparisons of college students' attitudes toward sexual behavior. *Adolescence, 25*(99), 615-627.

Yates, G., MacKenzie, R., Pennbridge, J., & Cohen, E. (1988). A risk profile comparison of runaway and non-runaway youth. *American Journal of Public Health, 78*(37), 820-821.

Zimet, G. D., Bunch, D. L., Anglin, T. M., Lazebnik, R., Williams, P., & Krowchuk, D. P. (1992). Relationship of AIDS-related attitudes to sexual behavior changes in adolescents. *The Journal of Adolescent Health, 13,* 493-498.

10

Adolescent Pregnancy and Too-Early Childbearing

Susan K. Flinn   *Jugna Shah*
Laura Davis   *Rachel Zare*
Shelby Pasarell

Pregnancy and childbearing among teenagers have been considered public health crises in the United States for over 20 years. Much has been learned about the antecedents of too-early pregnancy, effective prevention strategies, and other interconnected factors. This chapter describes current public health and policy views on teen pregnancy and childbearing and suggests curricula and programs that can effect positive change. Statistics and promising models are highlighted in illustrations. For the most part, this chapter will focus on prevention strategies targeting adolescent pregnancy rather than interventions for the pregnant teen. Greater efforts in preventing pregnancy will decrease not only the number of teen pregnancies but also the volatility of arguments about teen parenting and abortion. As with other public health issues, it is important to note that the same young people at risk for unintended pregnancy and too-early childbearing are also at risk of substance abuse, sex-

ual abuse, HIV/AIDS infection, and other health problems.

Introduction

Most pregnancy prevention strategies highlight the three Ds: disadvantage from pregnancy and too-early childbearing, disease from sexually transmitted infections, and potential death from HIV/AIDS. Both those who promote abstinence until marriage and those who favor prevention programs that include comprehensive information and health services have been trapped by the 3D model. Opponents use fear to encourage teens to abstain from the "evils" of sex altogether while proponents encourage teens to protect themselves from potential repercussions by using contraception and teaching negotiation skills. Both viewpoints use fear to change behavior and ignore sexuality as a fundamental part of life;

neither encourages youth to develop a healthy outlook about sexuality.

Sexuality and sexual expression are normal and healthy; the vast majority of people will have sexual relationships at some point in their lives. Adolescence is a time of negotiating the lengthy transition between childhood and adulthood. To help young people develop realistic and responsible sexual relationships, pregnancy prevention efforts must move away from the 3D model and toward more holistic intervention programs. Teaching teens to respect and cherish their bodies, providing information and skills, and acknowledging sexuality as normal and healthy would be more effective in promoting behavioral changes and responsible sexual decision making.

Teen pregnancy and too-early childbearing can have negative impacts, but expressions of sexuality or choosing to have a child are not inherently wrong. Prevention efforts need to recognize that both society and the individual have a role and responsibility in delaying teen pregnancies. This dual responsibility for prevention complicates most efforts to reduce teen pregnancy, which target only the adolescent. Society must provide the skills and opportunities for teens to take emotional, financial, and social responsibility for their decisions about sexuality. Only then can adolescents be expected to do so.

Adolescent Pregnancy and Childbearing: Mothers, Fathers, and Children

Two types of unintended pregnancy are of most concern to public health experts: pregnancies that are mistimed and those that are unwanted. About 60% of all pregnancies are unintended; over 80% of teen pregnancies are unintended (Institute of Medicine [IOM], 1995). Women facing an unwanted pregnancy are more likely to delay or fail to seek prenatal care. They are more likely to smoke and drink while pregnant; and their babies are at greater risk for low birthweight, infant mortality, and abuse (IOM, 1995). Teen pregnancies concern public health experts because adolescents' high rate of unintended pregnancy leads to negative consequences for this age group more often than for older women.

In addition to medical problems listed above, women under 20 face more physical difficulties during pregnancy, including increased rates of toxemia, anemia, cervical trauma, and premature delivery. Maternal mortality for mothers under age 15 is 60% greater than for mothers in their 20s (National Commission, 1988).

Furthermore, teen parents are usually unprepared to raise children. Future possibilities for teen mothers are often limited because they are more likely to drop out of school, be unemployed, and need public assistance to support their family (Moore, Miller, Glei, & Morrison, 1995). Teen mothers earn about half the lifetime income of women who delay childbearing until their 20s (Children's Defense Fund [CDF], 1987).

Even if they want to help support their child, teen fathers often face substantial economic barriers to providing any meaningful help (Brown, 1993). They are generally ineligible for federal social support programs, restricted from state social support programs, and ignored by family planning and parenting programs. Teen fathers are more likely to be high school dropouts and are only half as likely to complete college as their nonparenting peers (Marsiglio, 1987). The vast majority of teen fathers do not have frequent, ongoing contact with their children (Hardy, Duggan, Masnyk, & Pearson, 1989).

Children of teen parents are more likely to be of low birthweight, be hospitalized, die during infancy, and be abused than are babies born to older mothers. One study found that 50% of children born to teen parents began having sex before age 14; 64% had been suspended from school, and 45% repeated a grade. About 14% of those surveyed had been incarcerated, 25% reported major depressive symptoms, and 36% exhibited low self-esteem (Horowitz, Klerman, Koo, & Jekel, 1991). Children of teen parents also are more likely than other young people to become adolescent parents, continuing a cycle of poverty and low educational attainment (Kahn & Anderson, 1992).

Historical Perspectives on Adolescent Pregnancy and Its Outcomes

To better understand concerns about adolescent pregnancy today, it is important to examine historical perspectives on adolescent sexuality and childbearing. For many, the current "crisis" of teen pregnancy is one of definition: As one commentator queried, "Is the primary issue morality, fertility, or poverty?" This question, certainly relevant in the past, has taken on new meanings in contemporary debates about teen pregnancy (Lawson & Rhode, 1993).

The public perception of teen pregnancy as a problem is closely linked to the perception of both adolescence and nonmarital childbearing as problems. Teenagers have always been sexually active, become pregnant, and given birth, as evidenced by rising and falling rates of adolescent childbearing over 300 years of U.S. history. Although teen sexual activity has increased and individuals now engage in sexual intercourse at younger ages, it is important to recognize that teen sexual behavior has not changed as dramatically as portrayed by the media and politicians. What has changed is public perception of adolescence and the conflicting values attached to early, nonmarital childbearing and sexual activity.

Before the middle of the 19th century, adolescence was not conceptualized as a separate and distinct life stage. The profound economic and social changes of the late 19th century and the recognition that developmental and psychological changes occur specific to the adolescent years altered the public perception of adolescence. At the same time, illegitimacy became a more pressing social concern, due to financial concerns of families of unmarried women and the prevailing morality of the time. Young women of this era were often forced to marry in response to an unplanned pregnancy—in fact, many early homes for unwed mothers were founded as an alternative solution to marriage, and some were established to reform young prostitutes (Lawson & Rhode, 1993).

During the early to mid-20th century, changes in dating patterns, increased premarital sexual activity, and the availability of effective contraception shifted public perceptions of teen childbearing. It was not until the 1960s and 1970s, however, when large numbers of teens began having children out of wedlock, that teen childbearing took on the status of a social problem. The fact that many young unmarried teens have relied on federal, state, and local welfare programs only contributed to the public perception of teen childbearing as a crisis and an epidemic (Lawson & Rhode, 1993).

The links between marriage, childbearing, and poverty have been particularly evident in programs and policies targeting young women of color. Indeed, the long history of sterilization abuse, coercive contraceptive practices aimed at poor and minority women, and restrictions on contraception and abortion for young people point to the fact that sexual activity and childbearing have been conceived as "good" for some women and as "bad" for others. Pregnancy has been idealized for older, Caucasian, married, and wealthy women, yet demonized for women of color and young, single, poor women. For example, sterilization rates as high as 65% were once reported among Hispanic women in the Northeast (Nsiah-Jefferson, 1989). At the same time, many Caucasian middle-class women who sought sterilization were denied the service because they lacked a husband to consent to the procedure or were still able to give birth.

Contemporary debates about abortion, abstinence, and welfare continue to reflect these double standards. With its current social and economic crisis, the United States has continued to develop programs and policies that scapegoat certain groups, including adolescents, immigrants, poor women, and women of color. In considering this issue, the question to keep in mind once again is, "Is the primary issue morality, fertility, or poverty?" Using this question as a frame, this chapter seeks a more accurate picture of teen pregnancy. It untangles the statistics, spotlights the successes, and presents new challenges to consider as the 21st century approaches.

Current Statistics on Teen Pregnancy and Childbearing

Statistics on teen sexual activity, pregnancy, and childbearing indicate both promising and disturbing trends.

Approximately one million teens experienced a pregnancy in 1990. About 14% of these pregnancies were brought to term in births that were intended, 37% resulted in births that were unintended, 35% were terminated in abortion, and 14% ended in miscarriages (Alan Guttmacher Institute [AGI], 1994). Only 6% of pregnant, unmarried adolescents chose to place their baby for adoption (National Comittee on Adoption, 1989).

Far too many teens do not use contraceptives consistently, although the use of contraception, particularly condoms, increased considerably during the last decade. For young women whose first intercourse occurred between 1990 and 1995, 76% reported using a method of contraception during their first intercourse, up from 45% in 1982 (National Center for Health Statistics, 1997; Forrest, Singh, 1990). Contraceptive use among young men has also increased. More young men currently than in the past are reporting condom use during their most recent intercourse

(Kann, Warren, Harris, et al., 1996; Pleck, Sonenstein, Ku, 1993). These patterns are particularly important given the importance of condoms in protecting sexually active adolescents from HIV and other STDs.

Pregnancy and birth rates have decreased in recent years, in part due to increased contraceptive use among teens (See Figure 10.1). The birth rate for adolescents, ages 15 to 19, increased 24% between 1986 and 1991; however, from 1991 to 1996, the rate declined 12%. In 1996, the birth rate for adolescents was 54.7 births per 1000 females ages 15 to 19 (Centers for Disease Control and Prevention, 1997d).

Birth rates dropped in all adolescent subgroups between 1991 and 1996. There was a decrease of 14% in those ages 10 to 14, 12% for those ages 15 to 17 years, and 8% for those ages 18 to 19 (Centers for Disease Control and Prevention, 1997d).

Today, more births to teens and adults occur outside of marriage, although teens are more likely to be blamed for this phenomenon. The trend to marry later in life (if at all) is exhibited by both teens and adults. In 1960, only 15% of all births to women under 20 occurred outside of marriage, compared to 30% in 1970, 48% in 1980, and 71% in 1992 (Moore, Miller, et al., 1995) (see Figure 10.2).

Numerous studies indicate, however, that marriage is not a panacea for teen poverty. In fact, teen parents who are married are much less likely to receive (and may be ineligible for) public assistance. Teens who marry because of a pregnancy are more likely to complete less school than unmarried teens and to have a second child within 2 years of the first (Kalmuss & Namerow, 1994; Urban Institute, 1995). Many teen mothers who receive welfare do not see marriage as a realistic goal, citing the fact that eligible men are unable to support them (Maynard, 1994). Thus, although some argue that marriage is the first step in responding to teen childbearing, research suggests that marriage cannot be the sole solution.

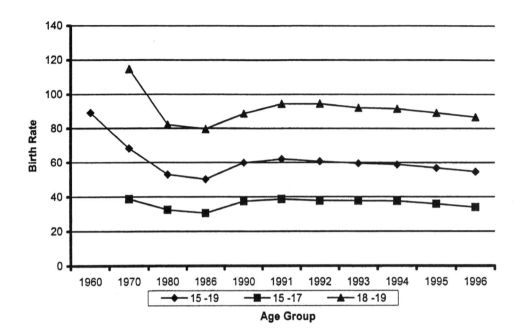

Figure 10.1.   Birth Rates (per 1,000 Females by Age Group, 1950-1992)

SOURCE: National Center for Health Statistics, 1993, 1994.

NOTE: Birth rates are calculated as the number of births per 1,000 females in the specified age group. Births prior to 1960 were adjusted for underregistration. Data for 1960-1966 and 1968-1971 are based on a 50% sample of births. Data for 1967 are based on a 20% to 50% sample of births. Data for 1972 to 1984 are based on 100% of births in selected states and on a 50% sample of births in all other states. Data are not available for subgroups ages 15 to 17 and 18 to 19 prior to 1966.

Many researchers and anthropologists view racial classifications as having little biologic or genetic explanatory value. Biological variation between races is limited, yet, health research continues to focus on it as one of the most important characteristics determining social identity, acceptance, and access to resources. Issues of race and ethnicity are difficult to separate from those of social and economic status, given that a disproportionate percentage of women of color live in poverty. Many researchers agree that race and ethnicity are less critical than class and life experience in determining risk for unintended pregnancy and too-early childbearing. The current use of race and ethnicity as primary factors in public health research means that most data available reflect these categorizations, and data presented in this chapter are, unfortunately, no exception (Shah, 1995).

Birth rates are higher for African American and Latina teens than for Caucasians, but rates of sexual activity are similar across race and ethnic groups. The age at which 50% of teens have had sex ranges from age 15 for African American men to age 17 for Caucasian and Latino males. For African American, Latina, and Caucasian women, 50% have had sex by age 16 and a half (AGI, 1994).

Rates of contraceptive use vary by race and ethnicity, affecting both pregnancy and childbearing rates. About 69% of Caucasian females report using contraception at first intercourse, compared to 54% of African American females and 53.9% of Latina females (Forrest & Singh, 1990). Among 15- to 19-year-old females, 8% of Caucasians experience a pregnancy, compared to 13% of Latinas and 19% of African Americans (AGI, 1994). The Caucasian birth rate in 1992 was 51.8 births for

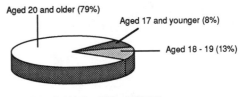

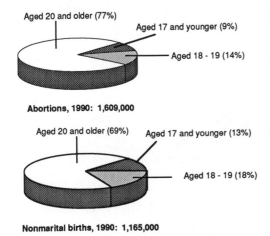

Aged 20 and older (77%)

Aged 17 and younger (9%)

Aged 18 - 19 (14%)

Abortions, 1990: 1,609,000

Aged 20 and older (79%)

Aged 17 and younger (8%)

Aged 18 - 19 (13%)

Unintended births, 1990: 1,796,000

Aged 20 and older (69%)   **Aged 17 and younger (13%)**

Aged 18 - 19 (18%)

Nonmarital births, 1990: 1,165,000

Figure 10.2. Teenagers, a Small Part of a Larger Problem
SOURCE: The Alan Guttmacher Institute, 1994; reproduced with permission.

every 1,000 15- to 19-year-olds, compared to 112.4 births for African American women that age (Latinas are categorized as Caucasian or African American) (Ventura et al., 1992).

Antecedents of Teen Pregnancy and Too-Early Childbearing

Public health experts recognize that the antecedents of adolescent pregnancy and childbearing are complex and diverse, including inadequate educational and health care services, developmental factors, social and economic issues such as poverty, disenfranchisement, sexual abuse, drug and alcohol abuse, violence, and family dysfunction. A comprehensive understanding of the needs of adolescents as well as the interconnectedness of psychosocial, economic, and developmental issues is critical in designing and implementing efforts aimed at changing adolescent behavior. Theories about factors related to teen pregnancy and prevention efforts can generally be categorized in three areas:

- Access to sexuality education and family planning services

- Psychological and developmental factors
- Environmental factors

Access to Sexuality Education and Family Planning Services

Traditional public health efforts have focused on teens' lack of access to accurate information about sexuality, as well as lack of access to the full range of family planning services. Teens typically receive information about sexuality from their peers, the media, and adults, including their parents. Peers too often provide information that is inaccurate (e.g., that pregnancy can't happen if sex occurs standing up). This country's sex-saturated media consistently present overly romantic visions of sexuality without information about the responsibilities and consequences of sexual intercourse. Young teens identify with characters on television and in the movies and can be greatly influenced by behavior portrayed on both the large and small screens. When young people see role models "swept away" romantically rather than planning for sexual interaction, they are influenced to act the same way.

Teachers and religious leaders are often unprepared and/or barred from addressing ques-

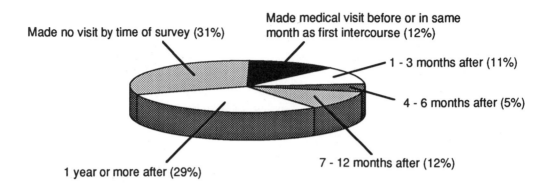

Figure 10.3. Delays Still Common
SOURCE: The Alan Guttmacher Institute, 1994; reproduced with permission.

tions about sexuality and pregnancy. Parents are very often nervous and uncomfortable talking with their children about sexual issues. Too often, health care providers are reluctant to ask adolescents about their sexual history and embarrassed when responding to teens' questions. Family planning has traditionally been viewed as the female responsibility, and males as family planning clients have been overlooked. Moreover, providers frequently fail to understand teens' specific needs and therefore fail to provide low-cost, convenient, and confidential family planning services. Without accessible services, teens do not stop having sex. Rather, they neglect to obtain and use contraception, and therefore experience high rates of unintended pregnancy (see Figure 10.3).

Psychological and Developmental Factors

Teen pregnancy has also been explained through numerous cognitive and behavioral theories. These theories hold that teens develop the physical capacity to reproduce before the emotional or psychological maturity to deal with the consequences. Thus, although teens are physiologically able to become pregnant, these theorists maintain that, without help building their skills, young teens may be unable to recognize the risks and unprepared to deal with the consequences of early and/or unprotected sexual activity.

These theories note that a lack of decision-making, assertion, negotiation, and problem-solving skills inhibits teens from making healthy, informed decisions about their sexuality. This is particularly a factor for younger teens, whose reasoning abilities reflect concrete rather than abstract thinking skills and who are therefore less able to assess the future consequences of high-risk behaviors. Because adolescence is a time of exploration and discovery, these teens are even more likely to engage in behavior that might, without the proper skills, place them at risk of negative outcomes.

Environmental Factors

Public health experts and researchers agree that although all sexually active teens are at risk for unintended pregnancy, the consequences of sexual activity and early childbearing are particularly severe for those who experience social, economic, educational, and environmental deprivation (Upchurch, 1993).

Poverty is increasingly recognized as a major antecedent of teen pregnancy and early childbearing, due to a number of factors. School failure, which often precedes teen childbearing, is high among low-income youth.

Substance abuse, physical and sexual violence, homelessness, and prostitution are increasingly endemic in urban communities with high rates of poverty and teen childbearing. Teens who live in rural areas, as well as those from economically distressed neighborhoods, are less likely to receive clinical and social services. Access to family planning, including contraception and abortion, is often limited or prohibitively expensive for these teens.

Adolescent sexual risk-taking behavior has also been linked to substance abuse. Teen sexual activity is often unplanned and frequently occurs after drinking and/or use of drugs (Hingson, Strunin, Berlin, & Heerin, 1990). Use of both legal and illegal drugs may impair adolescents' ability to make responsible and considered judgments about sexual activity and contraception (Hingson et al., 1990). This impairment places teens at increased risk of unplanned pregnancy and/or becoming infected with an STD, including HIV. The younger teens are when they first use drugs, the greater the likelihood of early sexual activity (Rosenbaum & Kandel, 1990). Adolescents who use marijuana are around three times more likely to be sexually active before 16 than their peers with no history of drug use (Rosenbaum & Kandel, 1990). One study of teens with unintended pregnancies found that almost half had been drinking and/or using drugs before the act of intercourse resulting in the pregnancy (Flanigan, McLean, Hall, & Propp, 1990).

Homelessness is also related to unintended pregnancy. Life on the streets necessitates risky strategies to find food, shelter, and clothing. Teens often turn to prostitution and are frequently paid more for sex without condoms. Street and homeless youth are additionally at increased risk for substance use and abuse, which is linked with early sexual activity and teen pregnancy (Mott & Haurin, 1988). Young people often become homeless after having fled an abusive family situation, which is also a risk factor for pregnancy.

Important research on sexual abuse and teen pregnancy has found that large numbers of young mothers have been forced to have sex with considerably older men. Child sexual abuse survivors are significantly more likely to become pregnant before age 18 than their nonabused peers. Surveys of pregnant and/or parenting teens have found that from 50% to 66% have a history of childhood sexual abuse (Boyer & Fine, 1992).

Recent studies have challenged the assumption that the male partner in teen births is an adolescent as well. In fact, research indicates that a significant number of births to teens were fathered by adult men, and the younger the female, the greater the age gap between parents (see Figure 10.4). In one national study, among mothers aged 15-17, approximately 27% had a partner who was five or more years older than themselves (Lindberg et al., 1997). The older man may be sexually abusing the teenage female, or the relationship may be consensual. Even in consensual relationships, such a great age difference creates a strong power differential between partners, affecting the females' choices and actions. Prevention programs must address both consensual and nonconsensual situations.

Gay, lesbian, and bisexual youth, although not traditionally targeted by pregnancy prevention programs, are also at risk for unintended pregnancy. These teens experience isolation and physical violence because of their sexuality, and many respond by abusing drugs or alcohol and by experimenting with unprotected heterosexual sex to mask their homosexuality (Cwayna, Remafendi, & Treadway, 1991).

Prevention and Promotion: Policy Goals

Serious policy efforts to reduce teenage pregnancy must commit adequate funding to proven solutions. Policymakers must abandon

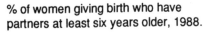

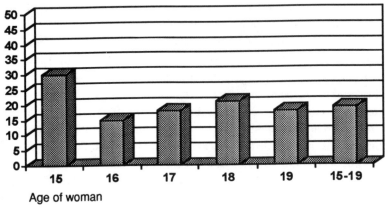

Figure 10.4.   The Older Man

SOURCE: The Alan Guttmacher Institute, 1994; reproduced with permission.

empty but popular political rhetoric and address the real reasons adolescents become pregnant and give birth. Resources and policies are needed to:

- Provide comprehensive sexuality education through K to 12 curricula and community-based programs
- Fund mentoring and developmental programs
- Improve economic opportunities
- Expand STD and HIV/AIDS prevention programs
- Increase access to health services, including mental health care
- Expand child sexual abuse prevention and intervention programs
- Increase access to and acceptability of teen contraceptive use and, when necessary, abortion

Policymakers can affect teenage pregnancies and birth rates by increasing support for family planning programs and reproductive health services, removing restrictions on comprehensive sexuality education, promoting programs to increase economic opportunities for low-income individuals, and encouraging government support for both behavioral and scientific research and evaluation. More effective contraceptive methods for both sexes must also be identified.

The goals of prevention policies must be realistic for a target population rather than a wishful projection of how adults want teens to behave. For example, an increase in how often sexually active teens use an effective contraceptive method is a more realistic goal than a 50% decline in teen pregnancy rates for the year.

The U.S. Department of Health and Human Services's *Healthy People 2000* sets national public health goals for the turn of the century. Teen pregnancy is included within the family planning priority area. (Specific goals are listed in the sidebar.) Because the Healthy People 2000 goals set an average national target, communities that are already near the goal will be able to reach it. Communities where rates are significantly higher will have difficulty reaching these goals. A recent report indicates that, although the Public Health Service is making progress in many areas of the Healthy People 2000 campaign, teen pregnancy rates have not been greatly affected (McGinnis & Lee, 1995).

Other priority area goals that will help reduce teen pregnancy include increased access to mental health services and the prevention of abuse and neglect. Efforts to decrease violence and rape among adolescents will increase teens' abilities to protect themselves. HIV/AIDS and STD infection prevention goals will affect teen pregnancy as they increase abstinence and barrier contraceptive use.

Because teen pregnancy is so complex, effective solutions cannot be one dimensional. They must be appropriate to the myriad circumstances surrounding teens and sexuality. Teen pregnancy prevention requires long-term, multimodal, comprehensive approaches that address female and male teens' self-esteem, sense of future opportunities, educational achievement, mental and physical health issues, and access to health care, contraceptive, and other community-based services. The particular needs and realities of specific populations being targeted by programs (such as out-of-school youth or preadolescents) must be foremost in the mind of program planners. At a minimum, priority must be shifted from a primary emphasis on intervention to a more holistic balance between treatment and prevention.

Prevention Strategies

Educational Programs

Teenagers who have information do make healthy decisions about sexuality (Howard & McCabe, 1990; Kirby, Barth, Leland, & Tetro,

1991). Education programs foster more open communication about sexuality and values (Advocates for Youth, 1990). Community programs that involve parents reinforce the message that adults do care about young people and want to reach out. Teens need information and skills to decide whether and when to engage in sexual intercourse and how to protect themselves from pregnancy and STDs. By discussing sexuality and reproduction openly, teens learn to accept sexuality as a normal part of the life cycle, but one that requires thought and responsibility. Skill-based education programs offer youth a means to clarify their own and their family values. Identifying values and building skills helps teens make more thoughtful decisions about sexual activity and contraceptive use. These programs are offered in a variety of settings, most notably schools, churches, youth services, and community-based organizations. Programming can be aimed directly at teens, teachers, parents, and other members of the community who play a role in adolescent development.

Although these programs vary greatly from one setting to the next, effective sexuality education should help teens build skills to choose abstinence until emotionally and physically mature enough to engage in sexual activity, along with skills to enhance contraceptive use when they do become sexually active. Guidelines for Sexuality Education (developed by SIECUS: the Sexuality Information and Education Council of the United States) provide a blueprint of age-appropriate goals and program components for sexuality education from kindergarten through high school. Comprehensive programs contain information on sexuality and reproduction, skills for refusing peer pressure and unwanted sexual intercourse, and practice in decision making and negotiating contraceptive use. Sexuality education is typically taught in high school, when many teens are already sexually active and programs to delay sexual initiation are less effective. Commitment to long-term educational programs that target young people before they start having sex will result in greater effectiveness.

Several specific types of programs offer education to young people and their families. Sexuality education programs are often provided in age-appropriate classes within schools and are often either mandated or recommended by the state legislature or board of education. All sexuality education programs include information about abstinence. Peer education programs use trained teen educators who serve to facilitate discussions and counsel their peers. Parent-child communication programs help parents and their children to talk about sexuality and reproduction. Counseling programs offer youth the opportunity to ask questions and discuss problems in a safe environment.

Although many sexuality education programs exist, few offer more than scant, short-term programming. Several studies indicate that the amount of time devoted to sexuality education varies greatly from one school district to another. The average North Carolina student receives less than 9 hours of family life education over 2 years (the North Carolina Coalition on Adolescent Pregnancy, 1989). New Jersey students receive an average of 24 hours of sexuality education, but 23% have 5 hours or less (Firestone, 1992).

Some mistakenly believe that comprehensive sexuality education might lead to adolescent sexual experimentation. In fact, a recent World Health Organization review of sexuality education programs found that participants engaged in neither earlier nor increased sexual activity (Baldo, Aggleton, & Slutkin, 1993). Studies consistently show that teens receiving sexuality education are more likely to report contraceptive use at first intercourse than teens not exposed to sexuality education (Marsiglio, 1986). Some programs have been proven to help delay sexual activity in younger adolescents but have little impact on reducing rates of teen pregnancy or the frequency of sexual intercourse for teens who are already sexually active (U. S. Congress, Office of Technology Assessment [OTA], 1991).

Health Service Programs

Studies document that most teens wait almost 1 year between starting to have sex and their first visit to a family planning clinic. One study found that over a third of sexually active teens surveyed first visited a family planning clinic because of a pregnancy scare (Zabin & Clark, 1981, 1983). To decrease this delay, programs exist to provide confidential family planning services for sexually active teenagers.

In addition to general health care services and contraception, family planning clinics provide information, counseling, and referrals. Services include pelvic and testicular exams, STD testing and treatment, contraceptives, pregnancy tests, options counseling, and information. Family planning services are provided through a variety of settings, such as private doctors, public health and Title X-sponsored clinics, school-based or -linked health centers, and hospitals.

School-based health centers are located within school settings and make general health care available to young people where they spend the majority of their time. School-linked health centers are a variation of the school-based model. Located near but not inside school grounds, school-linked centers often serve young people from several schools and other locations. School-based and school-linked health centers are designed to overcome obstacles teens face in receiving health care. With careful planning, these sites can succeed in reaching hard-to-reach populations as well, such as dropouts and runaways. Many school-based and -linked centers face restrictive policies regarding the type of family planning and reproductive health services and information that may be offered, however.

When contraceptives are recommended to teens, each individual's particular needs are taken into account. Teens consistently express concern about confidentiality, cost, and disapproval when they seek family planning services (Winter & Brechenmaker, 1991). Adolescents most at risk of unintended pregnancy, such as dropouts and runaways, are least able to afford private health care or to negotiate complicated family planning programs.

Evening and weekend hours; accessibility to public transportation; walk-in appointments; confidentiality; well-trained, multilingual, and friendly staff; explicit policies on serving teen clients; variety in family planning services; and reduced fees increase the likelihood that teens will use a program. Staff training in adolescent development and individual education sessions with teens increase adolescents' comfort at clinics as well. In-depth counseling on contraceptive options helps teenagers choose an effective method and continue to use it.

A crucial part of providing health services is the physical exam; but most teenagers are fearful about the examination and avoid clinics. The federal government has lifted its recommendation that women always receive a pelvic exam before obtaining oral contraceptives. Pelvics may be deferred if the woman has no indicated medical risk and has received counseling. Clinics have found that teens who use this option are somewhat more likely to continue care than those who do not (AGI, 1994; Moore, Miller, et al., 1995).

The availability of family planning services and contraceptives does not encourage teens to start having sex earlier or increase rates of sexual activity (Baldo et al., 1993). Providing family planning services for sexually active adolescents can lower pregnancy and childbearing rates (Winter & Brechenmaker, 1991). State data also seem to indicate that funding family planning programs is connected to reductions in the number of unintended teen pregnancies and lower rates of nonmarital childbearing by teens (Forrest & Singh, 1990; Moore, Miller, et al., 1995; Moore, Sugland, Blumenthal, Glei, & Synder, 1995).

Socioeconomic and Environmental Programs

Family planning programs increase contraceptive use among teens who are motivated to seek it, but for others, more comprehensive programs are required (U. S. Congress, OTA, 1991).

Life options programs encourage teens to delay childbearing by promoting positive alternatives to early parenting. Typically, these programs provide socially and economically disadvantaged youth with vocational skill training, career counseling, part-time employment, academic tutoring, and involvement in community service projects. Examples include Jobs Corps, Teen Outreach Program, and Youth Incentive Entitlement Pilot Project. Preliminary and anecdotal evidence suggests that these programs can help participants to delay childbearing (U. S. Congress, OTA, 1991).

Mentoring programs pair teenagers from high-risk situations with a positive adult or peer role model. Mentors expose adolescents to life and career options while providing them with social support, friendship, and tutoring. Mentors help in pregnancy prevention by raising their adolescent partners' educational and vocational goals.

Economic incentive programs focus on teens who are at high risk for pregnancy or repeat pregnancy and use cash payments, vouchers, and coupons to motivate teens to participate in weekly counseling sessions and delay additional childbearing. Evaluations show a lower repeat pregnancy rate for participants compared to the national average (Kates, 1990).

Multimodal Programs

Multimodal programs combine the strategies of educational, health service, and motivational programs to create a broader prevention strategy. An effective community-based program incorporates connections with businesses, religious leaders, the educational system, health care providers, recreational programs, and other programs in the area. Media involvement contributes a vital part of such a partnership, creating publicity about the program as well as community awareness about the need to address teen pregnancy with community-based strategies. Government agencies strengthen multimodal programs with funding as well as legislative approval and support.

Links with programs to serve youth in other high-risk situations increase the likelihood of success. Connections with runaway youth programs, confidential health care providers, HIV/AIDS prevention services, violence intervention, and academic attainment programs can help target and attract teens with the greatest need for services.

In many ways, the pregnancy prevention field is traversing its own rocky adolescence. Through trial and error, program planners, advocates, and researchers seek their way—sometimes hampered by powerful political interests, other times succeeding in advancing the field by leaps and bounds. The key to making this journey a bit less lonely, a lot more certain, and a great deal more enjoyable lies in the age-old notion of partnership.

Creating linkages and building bridges can be a daunting task in a world where turf battles abound, funds are scarce, and solutions few. Although there are no easy answers, it is critical to remember that the most successful programs result from the hard work, time, and resources of individuals, organizations, and communities working in concert.

Throughout this chapter, an effort has been made to highlight programs whose successes are attributable—at least in part—to the shared vision of agencies, the joint efforts of groups, and the critical voices and perspectives of young people. Indeed, it is the magic of these partnerships that lies at the heart of peer education and mentoring programs, parent-child communication programs, school-based health

centers, and community-wide media campaigns.

What Doesn't Work: Favoring the Stick Over the Carrot

Just as there is no single cause for adolescent sexual risk-taking behavior, there can be no single solution. Prevention programs must be comprehensive, sensitive to the needs of young people, and focused on the multidimensional nature of the problem. What fails to prevent pregnancy is the opposite of what succeeds: programs that give messages about fear and shame, distorted and incomplete information, commands to repress sexuality, inadequate health services, forced parental involvement, short-term educational programs, and censorship of young people's medical options.

Sexuality education programs that stress "just say no" are increasingly popular among educators and policymakers who shy away from controversy. Abstinence-only educational programs are based on the faulty premise that information about contraception and disease prevention will encourage youth to experiment sexually. These programs provide messages about the irreversible and inevitable negative effects of sexual expression and, for this reason, are also known as fear-based abstinence education. Abstinence-only programs often contain gender stereotypes and incorrect public health information: that females seek sex to obtain love, for example, or that a single abortion will cause infertility. Research indicates that teens tune out these messages and, without accurate information about family planning and encouragement to act responsibly, fail to protect themselves from pregnancy and STDs. Public health experts have not found abstinence-only programs to be effective in preventing teen pregnancy (Christopher & Roosa, 1990; Jorgensen, Potts, & Camp, 1993; Roosa & Christopher, 1990).

Many politicians are considering punitive measures designed to make teen childbearing less "acceptable." Unfortunately, these approaches are not grounded in sound research and are doomed to fail. Neither teens nor adults appear to seek pregnancy to qualify for a slightly higher welfare check. Nor will teens suddenly increase their ability to prevent pregnancies if the government refuses to provide support for children born to women under 18, a proposal currently before Congress. Such a strategy will only harm young women and their children and have severe repercussions in the future.

Perhaps the biggest reason programs are ineffective, however, is a lack of sustained public commitment. Without a long-term and continuous program, any reductions in pregnancy will be short-lived. Denmark-Olar, South Carolina, implemented a broad community-based program that contained a media campaign, sexuality education programs, and access to contraceptives through the school-based health centers. In 3 years, the pregnancy rate declined from 77 per 1,000 females to 37 per 1,000 females. Opposition to the family planning and educational components intimidated policymakers into abandoning the program in 1987. By 1988, teen pregnancy rates had risen to 66 per 1,000 (Koo, Cunteman, George, Green, & Vincent, 1994). The failure to address teen pregnancy and childbearing in the United States results less from a dearth of successful programming than from reluctance and inability to replicate and sustain these efforts on a broad scale.

Treatment and Coping Strategies: Services for Pregnant Teens

Pregnant women have only three options. If continuing the pregnancy, the teen can seek to place the baby into an adoptive home or become a parent. Alternatively, the teen can seek an abortion. Regardless of the teen's decision, certain services must exist for each to be a real option.

Parenting

Pregnant and parenting teens need a variety of interventions to help them care for their children and better plan future pregnancies. Health care—including early detection of pregnancy, complete prenatal and well-baby care, and ongoing child care services—is particularly crucial for this historically underserved population. Information on nutrition, childbirth, personal hygiene, child sexual abuse identification and intervention, child development, immunization, and parenting needs to be provided. Social services should include mental health and substance abuse services, housing, and assistance negotiating the welfare system. Access to these services can be dramatically increased if offered during flexible hours in a setting based in the home, school, or community health center. Follow-up intervention should stress school completion and vocational training. Although these programs traditionally target teen mothers, all should actively involve the fathers as well.

Adoption

Perhaps because of the complexity of the adoption system or concerns about the baby's welfare, few women place their children into adopted homes. Only 6% of pregnant, unmarried adolescents chose to place their baby for adoption (National Committee on Adoption, 1989). Nonetheless, adoption must be a feasible alternative for all women, including teens, facing an unplanned or mistimed pregnancy. Teens face complex legal issues related to paternity, open versus closed adoptions, and future access to information about the child. Youth-serving organizations should provide referrals to public and private agencies that facilitate adoptions and to reputable groups that independently arrange adoptions (if that is legal in the state). Teens who choose adoption also need services to ensure a healthy and safe pregnancy and delivery.

Abortion

Abortion is a safe and legal alternative to childbearing, and adolescents have the right to abortion counseling, referrals, and services. Currently, there are no abortion providers in 84% of counties nationwide, making it extremely difficult to locate and travel to a provider, particularly for teenagers (Henshaw & Van Vort, 1992). Restrictive laws such as waiting periods and forced parental consent for services add to the already considerable obstacles teens face when seeking abortion. About 91% of teen abortion decisions involve a parent or other adult, but confidentiality must be guaranteed for females whose parents will be unsupportive or abusive (Zabin & Sedivy, 1992). Access to clinics without the threat of violence or harassment, affordable procedures or funding assistance, counseling about the procedure, and follow-up care including contraceptive services must be available for teens seeking abortion.

Teaching Strategies: Other Program Considerations

Pregnancy prevention programs must be culturally relevant and account for the specific experiences, backgrounds, and identities of youth participants. To be effective, educational programs must be crafted in a culturally competent manner. Course content, instructor background and skills, teaching strategies, and location are important considerations in program design and implementation. Programs must account for diverse experiences and cultural backgrounds among youth with regard to beliefs about sexuality, health, and children; language and communication styles; sexual identity; family relationships; gender roles; religious background; immigration status; and level of acculturation.

Finally, programs and policies must reflect a solid understanding of the impact of racism, sexual abuse, poverty, sexism, heterosexism, and other forms of oppression in terms of the ability to access services and the right to healthy expressions of sexuality. Advocates for Youth's Life Planning Education curriculum, designed for high school students, provides experiential comprehensive life options education. Two teaching strategies are included as appendices to this chapter.

Conclusion

There is no "normal" path for human sexual development. Rather than following an idealized pathway from childhood through adolescence to adulthood, the course to maturity varies greatly from individual to individual and across communities. The task facing America is to provide the skills, opportunity, and information necessary for each individual to become a fulfilled and responsible member of society. Accepting sexuality as an important and normal part of the human condition will greatly further this ambition. Programs that seek to address adolescent sexual behavior without embracing this reality will fall short of their long-term goals to affect sexual relationships.

At the core of pregnancy prevention lies not only particular programs but, more important, the vital role played by parents and society. Before judging teenagers as irresponsible and immature because of their decisions about sexuality and reproduction, society must investigate whether an institutional commitment exists to provide young people with information and skills necessary to think critically, plan for an achievable future, delay sexual involvement, and access the means to prevent unintended pregnancy. One program in one setting cannot solve the myriad issues faced by teens as they seek to become healthy adults.

Shared resources and broad coalitions are required to make teen health a reality. Health care and family planning providers, community-based organizations, and others who wish to affect teen behavior must acquire expertise in adolescent-specific developmental issues and the unique youth perspective. Educational professionals and youth-serving organizations are skilled in these issues but need training and support in reproductive health issues. Shared information and resources can broaden the community understanding and commitment to effective programs. Continuity in funding from both public and private sectors and continued commitment from multiple organizations are essential to ensure that teen pregnancy prevention is adequately addressed.

It has taken years to understand the interconnected and complex factors that affect adolescent sexual behavior. The task now is to solidify support programs that work and to commit to replicating them; such resolution will make a world of difference for the adults of tomorrow. The difficult truths are that prevention is expensive and requires an honest discussion of sexuality and gender roles. Constant financial shortfalls and discomfort over sexuality have prevented models from being shared, promoted, and implemented across the country. But the costs of prevention are much less than the costs of intervention, and sexuality is an integral part of being alive. The time is long past due to stop castigating young people for normal behavior and start providing accessible, community-based settings to provide skills, information, opportunities, and services that help ensure that the sexuality of America's teens is truly freely chosen, responsibly considered, and, most of all, healthy.

Organizations and Resources

Advocates for Youth
Suite 200
1025 Vermont Avenue N.W.
Washington, DC 20005
(202) 347-5700
(202) 347-2263 FAX

Alan Guttmacher Institute
111 Fifth Avenue
New York, NY 10003
(212) 254-5656
(212) 254-9891 FAX

Associations of Junior Leagues International, Inc.
660 First Avenue
New York, NY 10016
(212) 683-1515
(212) 481-7196 FAX

Child Welfare League of America
Suite 310
440 First Street, N.W.
Washington, DC 20001
(202) 638-2952
(202) 638-4004 FAX

Children's Aid Society
Sexuality Training Center for the
 Children's Aid Society
350 East 88th Street
New York, NY 10128
Contact: Dr. Michael Carrera

THE DOOR: A Center of Alternatives
121 Sixth Avenue, 3rd Floor
New York, NY 10013
(212) 941-9090, ext. 215
Contact: Michaele P. White

ETR Associates
1700 Mission Street, Suite 203
P.O. Box 8506
Santa Cruz, CA 95061-8506
(408) 438-4060
(408) 429-9822 FAX

Girls Incorporated
30 East 33rd Street
New York, NY 10016
(212) 689-3700
(212) 683-1253 FAX

I Have a Future
Meharry Medical College
Department of Obstetrics and Gynecology
Box A-90
1005 D.B. Todd Boulevard
Nashville, TN 37208
(615) 327-6100
Contact: Lorraine Williams Greene, PhD

National Abortion Federation (NAF)
1436 U Street, N.W., Suite 103
Washington, DC 20009
(202) 667-5881
(202) 667-5890 FAX
(800) 772-9100

**National Coalition of Hispanic Health
and Human Services Organizations
(COSSHMO)**
1501 16th Street, N.W.
Washington, DC 20036-1401
(202) 387-5000
(202) 797-4353 FAX

National Urban League
The Equal Opportunity Building
500 East 62nd Street
New York, NY 10021
(212) 310-9214
(212) 593-8250 FAX

**National Center for Education in
Maternal and Child Health**
2000 15th Street North, Suite 701
Arlington, VA 22201-2617
(703) 524-7802
(703) 524-9335 FAX

**National Organization on Adolescent
Pregnancy, Prevention, Parenting, Inc.
(NOAPPP)**
4421A East West Highway

Bethesda, MD 20814
(301) 913-0378
(301) 913-0380 FAX

National Coalition of La Raza (NCLR)
810 First Street, N.E., Suite 300,
Washington, DC 20002
(202) 289-1380
(202) 289-8173 FAX

**National Network of Runaway and
Youth Services**
1400 I Street, N.W., Suite 330
Washington, DC 20005
(202) 682-4114
(202) 289-1933 FAX

Ounce of Prevention
188 West Randolph, Suite 2200
Chicago, IL 60601
(312) 853-6080

Plain Talk
The Annie E. Casey Foundation
1 Lafayette Place
Greenwich, CT 06830
(203) 661-2773
Contact: Sharon Lovick Edwards

**Planned Parenthood Federation of
America (PPFA)**
810 7th Avenue
New York, NY 10019
(212) 541-7800
(212) 245-6498 FAX
(800) 230-PLAN

Postponing Sexual Involvement
Grady Memorial Hospital
80 Butler Street, S.E.
P.O. Box 26158
Atlanta, GA 30335
(404) 616-3513
Contact: Marion Howard, PhD

Reducing the Risk
University of California at Berkeley
School of Social Welfare
Berkeley, CA 94720

(510) 642-8535
Contact: Richard Barth, MSW, PhD

The Self Center
(410) 752-1790
Contact: Rosalie Steett, MS, Former
Administrator

**Sexuality Information and Education
Council of the United States (SIECUS)**
130 West 42nd Street
New York, NY 10036
(212) 819-9770
(212) 675-1783 FAX

References

Advocates for Youth. (1990). *The facts: Parent-child communication about sexuality.* Washington, DC: Author.

Alan Guttmacher Institute. (1994). *Sex and America's teenagers.* New York: Author.

Baldo, M., Aggleton, P., & Slutkin, G. (1993, June 6-10). *Does sex education lead to earlier or increased sexual activity in youth?* Poster presented at the Ninth International Conference on AIDS, Berlin.

Boyer, D., & Fine, D. (1992). Sexual abuse as a factor in adolescent pregnancy and child maltreatment. *Family Planning Perspectives, 24,* 4-11, 19.

Brown, S. (1993). *Streetwise to sex-wise.* Hackensack: Planned Parenthood of Greater Northern New Jersey.

California Vital Statistics Section. (1992). *California resident live births, 1990, by age of father, by age of mother.* Sacramento: Department of Health.

Centers for Disease Control and Prevention. (1997). State specific birth rates for teenagers, United States, 1990-1996. *Morbidity & Mortality Weekly Report, 46,* 837-842.

Child Trends. (1996). *Facts at a Glance.* Washington, DC: Child Trends.

Children's Defense Fund. (1987). *Adolescent pregnancy: An anatomy of a social problem in search of comprehensive solutions.* Washington, DC: Author.

Christopher, F. S., & Roosa, M. (1990). An evaluation of an adolescent pregnancy prevention program: Is "just say no" enough? *Family Relations, 38,* 68-72.

Cwayna, K., Remafendi, G., & Treadway, L. (1991, July). Caring for gay and lesbian youth. *Medical Aspects of Human Sexuality,* 50-57.

Firestone, W. A. (1992). *Is playing it safe unsafe? Family life education in New Jersey.* New Jersey: Center for Education Policy Analysis, Rutgers University, and Center for Public Interest Polling.

Flanigan, B., McLean, A., Hall, C., & Propp, V. (1990). Alcohol use as a situational influence on young women's pregnancy risk taking behaviors. *Adolescence, 25,* 205-214.

Forrest, J., & Singh, S. (1990). Public-sector savings resulting from expenditures for contraceptive services. *Family Planning Perspectives, 22,* 6-15.

Hardy, J., Duggan, A., Masnyk, K., & Pearson, C. (1989). Fathers of children born to young urban mothers. *Family Planning Perspectives, 21,* 159-163, 187.

Henshaw, S., & Van Vort, J. (1992). Abortion services. In *Abortion factbook 1992: Readings, trends, and local tax data to 1988.* New York: Alan Guttmacher Institute.

Hingson, R. W., Strunin, L., Berlin, B., & Heerin, T. (1990, March). Beliefs about AIDS, use of alcohol and drugs, and unprotected sex among Massachusetts adolescents. *American Journal of Public Health, 80.*

Horowitz, S., Klerman, L., Sung Koo, H., & Jekel, J. (1991). Intergenerational transmission of school-age parenthood. *Family Planning Perspectives, 23,* 168-172, 177.

Howard, M., & McCabe, J. B. (1990). Helping teenagers postpone sexual involvement. *Family Planning Perspectives, 22*(1).

Institute of Medicine Committee on Unintended Pregnancy (IOM). (1995). *The best intentions: Unintended pregnancy and the well-being of children and families* (S. Brown & L. Eisenburg, Eds.). Washington, DC: National Academy Press.

Jorgensen, S., Potts, V., & Camp, B. (1993). Project Taking Charge: Six-month follow-up of pregnancy prevention program for early adolescents. *Family Relations, 42,* 401-406.

Kahn, J., & Anderson, K. (1992). Intergenerational patterns of teenage fertility. *Demography, 29,* 39-57.

Kalmuss, D., & Namerow, P. (1994, July). Subsequent childbearing among teenage mothers: The determinants of a closely spaced second birth. *Family Planning Perspectives, 26,* 149-153, 159.

Kates, N. (1990). *Buying time: The dollar-a-day program* (Case program for use at the Kennedy School of Government). Cambridge, MA: Harvard University Press.

Kirby, D., Barth, R., Leland, N., & Tetro, J. V. (1991). Reducing the risk: Impact of a new curriculum on sexual risk-taking. *Family Planning Perspectives, 23*(6).

Koo, H., Cunteman, G., George, C., Green, Y., & Vincent, M. (1994). Reducing adolescent pregnancy through a school and community based intervention: Denmark, South Carolina, revisited. *Family Planning Perspectives, 26,* 206-211, 217.

Lawson, A., & Rhode, D. (Eds.). (1993). *The politics of pregnancy: Adolescent sexuality and public policy.* New Haven, CT: Yale University Press.

Males, M. (1993). School-age pregnancy: Why hasn't prevention worked? *Journal of School Health, 63,* 429-432.

Marisglio, W. (1986). The impact of sex education on sexual activity, contraceptive use, and premarital pregnancy among American teenagers. *Family Planning Perspectives, 18,* 151-162.

Marsiglio, W. (1987). Adolescent fathers in the United States: Their initial living arrangements, marital experience, and educational outcomes. *Family Planning Perspectives, 19,* 240-251.

Maynard, R. (1994, July 29). *Teenage childbearing and welfare reform: Lessons from a decade of demonstration and evaluation research.* Statement for the Committee on Ways and Means, Subcommittee on Human Resources, U.S. House of Representatives, Hearing on Early Childbirth.

McGinnis, J. M., & Lee, P. R. (1995). Healthy People 2000 at mid decade. *Journal of the American Medical Association, 273,* 1123-1129.

Moore, K. A., Miller, B., Glei, D., & Morrison, D. (1995). *Adolescent sex, contraception, and childbearing: A review of recent research.* Washington, DC: Child Trends.

Moore, K. A., Sugland, B. W., Blumenthal, B. A., Glei, D., & Synder, N. (1995). *Adolescent pregnancy prevention programs: Interventions and evaluations.* Washington, DC: Child Trends.

Mott, F., & Haurin, R. J. (1988). Linkages between sexual activity and alcohol and drug use among American adolescents. *Family Planning Perspectives, 20,* 128-136.

National Center for Health Statistics. (1993). *Vital statistics of the United States, 1989: Vol. 1. Natality* (Tables 1-9). Washington, DC: Government Printing Office.

National Center for Health Statistics. (1994). *Monthly vital statistics report: Advance report of final natality statistics, 1992.* Washington, DC: Government Printing Office.

National Commission to Prevent Infant Mortality. (1988). *Death before life: The tragedy of infant mortality: Appendix.* Washington, DC: Author.

National Committee on Adoption. (1989). *Adoption factbook.* Washington, DC: Author.

North Carolina Coalition on Adolescent Pregnancy. (1989, March). *The myths—the facts—family life education in North Carolina schools.* Charlotte: Author.

Nsiah-Jefferson, L. (1989). Reproductive laws, women of color, and low-income women. In S. Cohen & N. Taub (Eds.), *Reproductive laws for the 1990s* (pp. 23-67). Clifton, NJ: Humana Press.

Roosa, M., & Christopher, F. S. (1990). Evaluation of an abstinence-only adolescent pregnancy prevention program: A replication. *Family Relations, 39,* 363-367.

Rosenbaum, E., & Kandel, D. B. (1990, August). Early onset of adolescent sexual behavior and drug involvement. *Journal of Marriage and the Family, 52.*

Shah, J. (1995). *The social construction of whiteness: Implications for epidemiologic research.* Unpublished manuscript, University of Michigan School of Public Health.

Upchurch, D. (1993). Early schooling and childbearing experiences: Implications for postsecondary school attendance. *Journal of Research on Adolescence, 3,* 422-443.

Urban Institute. (1995, June). *Welfare reform briefs.* Washington, DC: Author.

U.S. Congress, Office of Technology Assessment (OTA). (1991, November). Background and the effectiveness of selected prevention and treatment services. In *Adolescent health, Vol. 2.* Washington, DC: Author.

U.S. Public Health Service. (1988). *Vital statistics of the United States: Vol. 1. Natality.* Washington, DC: U.S. Department of Health and Human Services.

Ventura, S., Taffel, S., Mosher, W., & Henshaw, S. (1992, November 16). Trends in pregnancies and pregnancy rates, United States, 1980-88. *Monthly Vital Statistics Report, 41,* 1-11.

Winter, L., & Brechenmaker, L. C. (1991). Tailoring family planning services to the special needs of adolescents. *Family Planning Perspectives, 23.*

Zabin, L., & Clark, S., Jr. (1981). Why they delay: A study of teenage family planning clinic patients. *Family Planning Perspectives, 13,* 205-207, 211-217.

Zabin, L., & Clark, S., Jr. (1983). Institutional factors affecting teenagers' choice and reasons for delay in attending a family planning clinic. *Family Planning Perspectives, 15,* 25-29.

Zabin, L., & Sedivy, V. (1992). Abortion among adolescents: Research findings and the current debate. *Journal of School Health, 62,* 319-324.

11

Mental Health

Robert Friis
Sherry Stock

Definition and Statement of the Problem

Among the issues that confront educators, adolescent mental health problems pose immense challenges, and, on occasion, engender life-threatening crises. Mental illness symptoms, which may range from subtle to overt and dramatic, encompass a gradation of conditions from depressed mood/affect and eating disorders, substance abuse and other behavioral disturbances, to severe depression with suicidal symptoms and serious mental disorders such as schizophrenia. Among some afflicted persons, untreated mental illness carries the burden of profound loneliness, isolation, and stress vulnerability (Stoto, Behrens, & Rosemont, 1990). In contrast, positive mental health status refers generally to the absence of mental disorders as well as the ability to negotiate life's daily challenges and social interactions without experiencing cognitive, mental, or behavioral dysfunction. This chapter will provide an overview of mental health issues that are known to affect some teenagers and recommend methods for coming to terms with them.

The mental health services provider, whether located in a school or a community-based organization, is in a key position to provide early recognition of, and health promotion for, mental health problems and referrals to appropriate interventions. The provider may also be a central figure in furnishing social support to affected students and their families. Health care agencies and community organizations, including those that may not interact regularly with teenage clients, should nevertheless be aware of mental illness risk factors in order to collaborate more effectively with schools and other agencies.

The impact of adolescent mental health problems on the school and the community may be dramatic. Note the following example that was reported in the *Los Angeles Times* on February 26, 1995:

VICTORVILLE—How should a school acknowledge the traumatic loss of two 14-year-old girls who attended class Tuesday morning and had executed a mutual suicide pact by that evening? One opportunity came during a tear-filled funeral Saturday, when more than 200 grieving students and adults gathered at a Victorville church to bid farewell to Annette Sander. The teenager and her friend, whose family has asked that she not be identified, had composed more than 15 goodbye letters to

151

friends during the prior week, to be found later. On Tuesday, they dropped a note into a friend's locker with a map showing where to find their bodies, and then retreated into the desert, each with a handgun to complete their mission. School officials are struggling with how to allow Victor Valley High School classmates to mourn their loss—without giving the tragedy such attention that other troubled teenagers might be tempted to follow suit. (Gorman, 1995, p. 3)

The foregoing example demonstrates that high school suicides have a chilling effect on peers and organizations that serve them; other dramatic conditions that come to the attention of educators, mental health providers, and society less frequently include the psychoses, for example, schizophrenia and manic-depressive psychosis. However, a panoply of more subtle mental health issues and problems, for example, feelings of loneliness and isolation, post-traumatic stress disorders, conduct disorders, unrecognized depression, and eating disorders, may be equally troubling and need to be afforded the same level of attention as the more dramatic episodes.

Background/Historical Perspective/Causes

Given the tumultuous nature of adolescence and the challenges to the health care system that this developmental milestone presents, it is not surprising that the adolescent age group represents the only U.S. population subgroup whose health status has not improved in the past three decades. Mental health problems such as depression and suicidal behavior contribute significantly to the morbidity and mortality of adolescents and, within the past 30 years, appear to be occurring more frequently and earlier in life. In recent years, more than one tenth of high school students have been reported to suffer from clinical depression. Adolescent lifestyle and

risk-taking behaviors seem to play a role in substance abuse, depression, unplanned teenage pregnancy, and other major health problems. Violent death has replaced communicable diseases as the primary cause of juvenile mortality, with more than three quarters of adolescent deaths now caused by intentional and unintentional injury, suicide, and homicide.

Adolescent Development and Incidence of Mental Illness

In his classic work on adolescence, Jersild (1963) observed that this period of life is both a time of great possibility and a time of trial. The physical and mental impacts of adolescent development include changes in weight and height, increased ability to reason and deal with abstractions, and establishment of independence from parental control. Physical and hormonal changes lead to growth acceleration; among some adolescents, awareness of developing sexuality may be associated with guilt and anxiety as well as increasingly pessimistic attitudes, depression, and rebelliousness. At the same time that the typical adolescent is in the process of forming an autonomous identity, peer pressure increases. This latter factor, as well as media influences, may encourage the teenager to engage in potentially harmful and self-destructive behavior, for example, excessive alcohol and substance use, violence, and premature sexual activity. Not only are minor and major depression during the teenage years prevalent to varying degrees, but also some forms of severe mental illness, for example, schizophrenia, have a peak age of onset roughly during the mid- to late teenage years. About three-quarters of schizophrenia cases have an onset between the ages of 17 and 25 years (Torrey, 1988). Unmet goals, broken relationships, teenage pregnancy, the struggle for autonomy, and escalating societal violence are possible sources of stress, frustration, and disappointment that exacerbate the teenager's propensity for mental health problems.

Linkages Between Societal Violence and Mental Health

Let's focus on a potential contributor to adolescent mental health problems, societal violence, which has nearly doubled in the past 20 years in the United States, at the same time that the population has increased by only one-fifth. The media expose teenagers routinely to gratuitous violence; they may, themselves, become the targets of violence or witness violent acts in the community and in the media. For example, an ordinary western city reported the following representative incidents during a 6-month period: a hospital emergency room shooting, a violent confrontation at a family planning clinic, rival gang battles, an attack by an alleged serial rapist, and weekend rioting at a university.

One may ponder at the messages about society's sanction of violence that media reports communicate to adolescents. Regrettably, violence is an all too common feature of some adolescents' life experiences, one that surely has at least a minimal impact upon mental health status. According to most recently available data, one out of five teenagers were victimized by violence and about one out of four urban males were arrested at least once by the age of 16. In fact, homicide is the leading killer of African American adolescent boys. Firearm-related deaths account for more than 1 in 10 deaths among children and youth ages 19 years or younger. Recently, in Los Angeles high schools, nearly 11% of students had suffered at least one incident of violence—a weapon attack or an assault by other students; an additional 3% had been threatened with a weapon at school. Whereas youths in inner cities experience much higher rates of violence than do those in the suburbs, suburban youths experience more crime than do rural

youths. Obviously, violence directly impairs teenagers' ability to take advantage of life-enhancing educational and employment opportunities that provide preparation for adulthood (Adams, Gullotta, & Adams, 1994).

A second category of widespread, alarming violence occurs among families and predominantly affects women and children in the form of physical abuse. The emotional trauma remains long after the external bruises have healed; often, the severe emotional damage to abused children does not surface until adolescence or later, when many previously abused children become abusing parents. Low socioeconomic status, a history of physical abuse, and substance abuse are all factors that may engender aggression and violent conflict within households. Family violence tends to be perpetuated, because battered mothers' children also demonstrate in adulthood a propensity for stress-related physical problems, behavioral and developmental problems, and family violence. Not only does poverty correlate strongly with interpersonal violence (Stoto et al., 1990), but also the incidence of physical abuse and neglect is higher among the offspring of teenage parents who abuse alcohol and drugs than among those who do not (Bushong, Coverdale, & Battaglia, 1992). Other family violence factors include early unplanned parenthood and poor coping skills for stress. For the adolescent, the mental health consequences of family abuse include a poor self-image, inability to trust others, and aggressive and disruptive behavior (or the reverse, passive and withdrawn behavior).

Low Social Support Levels

Low social support levels or loss of social support may be linked to teenagers' mental health problems by engendering feelings of loneliness, isolation, and depression. Social support, which arises from friends and family members who are perceived as helpful, is regarded as a positive force in mental health. The changing nature of the American family, the impersonality of modern society, and the massive size of some secondary education systems are all variables that may contribute to loss of social support and to the individual's sense of isolation. Then, loss of social support may act as a contributing factor to depression and suicide, as well as to other adverse mental health outcomes. The loss of social support may also contribute, secondarily, to high-risk behaviors such as alcohol and drug abuse as well as gang participation.

Researchers report that gang members perceive themselves as unoccupied, disconnected, and alienated. The frightening result is numbing detachment from others and a self-destructive disposition toward the world. Because life without support, meaning, hope, and love breeds a cold-hearted, mean-spirited outlook that invalidates the self and others, the youth gang fills a void; it provides a sense of identity, belonging, power, protection, and security. Living in a high-risk environment without paternal protection, the young gangster lessens his insecurities by aligning himself with a gang, his surrogate family. In this sense, the gang provides social support that may be lacking from other sources.

High-Risk Behaviors:
Alcohol and Substance Abuse

Alcohol and substance abuse, both associated with adolescent depression, tend to follow rather than precede the onset of psychiatric disturbances. In comparison to those who report no substance abuse history, substance users are almost four times as likely to meet the diagnostic criteria for major depressive disorders. In some instances, the effects of alcohol abuse and illegal drugs mimic mental illness symptoms. Although it is not unusual for teenagers to experiment with alcohol and other drugs, most will stop or continue to use substances casually without significant prob-

lems. However, a minority will progress to habitual substance use, with varying physical, emotional, and social problems that, at the worst extreme, culminate in enduring drug-dependent, inwardly or outwardly directed violent behaviors. Because no method exists for predicting with certainty who will develop serious substance abuse problems, all adolescent substance use should be regarded as potentially problematic. Risk factors for substance abuse and consequent adverse mental health outcomes include a family history of substance abuse problems, early initiation of cigarette or alcohol consumption, and daily exposure to substances among friends, family members, or the drug culture. Trends for alcohol and substance abuse, an extremely prevalent phenomenon in almost every U.S. secondary school, are reported elsewhere in this book.

Stressful Life Events

Stressful life events encompass accidental injuries, loss of a friend or family member through violent death, incarceration, moving out on one's own, and pregnancy. Other stress-inducing situations include parental separation or divorce, family tension or violence, emotional abuse or neglect, breakup with a friend, academic problems, death of a family member or close friend, personal health problems or health problems of another family member, and sexual abuse. Although stressful life events may contribute to adolescent depression or other adverse mental health outcomes, inadequate social support resources may also increase vulnerability to stress.

Posttraumatic stress disorder refers to psychological consequences that result from experiencing, witnessing, or participating in an overwhelmingly violent or traumatic event (a natural event, e.g., earthquake, hurricane, tornado, fire flood; or a man-made event, e.g., the previously cited mutual suicide pact that occurred in Victorville, California). Traumatic events and violent acts may influence adolescents' mental health by creating many of the features of a posttraumatic stress syndrome, similar to the syndrome experienced by military personnel and residents of combat zones. Adolescents who are afflicted with this disorder sometimes report repeated episodes in which they experience and reexperience a traumatic event such as violence, rape, or murder. This syndrome, which may endure for years or for a lifetime, may impair the individual's mental health and functioning. Symptoms of the posttraumatic stress disorder include, but are not limited to, loss of concentration and irritability, behavior problems not typical for the teenager, physical symptoms (stomachaches, headaches, dizziness) for which a physical cause cannot be found, and withdrawal from family and friends.

Current Status

In this section, we will discuss the following examples of adverse teenage mental health conditions and outcomes: conduct disorders, learning disabilities and attention deficit disorders, depression, schizophrenia, manic-depressive psychosis, and eating disorders. Although this list is not exhaustive, the authors believe that it portrays a range of conditions that might affect adolescents. Perhaps, appropriate responses for coping with these and other mental health issues are early recognition and referral of the affected teenager to professional assistance. In illustration, a teenager who manifests depressive symptomatology, a risk factor for suicide, should be referred to professional help as soon as possible. According to vital statistics reports, U.S. adolescent suicide rates have increased steadily since 1950, with suicide the third leading cause of death in 1994 among the 15- to 24-year-old group. A second example is adolescent acting out behaviors (e.g., excessive truancy and rebelliousness), which may represent a cry for help that should be followed up. The practitioner/counselor needs to be aware of community and professional resources for intervention in mental health problems, such as depression and acting out behaviors, and needs to build bridges to family members in order to improve social support resources for students.

Conduct Disorders/Learning Disabilities/Attention Deficit Disorders

Adolescent conduct disorders form a complicated syndrome that is manifested typically as difficulty in following rules and maintaining socially acceptable behaviors. Afflicted teenagers are often viewed by peers, adults, and social agencies as bad or delinquent, rather than mentally ill. One of the features of the disorder is heightened expression of anger, characterized by physical and verbal interpersonal aggression; other aspects include prevarication, stealing, property destruction, sexual acting out/promiscuity, and antisocial deeds. Possible etiologic factors for adolescent conduct disorders include brain damage, child abuse, growth defects, school failure, and negative family and social experiences. Without early, intense, and continuing intervention (e.g., behavior therapy and psychotherapy), the prognosis of afflicted teenagers is likely to be poor; as adults, they will almost certainly have diminished capacity to adapt to the demands of interpersonal relationships, careers, and life in general.

Adolescent learning disabilities may lead to emotional problems such as low self-esteem and low frustration tolerance. Teenagers who are categorized as learning disabled are, as a group, usually bright and conscientious at home and school. They tend to lag behind academically, despite their strenuous efforts. In addition to difficulty in mastering elementary academic skills, other hallmarks of learning disabilities embrace difficulty understanding and following instructions, trouble remembering, poor coordination, misplacing of items, transposition of numbers and letters, and difficulty with the concept of time. Learning disabilities, which affect as many as 15% of all schoolchildren, are believed to be associated with impaired neural pathways for receiving, processing, and communicating information. Fortunately, learning disabilities are treatable; if not detected and treated early, they sometimes have a tragic snowballing effect, as in the case of acquiring mathematics or reading skills. For instance, a child who does not learn fundamental elementary school mathematics and reading will not, as a teenager, be able to comprehend high school algebra and literature instruction; frustration, low self-esteem, and mental health symptoms may result.

Attention deficit disorder (ADD) or attention deficit hyperactivity disorder (ADHD), a condition that is more common among boys than among girls, may also affect the adolescent's self-esteem by contributing to academic failure. The hyperactivity symptom component in ADHD may include extreme restlessness and disorganized, aimless, fidgety behavior. Other characteristics of ADD include poor organizing skills, easy distractibility, carelessness, impulsivity, and impatience. Without proper treatment, the afflicted teenager may suffer lowered self-esteem that results from school failure, lost friendships due to deficient social rapport, and family members' and teachers' criticisms. The therapeutic regimen for ADD and ADHD, both treatable conditions, may include counseling, medication, and special curricula.

Depression

Transient depressed mood or affect, common during adolescence in varying degrees, should be differentiated from major depressive episodes and clinically significant depression, which has a prevalence of about 5% in the general adolescent population. Although biological, organic, and genetic risk factors have been linked to depressive illness, psychosocial factors for adolescent depression include stress, loss experiences, and coexisting functional problems (e.g., learning disabilities, conduct disorders, and attention deficit disorders that were mentioned previously). These psychosocial instigators of depression include disappointment and frustration resulting from unmet goals, fractured relationships, struggles with parental control, parental divorce and remarriage with the formation of a new family, and events that bring about loss of social support such as moving to a new community. Although this does not always happen, protracted stressful situations are thought to increase risk of major depression, a severe and potentially life-threatening disorder. Due to its association with suicide, this form of depression, as well as lesser degrees of depression, needs to be recognized, diagnosed, and treated appropriately. Ironically, adolescent depressive symptomatology may be difficult to differentiate from normal behavior, because some nondepressed adolescents are sullen, irritable, and prone to mood swings, craving distance from parents. However, a number of behaviors distinguish depression from normal behavior:

- Depressed mood and poor self-concept taken together for a period of 1 month or longer
- Social withdrawal and isolation, fatigue, anorexia, loss of interest in family and work/school, heightened sensitivity to rejection in love relationships, suicidal ideation, and sleep difficulties
- Hostility, persistent periods of sadness, fear of failure, and an inability to experience a sense of efficacy
- Persistent periods of boredom and restlessness, fatigue, bodily preoccupation, as well as difficulty in concentrating
- Conduct disorders, hyperactivity, persistent periods of sadness, separation anxiety, and refusal to attend school
- Decline in school performance and a withdrawal from peer and extracurricular activities

TABLE 11.1. Warning Signs for Suicide and
              Depression in Teenagers

Persistent sadness and increased irritability

Change in eating and sleeping habits

Change in appetite, weight, level of activity

Withdrawal from friends and family and regular
    activities

Frequent absences from school or poor performance
    in school

Violent actions, rebellious behavior, or running away

Drug and alcohol use

Unusual neglect of personal appearance

Marked personality change

Persistent boredom, low energy, difficulty concentrating,
    or a decline in the quality of schoolwork

Frequent complaints about physical symptoms, often
    related to emotions, such as stomachaches,
    headaches, fatigue, and so on

Inability to enjoy what used to be favorite activities

Not tolerating praise or rewards

A teenager who is planning to commit suicide may also:

Talk, write, or hint about suicide

Have made previous attempts

Complain of being "rotten inside"

Give verbal hints with statements such as: "I won't
    be a problem for you much longer," "Nothing
    matters," "It's no use," "I won't see you again"

Put their affairs in order—for example, give away
    favorite possessions, clean out their locker,
    clean their room, throw away important
    possessions, and so on

Become suddenly cheerful after a period of depression

The teacher or practitioner may mistakenly attribute depressive symptomatology to more benign conditions, such as growing pains or minor somatic illnesses. Hence, youth who are experiencing one of the most common mental health conditions in the United States often do not receive needed and appropriate mental health services. This gap in services is unfortunate, because untreated depression may result in suicide.

Suicide

Depressed teenagers behave differently from depressed adults; note also that depression symptoms, like many of the suicidal symptoms, are cause for parents to talk to their affected teenager and to seek professional help if the concerns persist. (Refer to Table 11.1 for warning signs.)

Varying according to race, U.S. teenage suicide rates stand at two times higher for white and other minority adolescents than for African Americans, the respective rates for 15- to 19-year-olds being 11 per 100,000 among the former and 4.6 per 100,000 among the latter (U.S. Bureau of the Census, 1992, cited in Adams et al., 1994). With Native Americans two and one half times more likely than African Americans and twice as likely as whites to commit suicide, some Native American adolescents appear to have the highest suicide rates among all racial groups. Risk factors for adolescent Native American suicides include adoption outside the tribe, weakening of religious traditions, high unemployment, peer group support of excessive alcohol consumption, pent-up anger, and feelings of hopelessness, helplessness, and shame. Table 11.2 presents race and gender distributions of suicide ideation and attempts.

Schizophrenia

Each year from 100,000 to 200,000 Americans, mostly adolescents or young adults, develop schizophrenia. For nearly all, schizophrenia's onset produces severe consequences: possible temporary or long-term hospitalization and a life that is marred by recurrent psychotic episodes, impaired social relations, joblessness, and abject poverty. In the past, schizophrenia has been differentiated into three subtypes: hebephrenic or disorganized, paranoid (marked by delusions and hallucinations), and catatonic (characterized by somatic rigidity and mental stupor). The usefulness of the subtypes is limited, however, because many patients demonstrate symptoms that overlap the diagnostic categories (Torrey, 1988). Although much research remains to be done, it is now generally believed that schizophrenia

TABLE 11.2. Suicide Ideation and Attempts by Gender and Race/Ethnicity, U.S. Risk Behavior Survey, 1990

	Suicidal Ideation	Suicidal Ideation With a Plan	At Least One Suicide Attempt	Suicide Attempt Requiring Medical Attention
Gender				
Female	33.9%	20.2%	10.3%	2.5%
Male	20.5%	12.3%	6.2%	1.6%
Race/ethnicity				
Hispanic	30.4%	19.5%	12.0%	2.4%
White	28.1%	16.1%	7.9%	2.1%
Black	20.4%	13.5%	6.5%	1.4%
Total	27.3%	16.3%	8.3%	2.1%

SOURCE: CDC, 1991.

is a brain disease, associated with structural changes and impairment of neurotransmitters, that often runs in families. Medications are efficacious in treating some forms, whereas others are thought to be irreversible (Lindenmayer & Kay, 1992; Modrow, 1992).

Adolescents who are experiencing the onset of schizophrenia may demonstrate gradual behavioral changes, such as reduced enjoyment of social relationships, extreme shyness, withdrawal, sleeping more or less than usual, preoccupation with strange fears and ideas, and disorders of thinking. It should also be noted that parents should not worry about their adolescent's every quirk and eccentricity, because normal teenagers have also been known to be moody and withdrawn. The key issue seems to be whether the adolescent has shown a change in behavior from one pattern to another, for example, from outgoing to withdrawn. (See Table 11.3 for more information.)

Manic-Depressive Psychosis

About 1% of all adolescents suffer from manic-depressive psychosis, and one in six of those afflicted persons commit suicide (Holt, 1993). Manic depressive psychosis is less likely than schizophrenia to confront the practitioner, because it is one-third as prevalent (Torrey, 1988). Manic-depressive psychosis is characterized by periods of severe depression interspersed with episodes of uncontrollable elation, restlessness, racing thoughts, and delusions of grandeur. The manic-depressive patient may alternate rapidly between manic and depressed states, and, hindered by selective attention, may be unable to converse meaningfully or listen attentively. Other symptoms include ready distractibility by extraneous external or internal stimuli, rapid speech that lags behind the individual's thought process, and transitions from one subject to another without meaningful or obvious connection.

Eating Disorders: Anorexia and Bulimia

Anorexic individuals tend to deny themselves nourishment and engage in excessive

TABLE 11.3. Early Warning Signs in Adolescents With Schizophrenia

Trouble telling dreams from reality
Seeing things and hearing voices that are not real
Confused thinking
Vivid and bizarre thoughts and ideas
Extreme moodiness
Odd behavior
Ideas that people are "out to get them"
Behaving like a younger child
Severe anxiety and fearfulness
Confusing television with reality
Severe problems in making and keeping friends

TABLE 11.4. Anorexia Nervosa and Bulimia: Main Characteristics

Age	Victims are under the age of 25 when they begin to secretly limit the intake of food
Weight loss	They lose at least 25% of their ideal body weight
Distorted understanding of behavior	Victims, when confronted with their behavior, do not recognize the serious risks associated with it. They maintain that refusing food brings personal satisfaction. They seek and find pleasure in maintaining an extremely thin body image. They handle food in unusual or bizarre ways
Physical health	There is no medical explanation for the weight loss
Mental health	There is no known psychiatric condition to explain the weight loss
Appearance and behavior	Victims demonstrate at least two of these symptoms: (a) the inability to menstruate, if female; (b) soft, fine hair; (c) a constant resting pulse of 60 or less; (d) occasional periods of hyperactivity; (e) grossly excessive overeating; (f) induced vomiting (The last two symptoms are the two principal distinguishing characteristics of bulimia)

exercise, whereas bulimic persons may engage in unrestrained eating sprees only to purge themselves after overindulgence. About 1% to 3% of all adolescents suffer from eating disorders, which are found more often in upper-middle-income than lower income homes. Although both adolescent boys and girls have been diagnosed as anorexic or bulimic, young women afflicted with eating disorders outnumber young men by a factor of 10 to 20 times. White adolescent girls suffer more from eating disorders than do Hispanic, Asian, African American, and Native American girls. However, evidence suggests that African American and Native American teenagers experience eating disorders more frequently than do Hispanic and Asian teenagers. Activities that emphasize slender weight—for example, gymnastics, ballet, modeling, and certain sports—seem to attract especially high numbers of adolescent participants with eating disorders.

Although some reports have characterized these disorders as modern afflictions, anorexia nervosa and bulimia have existed for centuries, with one of the most famous anorexia cases documented in the mid-1400s. Italy's Saint Catherine, who at age 15 years developed anorexic symptoms that coincided with her sister's death, deprived herself of adequate nourishment and engaged in self-abusive behavior that contributed to her own demise at the young age of 33 years. An interpretation of Saint Catherine's alleged eating disorder is that it enabled her to control her own food intake, one of the few freedoms that a woman had in her time, and that it was akin to an ascetic, holy lifestyle.

Characteristic symptoms and warning signs of anorexia and bulimia increase the teacher/practitioner's index of suspicion for eating disorders. For example, the criteria for diagnosis of anorexia are shown in Table 11.4.

Several features characterize anorexia. Usually female, an anorexic teenager is typically a perfectionistic high academic achiever who, ironically, suffers from low self-esteem. Desperately wanting mastery over life, the anorexic teenager experiences a sense of control by negating the body's normal nutritional demands. Erroneously believing that she is overweight or even obese, regardless of how emaciated she becomes, the anorexic teenager engages in a relentless pursuit of thinness that results in self-starvation, often producing serious bodily damage, and, less commonly, death.

The symptoms of bulimia, different from those of anorexia nervosa, involve bingeing on huge quantities of high-caloric food and purging dreaded calories by self-induced vomiting and laxative use. These binges may alternate with severe calorie-restricted diets, resulting in dramatic weight fluctuations. The

TABLE 11.5. Healthy People 2000 Prevention/Promotion Goals

Objective Number	Objective	Baseline
6.1a	Reduce suicides among youth ages 15 through 19 to no more than 8.2 per 100,000	10.3 per 100,000 in 1987
6.2	Reduce by 15% the incidence of injurious suicide attempts among adolescents ages 14 through 17	Data available in 1987
6.3	Reduce to less than 10% the prevalence of mental disorders among children and adolescents	An estimated 12% among youth younger than age 18 in 1989
Risk Reduction Objectives		
6.6	Increase to at least 30% the proportion of people ages 18 or older with severe, persistent mental disorders who use community support programs	15% in 1986
6.7	Increase to at least 45% the proportion of people with major depressive disorders who obtain treatment	31% in 1982
6.8	Increase to at least 20% the proportion of people ages 18 and older who seek help in coping with personal and emotional problems	11.1% in 1985
6.9	Decrease to no more than 5% the proportion of people ages 18 and older who report experiencing significant levels of stress who do not take steps to reduce or control their stress	21% in 1985
Services and Protection Objectives		
6.12	Establish mutual help clearinghouses in at least 25 states	9 states in 1989
6.14	Increase to at least 75% the proportion of providers of primary care for children who include assessment of cognitive, emotional, and parent-child functioning, with appropriate counseling, referral, and follow-up, in their clinical practices	Data available in 1992

SOURCE: Adapted from U.S. Department of Health and Human Services (1991), pp. 99-100.
NOTE: Goals listed in *Healthy People 2000* reflect the federal government's interest in improving mental health.

purging of bulimia presents a serious threat to the individual's physical health, including dehydration, hormonal and electrolyte imbalance, the depletion of important minerals, and damage to vital organs. With intensive and continuing treatment that includes family and group therapy, medications, and personal counseling, some teenagers experience symptom relief and control. Nevertheless, with recovery rates limited to about 50%, bulimic teenagers frequently experience recidivism despite attempts at intervention and treatment. Perhaps, a more successful strategy for primary prevention of bulimia (and anorexia) would involve approaches that focus on the individual's self-esteem as well as work to change society's positive image of thinness.

Prevention/Promotion Goals

Goals posited in *Healthy People 2000* reflect the federal government's interest in improving adolescent mental health in the domains of health status, risk reduction, and services and protection (U.S. Department of Health and Human Services, 1991). (See Table 11.5 for a detailed list of the mental health goals.) With respect to mental health and mental disorders, the health status objectives call for a reduction to less than 10% in the prevalence of mental disorders among children and adolescents, a 20% reduction in suicides, and a 15% reduction in the incidence of injurious suicide attempts. The risk reduction objectives propose an increase in the use of community support programs by people who have severe, persistent mental disorders, as well increasing assistance programs for depressive disorders, personal and emotional problems, and significant stress levels. The services and protection objectives include the establishment of mutual help clearinghouses and increased involvement of primary care providers in the assessment, treatment, and referral of mentally ill people.

Prevention and Treatment/ Coping Strategies for Adolescent Mental Health Disorders

With respect to promoting teenage mental health, we have organized strategies along the lines of the venerable public health concepts of primary, secondary, and tertiary prevention; these types of prevention are directed toward interventions that may occur during the various phases of the natural history of disease (Friis & Sellers, 1996). Primary prevention of adverse mental health outcomes includes general mental health promotion, such as the provision of adequate social support and stress reduction in the home, the classroom, and society in general. Secondary prevention involves treatment programs that occur after mental illness onset; examples include psychotherapy, medication management, and group therapy programs. Tertiary prevention refers to efforts to rehabilitate the patient or to reduce the probability of a relapse, examples being halfway houses and protected living arrangements for the recovering mentally ill. The following discussion will elaborate on school-, family-, and community-based interventions for the primary, secondary, and tertiary prevention of psychiatric impairment among adolescents.

Primary Prevention

Previously, we suggested that the adolescent's loss of a sense of self-efficacy—the feel-

ing that one's actions have little effect on negative circumstances—is associated with malaise and, possibly, more severe adverse mental health outcomes such as depression. The family, the school, and society represent potential avenues for the primary prevention of mental illness through the emotional and social support that they provide. (A more detailed exposition of these concepts is also shown in the appendix: external assets—support, empowerment, boundaries and expectations, and time—and internal assets—educational commitment, values, social competencies, and positive identity.)

Creating support from various sources is a key element in the primary prevention of mental health impairments. Family social support levels and positive communication among parents and the adolescent create an atmosphere wherein the adolescent feels free to seek parental advice and counsel. Active parental involvement in school helps the adolescent succeed in academic pursuits. In addition to family social support, informal community support resources include extended/surrogate families and other adults, for example, caring relatives and neighbors, who reinforce parental social support. In addition, when the community shows that it values adolescents by providing them with useful roles, a sense of empowerment may be a fringe benefit. For example, the adolescent might perform community service, thereby developing a sense of security at home, at school, and in the neighborhood.

The school, dominant in many adolescents' lives, is potentially an important setting for preventing learned helplessness. A microcosm of society, the typical school could provide all students with multiple opportunities for competence in academic and extracurricular endeavors. To provide school personnel with a valuable mechanism for helping students, successful programs require a high level of commitment from school boards, principals, and community members. Following are some examples of school-based programs for primary prevention of mental health problems.

To encourage primary prevention of adolescent alienation from society, the school environment should help students to feel emotionally involved in social relationships and in the larger community. Beyond the traditional school activities—academic pursuits, athletics, and interest clubs—school personnel might consider ways to increase individualized contact among students, teachers, counselors, and other school staff. Increased opportunities for interaction would provide students with positive role models and increase potential sources of social support. Quality contact between students and school personnel could be achieved by scheduling regular small-group meetings that match a small number of students with one adult. These meetings, which could discuss career development, avocations, current events, and social dilemmas, might identify each student's strengths and problem-solving skills, thus enhancing self-esteem and self-efficacy.

Because peer pressure might be marshaled as a powerful primary prevention tool, student assistance programs could use peer pressure as a positive force for shaping and reinforcing an environment that supports teenagers' healthy choices, the opposite of what occurs in many schools. Typically, intense peer pressure for drug and alcohol use during the teenage years correlates with an individual's use of these substances. By recruiting student peers in both the design and implementation of drug and alcohol use prevention activities, a model program might use peer education to mentor at-risk students.

Secondary Prevention

The authors noted previously that factors associated with mental illness onset sometimes involve difficulty coping with the environment or low self-esteem; secondary prevention programs might focus on these factors. To give an example, the authors suggest that public schools should establish linkages with local community mental health centers and other agencies that provide adolescent mental health services. Schools could establish contracts with local agencies and selected mental health professionals (mental health liaisons) who are on call for consultation and referral. These agency and professional resources might offer individual and group therapy sessions that alleviate the sources of adolescent stress. Another example would be in-service training workshops for school personnel (teachers, guidance counselors, school administrators, and paraprofessionals) as well as parents in the recognition of adolescent self-esteem issues and mental illness symptoms. As a catalyst, the school mobilizes those community mental health resources that have the maximum likelihood of being culturally sensitive and appropriate.

A specific type of school-based secondary prevention, known as student assistance programs, focuses on school behavior and performance. Given that they rely on community agencies for assessment and treatment services, some student assistance programs represent a partnership between schools and community health agencies. They are modeled on employee assistance programs used at many workplaces, by screening students for alcohol, tobacco, and other substance use. Elements common to most student assistance programs include early problem identification, referrals to designated helpers, follow-up services, and in-school services, for example, support groups and individual counseling. Student assistance programs may also focus on identifying, referring, and assisting students with all issues that hinder development.

Assistance programs might also include training for school personnel regarding problem identification. However, staff are not expected to intervene personally, but to refer students to appropriate assessment and treatment resources. In some districts, school-based mental health professionals provide short-term intervention groups and crisis intervention services for depressed adolescents. Intervention groups should concentrate upon integrating or reintegrating adolescents into the school, in ways that enhance self-esteem and self-efficacy. Crisis intervention services should focus on stabilizing adolescents, their friends, and their families, as well as on making and monitoring referrals to mental health providers; school-based personnel might monitor a high-risk group for possible referral for more intensive treatment. Some community referral programs provide teenagers with problem-solving techniques to deal more effectively with school, peers, and developmental issues.

Several communities have established crisis referral and problem-solving telephone lines that are staffed by teenagers who have had crisis intervention and problem-solving training; ongoing training comes from certified counselors and psychologists who are familiar with adolescent concerns. Examples of talk lines include the Teen Pregnancy Information Center, the National AIDS Center, and suicide prevention centers. One talk line for teenagers received 7,000 calls during its first year; 23% of calls dealt with friendships, 26% with family relationships, 19% with dating issues, and 33% with other issues.

Beyond the realm of the school setting, possible community-based initiatives may include community forums on adolescent mental health, designation of social network resources, and identification of formal mental health resources: churches, community centers, ethnic associations, and self-help groups. Coordinating community resources with school-based and mental health center-based interventions maximizes the effectiveness of all interventions and enhances the community's empowerment to meet individual needs.

Tertiary Prevention

Although there is some overlap among all levels of prevention, tertiary prevention is more concerned with monitoring and rehabilitating students who have already developed mental health problems, with the objective of stemming subsequent functional deterioration. Considering their almost daily contact with adolescents, school-based personnel can play a major role in observing students under treatment in order to prevent a recurrence or relapse; for example, timely recognition of depressive episodes serves as an essential, life-saving resource, should a suicide attempt be prevented. By monitoring adolescents who are receiving treatment for depression or other mental health problems, school personnel function as the eyes and ears of mental health professionals. Schools could also enhance a teacher's monitoring role by matching one or two peer contacts with an adolescent who has been diagnosed with depressive or other mental health symptoms.

School-based personnel may also facilitate the reintegration of treated mentally ill teenagers into the school community. The contact person assigned to monitor the adolescent's progress might convene a meeting of involved teachers, counselors, aides, and mental health professionals, as well as parents and other family members; jointly, they could discuss the adolescent's current status and plan for reintegration. Such reintegration efforts optimize the mentally ill adolescent's recovery chances, especially when the stigma that often accompanies episodes of severe psychiatric disturbance is minimized.

Conclusion

The authors of this chapter advocate a multifaceted and community-oriented plan that identifies adolescents who are afflicted with mental health problems. Schools represent a major resource in identifying these problems, preventing their recurrence, and limiting their adverse effects. Those who work closely with adolescents, whether in a school- or a community-based organization, are in a key position to provide primary prevention of mental health problems, their early recognition, and referrals to appropriate interventions; they may also be central in furnishing social support to affected students and their families. Health care and community organizations, including those that do not work with adolescents routinely, should nonetheless be aware of mental illness risk factors and be able to collaborate with the school and the mental health system. A successful approach to adolescent mental health problems is most likely to result from collaboration between the school and the community in designing primary, secondary, and tertiary prevention strategies.

References

Adams, G. R., Gullotta, T. P., & Adams, C. M. (1994). *Adolescent life experiences* (3rd ed.). Pacific Grove, CA: Brooks/Cole.

Bushong, C., Coverdale, J., & Battaglia, J. (1992). Adolescent mental health: A review of preventive interventions. *The Journal of Texas Medicine, 88*(3), 62-68.

Friis, R. H., & Sellers, T. A. (1996). *Epidemiology for public health practice.* Gaithersburg, MD: Aspen.

Gorman, T. (1995, February 26). Dealing with grief: Some experts say establishing memorials for young suicide victims is healthy, but others fear it prompts imitations. *Los Angeles Times,* p. 3.

Holt, L. (1993, November 10-16). The adolescent in accident and emergency. *Nursing Standards, 8*(8), 30-34.

Jersild, A. T. (1963). *The psychology of adolescence.* New York: Macmillan.

Lindenmayer, J. P., & Kay, S. R. (Eds.). (1992). *New biological vistas on schizophrenia.* New York: Brunner/Mazel.

Modrow, J. (1992). *How to become a schizophrenic.* Washington, DC: Apollyon Press.

Search Institute. (1996). *Developmental assets among Minneapolis youth: The urgency of promoting a healthy community.*

Stoto, M. A., Behrens, R., & Rosemont, C. (Eds.). (1990). *Healthy People 2000.* Washington, DC: National Academy Press.

Torrey, E. F. (1988). *Surviving schizophrenia: A family manual.* New York: Harper & Row.

U.S. Department of Health and Human Services. (1991). *Healthy People 2000: National promotion and disease prevention objectives.* Washington, DC: Author.

APPENDIX: 40 Developmental Assets

Asset Type	Asset Name	Definition
Support	1. Family support	Family life provides high levels of love and support
	2. Positive family communication	Parents and child communicate positively; child is willing to seek parents' advice and counsel
	3. Other adult relationships	Child receives support from three or more nonparent adults
	4. Caring neighborhood	Child experiences caring neighbors
	5. Caring school climate	School provides a caring, encouraging environment
	6. Parent involvement in schooling	Parents are actively involved in helping child succeed in school
Empowerment	7. Community values youth	Child perceives that community adults value youth
	8. Youth given useful roles	Youth are given useful roles in community life
	9. Community service	Child gives 1 hour or more per week to serving in his or her community
	10. Safety	Child feels safe in home, school, and neighborhood
Boundaries and expectations	11. Family boundaries	Family has clear rules and consequences and monitors whereabouts
	12. School boundaries	School provides clear rules and consequences
	13. Neighborhood boundaries	Neighbors would report undesirable behavior to family
	14. Adult role models	Parent(s) and other adults model prosocial behavior
	15. Positive peer influence	Child's best friends model responsible behavior
	16. High expectations	Both parents and teachers press child to achieve
Time	17. Creative activities	Involved 3 or more hours per week in lessons or practice in music, theater, or other arts
	18. Youth programs	Involved 3 hours or more per week in sports, clubs, or organizations at school and/or in community organizations
	19. Religious community	Involved 1 or more hours per week
	20. Time at home	Out with friends "with nothing special to do" 2 or fewer nights per week
Educational commitment	21. Achievement motivation	Child is motivated to do well in school
	22. School engagement	Child is actively engaged in learning
	23. Homework	Child reports 1 or more hours of homework per day
	24. Bonding to school	Child cares about her/his school
	25. Reading for pleasure	Child reads for pleasure 3 or more hours per week
Values	26. Caring	Child places high value on helping other people
	27. Equality and social justice	Child places high value on promoting equality and reducing hunger and poverty
	28. Integrity	Child acts on convictions, stands up for her or his beliefs
	29. Honesty	Child "tells the truth even when it is not easy"
	30. Responsibility	Child accepts and takes personal responsibility
	31. Restraint	Child believes it is important not to be sexually active or to use alcohol or other drugs
Social competencies	32. Planning and decision making	Child has skill to plan ahead and make choices
	33. Interpersonal competence	Child has empathy, sensitivity, and friendship skills
	34. Cultural competence	Child has knowledge of and comfort with people of different racial backgrounds
	35. Resistance skills	Child can resist negative peer pressure
	36. Peaceful conflict resolution	Child seeks to resolve conflict nonviolently
Positive identity	37. Personal control	Child feels she/he has control over "things that happen to me"
	38. Self-esteem	Child reports high self-esteem
	39. Sense of purpose	Child reports "my life has a purpose"
	40. Positive view of personal future	Child is optimistic about his/her personal future.

Search Institute (1996). With the support of Lutheran Brotherhood, the Cargill Foundation, and Norwest Bank Minnesota.

12

Youth Violence

Mohammed R. Forouzesh
Daria Waetjen

Violence is a major contributor to premature death, disability, and injury to youth. In addition, it is an epidemic that threatens not only our physical health, but the integrity of our social fabric, the family, and the community. Violence affects all sectors of our society; no one is immune. The fear of violence infringes on the individual freedom of all and interferes with one of a child's basic needs, the need to be safe. Youth, whether perpetrators or victims, are often the most adversely affected by violence.

The term *violence* refers to a specific set of behaviors that cause injuries. The National Academy of Sciences has adopted as its definition of violence: behaviors by individuals that intentionally threaten, attempt, or inflict physical harm on others (National Research Council, 1993).

The prevention of violence is now one of the most important public health challenges facing our society (For a description of federal goals in this area, see Table 12.1). Public health brings forward a new vision of how to address this multifaceted and complex problem. Schools cannot address the issue of youth violence alone. Violence is rarely isolated. What exists in the neighborhood spills into the schoolyard. The existence of this reality has changed the school climate in which we expect our children to learn, grow, and become productive citizens. A host of factors, including media influence, peer pressure, drugs and alcohol, availability of weapons, domestic violence, prejudice, gangs, poverty, anger, and lack of communication, contribute to the spread of violence.

The Scope of Youth Violence

Youth violence is escalating at an alarming rate. Statistics on juvenile homicides, the number of youth carrying weapons, and youth gang membership are staggering. The age at which youth engage in violent crime is lower every year. In 1993, nearly 50% of the estimated 4.2 million nonfatal crimes of violence in the nation were committed by offenders between the ages of 12 and 19 (Stephens, 1994).

TABLE 12.1. Healthy People 2000 Objectives

Healthy People 2000 is a national initiative to improve the health of all Americans through prevention. It is driven by 300 specific national objectives targeted for achievement by the year 2000. Following are eight priority areas related to youth violence:

- Reduce homicides
- Reduce weapon-related deaths
- Reduce assault injuries
- Reduce physical fighting among youth
- Reduce weapon-carrying by youth
- Reduce inappropriate storage of weapons
- Improve school programs for conflict resolution skills
- Increase violence prevention programs

The average age of the first arrest for a juvenile in a state institution is 12.8 years, and the average age of incarcerated youth is 15.4 years, not yet old enough for a driver's license (Sheahan, 1991).

The United States now has the highest incidence of interpersonal violence among all industrial nations, with police reports illustrating that teenagers are involved in 30% of all crimes.

- Homicide is now the nation's third leading cause of death for elementary and middle school children, with a death toll of nearly 50,000 between 1979 and 1991, equivalent to that of the Americans killed in the Vietnam War. It is estimated that by the year 2000, over 8,000 teenagers will be victims of violence every year (Children's Defense Fund, 1995).

- The number of crimes committed by youth has climbed drastically; between 1984 and 1993, the number of juveniles arrested for violent offenses increased nearly 68% (U.S. Department of Justice, 1995a). In California alone, the arrest rate has increased 53%, and it is expected to increase as much as 29% over the next 10 years (Hill, 1995).

- Violence committed by youth is no longer isolated to urban areas. The California De-

partment of Justice reports that gang membership has increased in rural and suburban neighborhoods. It also reports that in Los Angeles, there are 175,000 known gang members making up 2,000 gangs (California Department of Justice, 1994).

- The dramatic escalation of violence is psychologically affecting students and reducing the quality of their education. Of 65,000 American youth surveyed, 36% said they do not feel safe at school, 42% avoid restrooms out of fear, 7% of 8th graders reported staying home at least once during the previous month because of concerns for their physical safety, and 63% say they would learn more if they felt safer (Stephens, 1994). Students at times join gangs to seek protection and to be left alone.

- In a survey of 10 high schools in four states, 15% of inner-city high school students said they were scared at school almost all of the time (Sheley, McGee, & Wright, 1992). Of 10,000 students surveyed, 9% of students age 12 to 19 were crime victims in or around their school during a 6-month period; 2% reported experiencing one or more violent crimes, and 7% reported at least one property crime (U.S. Department of Justice, 1991).

The most frequently reported types of violent incidents on school campuses reported by both suburban and urban superintendents and principals included: girls fighting, violence involving guns, alcohol and other drugs, school bus violence, vandalism, graffiti, sexual fighting, and sexual assaults (Institute for Educational Leadership, 1994).

For youth of color, violence is a greater reality. In 1990, compared to whites, blacks were 41% and Hispanics 32% more likely to be victims of violent crime. Ethnic differences, age, and gender patterns combine to make blacks 20 times more likely to be victimized. Homicide rates are also highest for minorities: Black homicide is 5 times greater than the white rate, and rates for Native Americans are double the rate of the entire population (National Research Council, 1993).

Cost of Violence

Not including the lives lost to violence, the direct cost of medical expenditure, emergency service, and claims processed for the victims of gun violence nationwide totaled about $3 billion (The Carter Center, 1994). Other studies place the societal cost of firearm injuries at about $20 billion (Rice & McKenzi, 1989). The National Institute of Justice places the cost of violent injuries, including medical treatment, physical and psychological rehabilitation, and lost productivity of victims, in addition to the criminal justice response, at an estimated $60 billion annually (U.S. Department of Justice, 1995b).

Drugs and Alcohol

Drugs and alcohol are often involved in all forms of violence, and alcohol and drugs are readily available and accessible to the youth in our society. One fourth of all the students surveyed reported that beer, wine, liquor, and marijuana were easy to obtain at school or on school grounds, and 24% of 16,000 students, Grades 9 to 12, reported that they were offered, sold, or given an illegal drug at school in the previous year (CDC, 1993).

Handguns

The problem of violence is exacerbated by the presence of handguns on school campuses. Weapon-carrying practices have changed dramatically in our society, and too often adult practices affect children. In a Louis Harris national poll, it was found that 59% of the students surveyed nationwide said guns are easily obtainable whereas 35% said it would take 60 minutes to get one (Fulwood, 1993).

In one U.S. city, half of 11th-grade students who owned handguns said they got the gun from their parents or from friends. About 29%, or one in three ($n = 209$), said that they could easily get a handgun if they wanted one. Students who said they could easily obtain a handgun were most likely to get the gun from friends, rather than on the street (Callahan & Rivara, 1992). In a recent study of homicides, it was found that having guns in the home increased the likelihood of homicide three-fold (Kellermann, Rivara, Rushforth, Banton, & Reay, 1993).

High schools experienced the greatest increase, but more guns were found at all grade levels, including elementary school. Most of the students who carry guns to school say that they do so for protection on their way to and from school. On any given day, the odds are that at least one of the students in any urban high school classroom is carrying a gun (National Center for Education in Maternal and Child Health, 1992).

About 26% of students in Grades 9 to 12 reported having carried a weapon during the past 30 days (CDC, 1993). The number of guns confiscated in California public schools doubled from 1985 to 1988. In 1990, 4,941 children in the United States under age 19 died from gunshot wounds, and 538 of these children were shot accidentally (The Carter Center, 1994).

Laws in recent years have changed to make parents responsible for keeping weapons and ammunition locked and away from children. It is estimated that half of all American households have guns (National Center for Education in Maternal and Child Health, 1992). About 16% of students reported having access to a handgun at home, and 8% of 12th graders reported bringing a weapon to school at least once during the previous month.

These facts and figures related to youth violence illustrate that many social issues directly or indirectly affect violence. Solutions are often multidimensional in scope and require the coordination of many educational and prevention programs.

Preventing Violence: Applied Models

Violence is the number one public health threat facing our nation today (Prothrow-Stith, 1991). Violence is a multifaceted problem and involves a complexity of issues. Violence has many faces: homicide, domestic violence, child abuse, suicide, gang violence, guns and weapons, and unintentional injuries. Violence affects all ages and socioeconomic groups.

Prevention programs can be most effective when focused at a very young age. No one method of intervention and/or approach could be solely offered as a solution. Interventions need to be viewed from both the micro and macro level. It is believed that a key component in the prevention of adolescent violence is delinquency prevention. Not only would delinquency prevention reduce the risk of violence among delinquency-prone subgroups, but the risk of violence for other groups in proximity to delinquents should be reduced as well (Lauritsen, Laub, & Sampson, 1992). These researchers believe that intervention strategies, such as alternative dispute resolution programs, are the most promising path for reducing adolescent violence. Finding ways to challenge the cultural and social norms that support violent behavior must become the central issue of violent prevention efforts (Noguera, 1995).

On a larger scale, social and economic opportunities, employment and career training, and multicultural programs need to be part of any proposed solution. School policies, such as school uniforms, suspension, and expulsion, are only part of the equation. Such interventions cannot be used as the only means to solve this problem but must be integrated with a comprehensive approach.

Public Health Approach

The CDC (1992) has made the prevention of violence one of its highest priorities. Public health brings a systematic approach to reducing the burden of illness, suffering, and premature death among the human population. The traditional public health approach consists of health event surveillance, epidemiologic analysis, intervention design, evaluation, and focus on a single clear outcome to prevent a particular illness or injury. The traditional public health model suggests that injury, like infectious disease, can be conceptualized as an interaction between agent, host, and environment. It has been accepted that the public health model could be easily applied to a violence prevention approach in our society.

The agent is the mechanism of injury. Firearms have been identified as the mechanism of injury in 50% to 70% of homicides. The host may be either the perpetrator or victim of the injury. Compared to white males, Latino and African American males are about three and six times more likely to be victims of homicides, respectively. Environmental factors are also critical in violence prevention efforts. Environmental factors are physical, economic, and social. Violence has been found to be highest among those who live under the most adverse socioeconomic conditions. These include (a) limited social, recreational, educational, and employment activities; (b) unplanned pregnancy; (c) single-parent households; (d) household size; (e) poverty; (f) poor housing conditions; (g) unemployability of young males; (h) fear, hopelessness, and racism; (i) low self-esteem; (j) limited social support systems; (k) the nonexistence of traditional institutions such as family and church; and (l) ineffective schooling (Mercy & O'Carroll,

1988; Pacific Center for Violence Prevention, 1993; Steinberg et al., 1992).

Ecological Model in Developing Effective Violence Prevention Programs

One way to deal with youth violence is to view the problem from an ecological perspective. This assumes that human behavior is determined by the interaction of individual and environmental characteristics. Apter and Popper (1986) describe this ecological principle based on the following assumptions.

- Each child is an inseparable part of a small social system.
- Disturbance is viewed not as a disease, but rather as a lack of balance.
- This lack of balance is defined as a disparity between an individual's abilities and the demands or expectations of the environment.
- The goal of the intervention is to make the system work ultimately without the intervention.
- Improvement in any part of the system can benefit the entire system.

The ecological model gives rise to three major areas of intervention: changing the child, changing the environment, and changing attitudes and expectations. Ecological orientation stresses the importance of looking at the entire system surrounding each child. In the process of developing effective prevention programs, the following factors need to be considered carefully:

- The economic situation within the community, that is, poverty, unemployment, and underemployment
- The public health model—agent, host, environment—as applied to the community
- The level of domestic violence, sexual assault, rape, and acquaintance rape
- Violence as related to economic, racial, cultural, sexual, and age-based inequities
- Gun availability
- The involvement of males in the solution

- The inclusion of adults, particularly parents and other caregivers, as part of the solution
- Youth as part of the solution
- Recognition of posttraumatic stress needs to be applied to inner cities
- Relationship of alcohol and other drugs to violence
- Media and their impact on violence
- The effective evaluation of violence prevention programs
- Stress and turnover ("burnout") among staff in the field of violence prevention programs
- Increased empowerment including self-esteem and skill development

Community Mobilization and Coalition Building

Mobilizing the community around the issue of violence prevention is a very powerful strategy to address this problem. The National Center for Education in Maternal and Child Health (1992), in "Violence as a Public Health Problem," made the following recommendations:

- Organize parents and grassroots neighborhood efforts that involve community organizations and individual residents in the leadership
- Establish coalitions that have political input to combat racism, sexism, and other social and cultural issues, to promote cooperation, and to reject violence
- Challenge teachers and school administrators to make a personal commitment to organize communities and work through existing groups, such as the PTA

The establishment of a community coalition is one way to bring the community together around the issue of violence. By definition a coalition is "an organization of individuals representing diverse groups or constituencies who agree to work together in order to achieve a common goal" (Feighery & Rogers, 1989). Health promotion practitioners stress the importance of coalitions to target the behavior of individuals by intervening at numerous social levels that can affect behavior and in turn affect health status (Hawkins, 1994; McLeroy, Bibeau, Steckler, & Glanz, 1988; Minkler, 1989). The development of a coalition can enable organizations to become involved in new, wider range issues, without having the sole responsibility for overseeing those issues. The coalition could be used to demonstrate and develop widespread public support for issues, actions, or unmet needs of the population.

Coalitions also have the ability to maximize the power of individuals and groups through collaboration and joint action (Brown, 1984). Coalitions mobilize broad talents, resources, and approaches in the community, exercising more influence on an issue than any single organization could achieve (Roberts-De Gennaro, 1986). Most important, coalitions are able to recruit participants from a number of diverse constituencies, such as political, business, human services, social, and religious groups, as well as less organized grassroots groups and individuals, which leads to an extremely influential, unique conglomerate of people and resources with which to identify problems and implement practical solutions (Black, 1983; Feighery & Rogers, 1989). School and community linkages and interagency collaboration are a critical ingredient in finding viable solutions to youth violence.

Violence Prevention in Schools

School can play a significant role in the reduction of youth violence. School staff should begin addressing this issue by becoming informed through awareness education. It is critical to set standards of nonviolence, enforce policies, and educate students and their families on strategies to build peace and resolve conflict peacefully. Prevention curriculum and prosocial skill development also build student resilience. Schools can begin this task by:

- Becoming informed through awareness education
- Implementing prevention and content-based curriculum
- Reinforcing children's success and achievement
- Involving children in the solutions

Policy Development

Campus-based prevention programming begins with setting policy at an administrative, district, and site level. Policy development should begin with a planning component. Planning steps should include:

- A thorough needs assessment should establish baseline information and clearly define the level of violence on campus. These data should also reflect parent and student concerns, fears, and attitudes as related to violence. This information can later be used to evaluate program effectiveness.
- Action planning should follow and involve all stakeholders. The needs assessment should be reviewed and goals developed from the determined needs. Staff development, student and parent awareness, community partnerships, focus groups, and advisory boards should then be used to plan appropriate activities.
- Implementation of the agreed-upon plan should be initiated at the district or at the site level. Community, parent, and staff support should be enlisted to help make the program activities a success.
- Evaluation should be ongoing, with the constant collection of relevant data. Review of data assists in the evaluation of program effectiveness and can influence future program planning.

(See appendix for a model policy statement developed by the American Medical Association's National Coalition on Adolescent Health.)

Strategies for School-Based Violence Prevention Programs

Specific strategies assist in the development of a comprehensive school-based violence prevention program. These strategies should focus on building resiliency in youth. Consideration of the inclusion of the programs/factors described below is critical in the development of an effective comprehensive plan. The following continuum of responses to violence allows schools and policymakers to address campus safety issues.

Continuum of Responses to Violence

1. Responding to emergency
   — a. crisis management plan
   — b. student conduct codes
   — c. search and seizure
   — d. surveillance and security
   — e. student identification, dress codes, and restricted access
   — f. suspension, expulsion, and referral to law enforcement
2. Moving away from crisis
   — a. conflict resolution and violence prevention curriculum and training
   — b. multicultural education
   — c. character education
   — d. law-related education
   — e. counseling
   — f. staff development
   — g. alternative education programs
   — h. student assistance programs
   — i. support groups
3. Preparing today for the future
   — a. family/home support programs
   — b. early childhood education
   — c. peer-helper programs
   — d. job-skills training/employment opportunities
   — e. community service projects, implementation of violence prevention curriculum, or life coach program (Linquanti & Berliner, 1994)

Early Intervention

Early intervention needs to focus on prevention rather than suppression. The earlier you intervene, the better the result. Research has shown that dealing with adolescents once they have exhibited problem behavior has shown only modest success (Hawkins, 1994). Spergel and his colleagues support Hawkins with findings from a nationwide assessment of approaches aimed at youth gangs. They found that in communities with emerging gang problems, suppression strategies were not reported to be particularly effective, except in conjunction with other approaches (Bastian & Taylor, 1991). Effective prevention programs directed at youth could focus on conflict resolution, social responsibility, decision making, refusal skills, tolerance, and other related issues. These personal approaches are costly because programs must be directed individually at each person with a problem, and even a large investment in treatment does nothing to break the cycle of the problems spreading to other young people through a peer network. It is as if we were providing expensive ambulances at the bottom of a cliff to pick up the youngsters who fall off, rather than building a fence at the top of the cliff to keep them from falling off in the first place.

Family Involvement

A successful intervention requires extensive family involvement and family management practices. The prevention model that is recommended by Hawkins (1994) is known as a *risk-focused prevention model*. In this model the family involvement includes family management, problem solving, and identification of risk factors.

Family management problems include a lack of clear behavioral expectations, failure of parents to supervise and monitor their children (knowing where they are and whom they are with), and excessive, harsh, or inconsistent punishment. Other researchers support Hawkins's findings that successful intervention programs need to involve parental training in behavioral strategies, modeling, rehearsal, and feedback (Blythe, Tracy, Kotovsky, & Gwatkin, 1992; Denicola & Sandler, 1980). Today, escalating gang association and violence among our youth often stem from the rage in children whose basic needs for protection, safety, and affiliation are not being met.

Teaching Strategies

When teaching violence prevention to students, an important concept to keep in mind is that students and adults view violence from very different perspectives. Many students view gang membership, weapon carrying, and engaging in violent activity as a way to gain respect or protect themselves. For example, if you ask your students what they think about when they hear the word *gang,* you will often hear words such as *power, control, respect, belonging,* and even *money* (Hochhaus & Sousa, 1988). However, when you pose the same question to a group of adults, you hear words such as *fear, loss of control, lack of safety and security,* and even *anger.*

Comparing these two lists, you will find that often the student list contains positive ideas whereas the adult list contains negative associations. It is critical to keep this in mind while teaching violence prevention to youth. Instruction should begin early. It should be integrated into existing curriculum when possible and be delivered by significant people in the student's life. Instruction should not be a one-time event/delivery by a person the students do not know (assembly format). Little behavioral change is indicated in this approach (Project Yes!, 1993). Table 12.2 outlines teaching strategies for implementing violence prevention into the classroom.

What to Teach?

Specific content has been found to be effective in addressing issues pertaining to violence, substance abuse, gang involvement, and other high-risk behaviors (Project Yes!, 1993). Infor-

TABLE 12.2. Teaching Strategies for Implementing Violence Prevention Into the Classroom

Integrate prevention content into existing curriculum content
Present meaningful content
Practice strategies applicable to everyday life of the students
Reinforce content through role playing, written expression, and open discussion
Use reasoned decision-making skills
Use cooperative learning strategies
Avoid judgment and lecturing

mation, as well as specific learning strategies, can assist youth in making positive, reasoned decisions when faced with negative peer pressure. The following topics have been found to be effective themes in violence prevention education.

- Responsible citizenship including character and legal education
- Value of diversity (multiculturalism)
- Recognition and control of emotions through anger management and conflict resolution
- Understanding about choices and consequences
- Refusal skills
- Goal setting

Gang Membership and Affiliation at School

Awareness education for school personnel can help to more clearly assess the situation in a school or classroom. According to a California Department of Justice (1994) report, gang involvement can begin as early as elementary school. Children as young as 7 or 8 years old have been recruited to work for gangs.

Early recognition of gang affiliation and high-risk association can assist in planning an effective and realistic program. Identifying the signs and symptoms of gang involvement empowers the educator to knowledgeably address the situation. Specific characteristics of

TABLE 12.3. Why Do People Join Gangs?

Peer pressure
Protection
Gang associates
Money
Self-esteem
Unhappy home life
Family violence
Lack of a significant adult in their life
Hopelessness and helplessness
Unsafe school or neighborhood
Power
Status and respect

TABLE 12.4. Warning Signs of Gang
Involvement and Activity

Wearing colors associated with local gangs
Wearing pants that sag on hips or waist or oversized clothing
Wearing an excessive amount of jewelry
Using gang slang
Withdrawing from family members
Being truant
Staying out late without accounting for whereabouts
Desiring much privacy
Developing attitude problems with parents, teachers, or other authority
Smoking cigarettes, drinking alcohol, and using drugs
Carrying and receiving unexplained amounts of money and other articles without permission
Experiencing sudden drop in grades and changes in behavior
Associating with known gang members and/or change of friends

gang association include clothing and style of dress, such as sagging or baggy style, color selection, hand signs, common language or use of slang, tattoos, and weapon-carrying practice. Additional clues may include truancy, desire for privacy, unexplained money or possessions, and withdrawal from family and school.

Students may choose to affiliate with gangs for a variety of reasons (see Table 12.3). A history of family involvement, neighborhood membership, and disenfranchisement from school and/or the community are often precipitating factors. Peer pressure and the glamorous media portrayal of violence often influence youth. Youth who feel helpless and out of control may also turn to the gang for protection or a sense of identity. The lack of significant positive adults or role models may also create a void that the gang can appear to fill. Educators and parents who can profile the gang member and address the root causes of affiliation and violence are more likely to implement an effective comprehensive prevention strategy (White, 1995).

What Are the Warning Signs of Gang Involvement?

The California Department of Justice (1994) report, *Gangs: A Community Response,* encourages parents and educators to watch for signs

that their children or students may be involved with gangs. The report cautions parents and teachers not to jump to hasty conclusions about their children and gangs. The warning signs of gang involvement can be similar to normal behavior during adolescence. The key is to question the behavior if it appears to go beyond the norm. Table 12.4 lists some of the most common warning signs of gang involvement and activities.

Gang and Violence Discussion Topics

One of the best ways to initiate a dialogue related to gang violence with students is to ask questions to engage the youth in the discussion. This interactive exchange is useful to get the students to think about the consequences of their behavior and their gang involvement. The following questions could be useful to guide classroom discussion:

As a gang member, would it be safe to move into another part of the city?

Do gang members use alcohol and drugs?

Do gang members usually carry knives, guns, and other weapons?

Do you make loyal friends when you join a gang?

Do you gain or lose your freedom when you join a gang?

Could you avoid using drugs or alcohol when you are in a gang?

Could you get into trouble when you choose to join a gang?

If you get arrested by the police for being a gang member, could it ruin your future?

How do gang members get their money?

Are there only boys in a gang?

Do people join gangs to protect their neighborhood?

How could your family members be affected by your joining a gang?

What would you do if you found out that your best friend is carrying a weapon to school?

Conclusion

To bring about a positive change and create lasting solutions to this problem, schools, law enforcement, health care providers, parents, and youth must collaborate. Policy formulation, ongoing data collection, physical and structural modification, strict adherence to standards and the law, broadened cultural understanding, and curriculum are key elements in the development of a comprehensive violence prevention program (see Table 12.5).

Resource Guide

Violence Prevention Resources

A. Violence prevention curricula: The following are samples of curricula available for schools to address the issue of youth violence.

Conflict Resolution; Community Boards
Description: Classroom curriculum teaching students to be conflict managers

TABLE 12.5. Practical Plans or Getting Started

What can schools and communities do to effectively deal with violence on their school campus?

1. Obtain a commitment from top-level school district official to make violence prevention a priority
2. Promote clear guidelines, procedures, and protocols related to incidents of violence on campus, for example, zero tolerance for weapons
3. Create staff counselor positions to provide support to students affected by violence
4. Create or strengthen alternatives to expulsion
5. Strengthen lines of communication between school and home
6. Increase family participation through parent contracts and other methods
7. Promote respect for cultural diversity
8. Sponsor school-based events with violence prevention and cultural celebration themes, for example, Violence Prevention Month
9. Create student "Bill of Rights" where it does not already exist
10. Create or expand student assistance programs that encourage young people to work together to improve the school
11. Establish a partnership between the school and the business community
12. Develop a mentorship program
13. Repeatedly communicate school policies to parents
14. Strict enforcement of school policies and the rules

SOURCE: Contra Costa County Health Services Department, 1995.

by developing communication leadership, problem-solving, and mediation skills for Grades K through 12.
Publisher: The Community Board Program
1540 Market Street, Suite 490
San Francisco, CA 94102
(415) 552-1250
EVALUATION: Copies of report and demonstration project available upon request.

Get Real About Violence
Description: Violence prevention curriculum for students in Grades 6

through 8. Based on risk reduction research and social development strategy, which focus on encouraging nonviolent norms.
Publisher: Comprehensive Health
    Education Foundation
22323 Pacific Highway South
Seattle, WA 98198-5104
(800) 323-2433(30-day preview)

Sane: Gang Curriculum
Description: A gang prevention curriculum designed to be delivered by a teacher and a deputy sheriff for Grades 4 through 6.
Publisher: Los Angeles Sheriff's
    Department
211 West Temple Street
Los Angeles, CA 90012
(310) 946-7236

Second Step
Description: A violence prevention curriculum aimed at reducing impulsivity and aggressive behavior through the development of pro-social skills. This program is available for preschool through Grade 8.
Publisher: Committee for Children
Airport Way South, Suite 500
Seattle, WA 98134-2027
(800) 634-4449
EVALUATION: Pilot study completed on curriculum, available upon request.

Star: Straight Talk About Risks
Description: Curriculum focusing on educating children about gun risks, thus enabling them to recognize threatening situations, identify trusted adults, make safe choices, and resolve conflict peacefully.
Publisher: Center to Prevent Handgun
    Violence
1225 I Street, NW, Suite 110
Washington, D.C. 20005
(202) 289-7319

Violence Prevention for Adolescents by Deborah Prothrow-Stith
Description: Curriculum-based activities that promote solving problems nonviolently between peers. Ten lessons included and video available.
Publisher: Education Development
    Center, Inc.
55 Chapel Street
Newton, MA 02140
(617) 969-7100

Project Yes! Yes to Education and Skills
Description: A primary gang violence and drug prevention curriculum for Grades 2 through 6. An integrated thematic model focuses on responsible citizenship, refusal skills, cultural diversity, and reasoned decision making.
Publisher: Orange County Department of
    Education
200 Kalmus Drive
Costa Mesa, CA 92628-9050
(714) 966-4473
EVALUATION: Pre- and posttest survey results available on request.

B. Media Related Resources

TV Alert
Description: A user friendly resource containing ideas and activities to help classes and groups recognize and evaluate the subtle impact of TV in everyday life.
Publisher: Center for Media Literacy
1962 South Shenandoah Street
Los Angeles, CA 90034
(800) 226-9494
Fax: (310) 559-9396

C. Parenting Resources

Active Parenting
Description: Parents learn how to identify parenting styles and become active rather than reactive. Additional

skills are developed to increase
consistency and create an atmosphere of
mutual respect, trust, and teamwork.
Publisher: Harper and Row
10 East 53rd Street
New York, NY 10022
(800) 825-0060

Discipline With Dignity
Description: A program offering essential
skills and strategies for dealing with
angry and disruptive behavior while
positively affecting the lives of youth.
Publisher: National Educational Services
P.O. Box 8
Bloomington, IN 47402
(800) 733-6786

Effective Black Parenting
Description: Program offering African
American parents skills and strategies to
direct youth to pathways of success.
Publisher: National Parenting Instructors
  Association
11331 Ventura Boulevard, Suite 103
Studio City, CA 91604-3147
(800) 325-CICC

CICC's Confident Parenting
Description: Participants learn to use
observation skills, to effectively praise
and ignore, and to offer social
disapproval and incentives.
Publisher: National Parenting Instructors
  Association
11331 Ventura Boulevard, Suite 103
Studio City, CA 91604-3147
(800) 325-CICC

CICC's Los Ninos Bien Educados
Description: Program offering assistance
to Spanish-speaking and Latino origin
parents to effectively provide social skill
development and assist with academic
success.
Publisher: National Parenting Instructors
  Association

11331 Ventura Boulevard, Suite 103
Studio City, CA 91604-3147
(800) 325-CICC

The Parent Project
Description: This project is designed to
address critical issues of parenting today
through multilevel instruction, self-help
parent groups, and behavioral
interventions with destructive adolescent
behavior.
Publisher: Alternative Resources
2848 Longhorn Street
Ontario, CA 91761
(800) 897-0219

D. Community Resources

National School Safety Center
Description: Publications, resources, and
consultation on the promotion of safe
campuses.
4165 Thousand Oaks Boulevard,
  Suite 290
Westlake Village, CA 91362
(805) 373-9977
Ron Stevens, Director

Appendix

Guide to Policy Development

The American Medical Association
(AMA) created the AMA National Coalition
on Adolescent Health in 1987 as a forum
for multidisciplinary, coordinated activities
on behalf of youth in the United States. This
policy statement was developed by survey-
ing numerous national organizations. The
result of this survey is presented as part of
the Policy Compendium on Violence and
Adolescents: Intentional Injury and Abuse.
This policy statement is an excellent model
statement for organizations who wish to
draft policy recommendations on violence
(American Medical Association, 1993).

Model Policy Recommendations on Violence and Adolescents: Intentional Injury and Abuse[a]

WHEREAS violence is considered to be a public health problem in the general population and among adolescents; and

WHEREAS violence produces deleterious short-term and long-term effects on the physical and mental health of adolescents; and

WHEREAS adolescent victims and perpetrators of violence and abuse have health care needs which are specific to their age and developmental status; and

WHEREAS physicians and other health care providers have a critical role to play in the prevention of violence, and in the screening and treatment of adolescent victims of violence; and

WHEREAS health and social service providers have a responsibility to advocate on behalf of adolescents to reduce their risk of being victims or perpetrators of violent behaviors, and the detrimental effects associated with these violent acts; and

WHEREAS insufficient data exist on the causes and correlates of violence, the prevention of violence, and the effectiveness of violence prevention programs; therefore be it:

Resolved That:

1. The prevention of violence which affects the adolescent population should be a primary concern of adolescent health care professionals.

2. Protocols which address the health needs of adolescent victims and perpetrators of violence should be developed and disseminated to medical, education, and allied health professionals who work with youth. Protocols for the prevention of violence should also be developed.

3. Health and social service professionals should receive training to develop the skills necessary for the identification, assessment, and treatment of adolescent victims of violence and their perpetrators.

4. Health care providers, social service professionals, and educators have an obligation to report incidents of abuse involving adolescents and to ensure that follow-up is done in a coordinated, conscientious way which is sensitive to the developmental and individual needs of adolescents.

5. Multidisciplinary and multiagency efforts which effectively meet the physical, mental health, social, and legal needs of adolescent victims and perpetrators of violence should be systematically coordinated.

6. National, state, and local surveillance systems should be developed which monitor the prevalence of violent acts involving adolescents. Information from these systems should be used to promote the effective delivery of services to adolescent victims and perpetrators of violence.

7. Research must be conducted to identify various strategies to prevent violence against adolescents, and treat adolescent victims of violence. Similar efforts should be made to find strategies which help to deter adolescents from perpetrating violence, and treat adolescents who engage in violent behaviors. Implementation of successful strategies should be actively promoted by medical, public health, social service, juvenile justice, and education professionals.

8. Minors' unsupervised access to and use of firearms and other weapons are not supported.

---

a. The model policy statement is presented for organizations who wish to draft policy recommendations on violence. It does not represent or imply endorsement by any of the organizations affiliated with the AMA National Coalition on Adolescent Health.

9. Youth should not be subjected to corporal punishment or other forms of abuse in schools, mental health facilities, detention centers, or other community institutions which serve adolescents.

10. Efforts should be made to eliminate media presentations which depict excessive violence, glamorize violent acts, or encourage violent behaviors. Media presentations which portray positive, nonviolent conflict resolutions should be promoted.

11. Adequate funding should be allocated for training, research, and program development in violence prevention affecting adolescents. Training, research, and violence prevention programs should take into account alcohol, substance abuse, and other factors which are associated with many acts of violence and abuse. Efforts should be made to implement exemplary programs in other communities.

12. Legislation and regulations on violence should consider and address the needs of adolescents.

References

American Medical Association. (1993). *Policy compendium on violence and adolescents: Intentional injury and abuse* (J. E. Gans & K. L. Shook, Eds.). Chicago: Author.

Apter, S. J., & Popper, C. A. (1986). Ecological perspective on youth violence. In S. J. Apter & A. J. Goldstein (Eds.), *Youth violence, program, and prospects* (pp. 140-159). New York: Pergamon.

Bastian, L. D., & Taylor, B. M. (1991). *School crime—A national victimization survey report* (NCJ-131645). Washington, DC: U.S. Department of Justice.

Black, T. (1983). Coalition building: Some suggestions. *Child Welfare, 62,* 263-268.

Blythe, B. J., Tracy, E. M., Kotovsky, A., & Gwatkin, S. (1992). Organizational supports to sustain intensive family preservation program. *Families in Society, 73*(8), 463-470.

Brown, C. R. (1984). *The art of coalition building: A guide for community leaders.* New York: The American Jewish Committee.

Bush, G. B., et al. (1990). Adolescents who kill. *Journal of Clinical Psychology, 46*(4), 472-485.

California Department of Justice. (1994). *Gangs: A community response.* Sacramento: Office of the Attorney General.

Callahan, C. M., & Rivara, F. P. (1992, June 10). Urban high school youth and handguns: A school-based survey. *Journal of the American Medical Association, 267*(22), 3038-3041.

The Carter Center. (1994). *Uniting to wage peace: Scholastics' annual summit of youth violence.* Atlanta, GA: Author.

Centers for Disease Control. (1992). Position papers from the Third National Injury Control Conference: Setting the national agenda for injury control in the 1990s. Atlanta, GA: Author.

Centers for Disease Control and Prevention. (1993). *Adolescent health: State of the nation: Mortality trends, causes of death, and related risk behaviors among U.S. adolescents* (Monograph Series No. 1, CDC Publication No. 099-4122). Atlanta, GA: Author.

Children's Defense Fund. (1995). *The state of American children yearbook.* Washington, DC: Author.

Contra Costa Health Services Department. (1995). *Preventing violence in Contra Costa County: A countywide action plan.* Available from author at 75 Santa Barbara Road, Pleasant Hill CA 94523. (510) 646-6511; Fax (510) 646-6520.

Denicola, J., & Sandler, J. (1980). Training abusive parents in child management and self-control skills. *Behavior Therapy, 11*(2), 263-270.

Feighery, E., & Rogers, T. (1989). *Building and maintaining effective coalitions* (Guide No. 12 in the series How To Guides on Community Health Promotion). Palo Alto, CA: Stanford Health Promotion Resource Center.

Forouzesh, M. R., & Watjen, D. (1993). *Project Yes! Evaluation report.* Unpublished report, Orange County Department of Education, Costa Mesa, CA.

Fulwood, S. (1993, July 20). 59% of the school children surveyed say handguns are easy to get. *Los Angeles Times.*

Garbarino, J., Dubrow, N., Kostelny, K., & Pardo, C. (1992). *Children in danger: Coping with the consequences of community violence.* San Francisco: Jossey-Bass.

Hawkins, D. J. (1994). *Communities that care: Advocating communities to reduce risks for health and behavior problems.* Available from University of Washington, Proceeding of the workshop E1, DRP, Inc., 130 Nickerson, Suite 107, Seattle, WA 98109. (800) 736-2630, Fax (206)286-1462. (Need permission to print)

Hill, E. (1995). Juvenile crime: Outlook for California. Sacramento: Legislative Analyst's Office.

Hochhaus, C., & Sousa, F. (1988). Why children belong to gangs: A comparison of expectations and reality. *The High School Journal, 71*(2).

Institute for Educational Leadership. (1994, January 24). *Sad statistics.* Sacramento: EDCAL, Association of California Administrators.

Kellermann, A. L., Rivara, F. P., Rushforth, N. B., Banton, J. G., & Reay, D. T. (1993, October). Gun ownership as a risk factor for homicide in the home. *New England Journal of Medicine.* pp. 1084-1091.

Lauritsen, J. L., Laub, H. H., & Sampson, R. J. (1992). Conventional and delinquent activities: Implications for the prevention of violent victimization among adolescents. *Violence and Victims, 7*(2), 91-105.

Linquanti, R., & Berliner, B. (1994). *Rebuilding schools as safe havens: A topology for selecting and integrating violence prevention strategies.* San Francisco: Western Regional Center for Drug-Free Schools and Communities.

McLeroy, K., Bibeau, D., Steckler, A., & Glanz, K. (1988). An ecological perspective on health promotion programs. *Health Education Quarterly, 15,* 351-377.

Mercy, J. A., & O'Carroll, P. W. (1988). New directions in violence prediction: The public health arena. *Violence and Victims, 3,* 285-301.

Minkler, M. (1989). Health education, health promotion and the open society: An historical perspective. *Health Education Quarterly, 16,* 17-30.

National Center for Education in Maternal and Child Health. (1992). *Firearms facts: Guns in schools.* Washington, DC: Author.

National Research Council. (1993). Summary. In A. J. Reiss, Jr., & J. A. Roth (Eds.), *Understanding and preventing violence* (pp. 1-27). Washington, DC: National Academy Press.

Noguera, P. (1995). *Reducing and preventing youth violence: An analysis of cause and assessment of successful program.* Berkeley, CA: The California Wellness Foundation.

Pacific Center for Violence Prevention. (1993). *Preventing youth violence: Reducing access to firearms.* Policy paper, Preventing Handgun and Violence Against Kids: A Public Education Campaign, 454 Las Gallinas Avenue, Suite 177, San Rafael, CA 94903 (415) 331-3337.

Project Yes! (1993) *Gang violence and drug prevention curriculum K2-7* (Funded by the Governor's Office of Criminal Justice Planning). Costa Mesa, CA: Orange County Department of Education.

Prothrow-Stith, D. (1991). *Deadly consequences: How violence is destroying our teenage population and a plan to begin solving the problem.* New York: HarperCollins.

Rice, D. P., & McKenzi, E. J. (1989). *Cost of injury in the United States: A report to Congress.* San Francisco: Institute for Health and Aging; and Baltimore, MD: Johns Hopkins University.

Roberts-De Gennaro, M. (1986, July/August). Building coalitions for political advocacy. *Social Work,* pp. 308-311.

Rosenberg, M. L., & Mercy, J. A. (1991). Introduction. In M. L. Rosenberg & M. A. Fenley (Eds.), *Violence in America: A public health approach* (pp. 3-13). New York: Oxford University Press.

Sheahan, P. M. (Ed.). (1991). *Health care of incarcerated youth: Report from the 1991 tri-regional workshops —Executive summary.* Washington, DC: National Center for Education in Maternal and Child Health.

Sheley, J. F., McGee, Z. T., & Wright, J. D. (1992). Gun-related violence in and around inner-city schools. *American Journal of Diseases of Children, 146,* 677-682.

Spergel, I. A., Curry, D., Ross, R., & Chance, R. (1990). *Survey of youth gang problems and programs in 45 cities and six sites.* Chicago: University of Chicago.

Steinberg, J. B., et al. (1992). *Urban America: Policy choices for Los Angeles and the nation.* Santa Monica, CA: Rand.

Stephens, R. D. (1994). Gangs, guns, and school violence. *USA Today Magazine, 122*(2584), 29-32.

U.S. Department of Justice. (1991). *School crime: A national crime victimization survey report* (NCJ-131645). Washington, DC: Author.

U.S. Department of Justice. (1995a). *Guide for implementing the comprehensive strategy for serious, violent, and chronic juvenile offenders.* Washington, DC: Author.

U.S. Department of Justice. (1995b). *National Institute of Justice: Research in action.* Washington, DC: Author.

White, J. A. (1995). Violence prevention in school: Teaching ideas. *Journal of Health Education, 26*(1), 52-53.

13

Family and Dating Violence

Judy Kaci
Harvey Morley
Therese Morley

Definition and Statement of the Problem

In 1985, the Surgeon General of the United States identified domestic violence as a major nationwide health problem. Despite the resulting awareness of violence as a nationwide public health concern, support for an integrated multiple agency attack on the problem has been difficult to find. In a 1994 editorial for the *Journal of the American Medical Association,* Christoffel wrote that "[not only does violence] deserve more attention . . . [but it] poses a disproportionate current and future burden [on society]" (pp. 539-542). Its prevalence enables it to be categorized as a chronic danger affecting the physiological, psychological, and sociological development of families in general and adolescents in particular (Garbarino, Kostelny, & Dubrow, 1991, pp. 376-382). Often, as a result of family violence, the "innocence of youth" is turned into the fight for survival.

Since 1976, the number of adolescents categorized as maltreated has continued to rise (Oreskovich & ten Bensel, 1991, p. 358). Although this is easily attributable to an increase in simple assault rates (Moone, as cited in Office of Juvenile Justice and Delinquency Prevention, 1995), the problem is far more complex. Something is happening, and adolescents are being affected. One explanation is that adolescents are often caught behind walls of darkness. The walls may be erected intentionally. In more instances than not, they are the product of culturally initiated moral codes that contribute to the cycle of violence. As a result, family members' actions against teens can be easily shielded from the eyes of outsiders, often with devastating consequences.

Adolescents have been called the missing persons of the family violence literature (Gelles, 1987). This chapter will assist those that are involved with teenagers in identifying adolescents who are victims of violence in family and dating relationships. The recognition that a problem exists is the first step in correcting a grievous error that has been perpetuated through the history of this country.

Background

Even a cursory look at U.S. history clearly illustrates the fact that violence, initiated by groups and individuals, has been an inherent part of its development. The Boston Tea Party, categorized by most historians as an orchestrated response against an intolerable set of conditions, is clearly a classic example of group violence. Less overt yet equally aggressive acts, deemed acceptable at the time, commonly occurred against women, children, and other segments of the population.

Gustave LeBon, one of the first theorists of human behavior, identified these violent acts by groups of normally peaceful people as a phenomenon where individuals "[misplaced] their sensibilities, *forfeited their mind to the crowd* [italics added] and lost their sense of reason. Even educated people [under specific conditions] become simple minded and irrational in its influence" (LeBon as cited in Bartol, 1991, p. 240). Acts that most people now look upon with disdain were common. Forays against Native Americans, designed to eliminate their presence (if not their total existence) in specific areas of the country, were frequent occurrences. Similarly, African slaves, some of whom appeared in Virginia as early as 1619, continued to be subjected, collectively as well as individually, to various forms of violence (Wood, 1993, p. 19). Throughout the country, violence against women, children, the elderly and infirm, and the mentally ill occurred on a regular basis.

Slowly the lack of recognition that violence within the family unit was a cause for concern began to change. In the early 1870s, shortly after family violence was identified as a social problem, wife beating became illegal. Organizations already dedicated to assisting children expanded their focus to encompass wife abuse (Glazer, 1993, p. 179). Yet, despite these advances, the plight of adolescents still went unrecognized.

Tides of immigrants sweeping across the United States made the creation of less violent norms more difficult. Individuals from many countries brought not only the customs of their homelands and cultures, but patterns of behavior approved in their cultures. Some of these were not considered acceptable in their new country. This fact, along with the extreme ethnocentrism and religious prejudice confronting emigres, set the stage, in many instances, for acts of violence in the home, on the job, and within the community. Many of these issues still confront our multicultural society.

We can say, with a reasonable amount of certainty, that a portion of the problem associated with family violence is attributable to changes within our society. As illustrated in Figure 13.1, several factors contribute to this phenomenon.

Changes may affect a family either directly or indirectly. As an example, the loss of a job may create a stressful atmosphere conducive to violent behavior. Similarly, an indirect cause of violence may be as basic as an unpopular political decision. Social, economic, political, and technological changes with impact at the local, state, and national levels eventually affect the family unit. In addition, seemingly independent changes may affect one another.

Three possible outcomes of change agents on the family unit exist. First, the family may react in a supportive manner. Second, there may be no reaction. Third, there may be a direct and violent effect focused on vulnerable family members. According to Belsky's *ecologically integrative model of child abuse,* an indirect result of this violence may be negative behavior on the part of an adolescent (Oreskovich & ten Bensel, 1991, pp. 365-366). Figure 13.1 presents examples of change agents that may contribute to this syndrome.

No location is immune from violence, whether it be the workplace, where violence has reached unprecedented levels, or a high school campus. Throughout today's society,

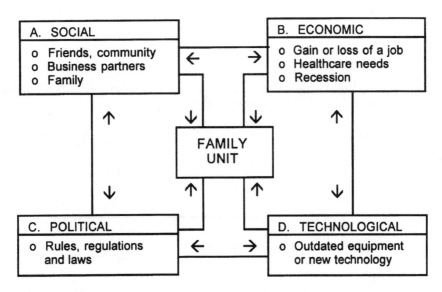

Figure 13.1. Changes Affecting the Family Unit

SOURCE: Developmental Research and Programs, Inc., as cited in Hawkins, 1995.

violence is constantly present, prompting some to say that "violence has [now] reached epidemic proportions, requiring all of us to fundamentally change the way we run our lives, because we now feel insecure about our physical safety and the well-being of our families" (Biden, 1994, pp. 322-325). Roth (1994) expressed it in this manner: "No statistics fully capture the devastating effects of violence on local communities—their economies, neighborhoods, and the quality of life" (p. 4). One must question how much of this is due to actions that were previously condoned or ignored that have now taken on a new meaning.

Family Violence

A few teens will report being abused by family members; most will not. Some are in a state of denial; others have been threatened with dire consequences if they tell; many are too embarrassed to admit being abused. Victims who are confronted may lie about the cause of their injuries and/or who inflicted

them. For these reasons, it is important that family members, teachers, health care professionals, youth workers, police, and others who interact with teens be aware of both physical and behavioral indicators of family and dating violence. For example:

A high school teacher noticed a student with a black eye and asked what happened; the student replied that his father hit him because he failed a math test.

A guidance counselor noticed bruises and inquired what caused them; the student reluctantly replied that her boyfriend hit her when she refused to have sex.

A recreation leader noticed a girl had on unusually heavy makeup, which poorly concealed a bruised cheek and asked what was wrong; the girl replied her mother hit her because she came home too late after a date.

A coach noticed a boy having difficulty throwing a football and asked how he injured his shoulder; the boy replied that he tried to protect his mother from being hit by her abusive boyfriend and was slammed into a wall.

A caseworker interviewing a pregnant teen who was applying for food stamps learned the girl was a victim of date rape.

Characteristic	Application	Potential Outcome
Time at risk	• Family members spend more time with each other than with nonfamily members	• Increased potential for stress and violent outbursts
Range of interests and impinging activities	• Numerous shared activities in which members must accommodate each other's interests	• Conflict, resentment, and anger
Intensity of involvement and knowledge of social biography	• Quality of involvement results in members knowing each other's strengths and weaknesses	• Increased ability to inflict severe emotional pain; heightened sensitivity to insults
Right to influence	• Opinions of some members, usually the parents, are considered more important	• Ability to control behavior of others may lead to resentment and violent outbursts
Ascribed roles	• Society assigns roles in family based on traditional stereotypes	• People may assume roles for which they are not suited
Privacy	• Many activities occur "behind closed doors"	• Ability of outsiders to intervene when crisis occurs is limited
Involuntary membership	• Family membership is based on biology or marital relationship of adults	• Individuals who are not compatible may be forced to live together

Figure 13.2.   Characteristics of the Family That Contribute to Domestic Violence
SOURCE: Modified from Gelles and Straus (1979).

A doctor questioned a boy after blood tests revealed he had an STD; the doctor learned that the boy's father had been forcing him to have sex with him for several years.

All of these examples have two things in common: someone became aware of the symptoms of abuse, and that person took the time to find out what had happened.

One of the problems in working with family violence and associated problems is that the terminology varies with the discipline that is studying it. For example, criminal law applies the word *incest* to cases of sexual intercourse between two people who are within the same blood line, but the therapeutic community uses the same term to include all forms of sexual contact between a child and an adult member of the household and extended family. For the purpose of this chapter, the following definitions will be used:

Physical abuse: Any use of force against a teen by an adult who is a member of the family or household that results in physical injuries. Physical abuse, as used here, does not include sexual assaults.

Incest: Sexual contact with a juvenile by any member of the family, including stepparents and unrelated adults living in the household.

Sibling abuse: Physical force used between children living in the same home except in self-defense. Sexual contact between siblings is included in incest.

Structural Aspects of Families That Make Them Susceptible to Violence

The family is a unique social institution. Ideally, it forms the basis for a warm, intimate, and supportive environment. Despite this, the potential for violence in the family is ever present. Ironically, many of the same features that give the family the ability to nurture can also trigger violence. Figure 13.2 shows how these characteristics of family life contribute to physical abuse.

The second National Family Violence Survey, conducted in 1985, involved a representative sample of 6,002 households (Straus & Gelles, 1988). *Violence* was defined to include intentional acts ranging from push-

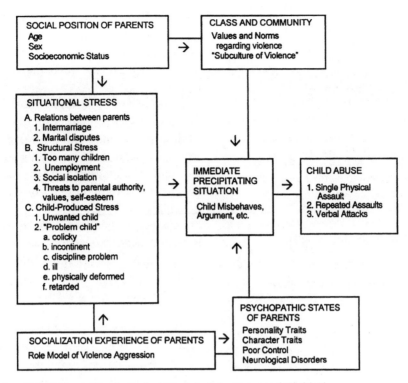

Figure 13.3. Gelles's Social Psychological Model of the Causes of Child Abuse

SOURCE: Based on Gelles (1973). Reprinted with permission from Richard Gelles and from the *American Journal of Orthopsychiatry.* Copyright 1973 by the American Orthopsychiatric Association, Inc.

ing, shoving, slapping, or spanking to using a knife or gun. *Severe violence* included acts beyond the range of reasonable child discipline that have a relatively high probability of causing injuries: kicking, biting, punching, hitting with an object, scalding, threatening with or using a knife or gun. Parents in 340 out of 1,000 households used violence at least once during the preceding year against children ages 15 to 17; the corresponding figure for severe violence was 70 out of 1,000 households.

Teens as Victims

Human nature is so complex that behavioral research rarely, if ever, establishes one-to-one relationships. It is not surprising, therefore, that family violence studies have not found that everyone who is raised in a home

where one parent physically abused the other grows up to abuse his/her spouse. Similarly, it has not been established that every child who was the victim of incest or other sexual abuse becomes a child molester in adult life. Some studies have shown, however, that a higher than expected proportion of wife beaters grew up in homes where the father physically abused the mother (Smith & Williams, 1992); an unusually high number of sexual predators who target children were sexually abused during their childhood (Finkelhor, 1986, pp. 117-118).

Gelles (1973) postulates that incidents of child abuse are the result of six factors: situational stress, socialization experience, psychopathic states, social position of parents, class and community, and the immediate precipitating situation. Figure 13.3 shows how these factors interrelate.

Color	Time Lapse After Impact
Red	First 6 hours
Blue	6-12 hours
Black-blue	Begins 12-24 hours after impact and lasts several days
Dark green tint	4-6 days
Pale green	5-7 days
Yellow/orange	7-10 days
Brown	10-14 days

Figure 13.4. Determining the Age of a Bruise
SOURCE: Mead, Balch, and Maggio (1985).

Physical Abuse of Adolescents

Statistics indicate that infants and toddlers are the most common victims of child abuse; teenagers rank second. Rebelliousness, poor school performance, and arguments over dating and curfews lead to conflicts in which physical force may be used against them. Parents whose main method of discipline is spanking do not automatically stop as the child grows older. Greater amounts of force are often used to "get the attention" of unresponsive teens. Although reasonable force may be used for disciplinary purposes, parents sometimes cross the line and go beyond what is acceptable. In addition to misguided attempts at discipline, teens may also be the victims of unprovoked attacks by adults or siblings living in the household.

Physical indicators. Bruising is the most obvious indicator of physical abuse. A single bruise may be easily explained. Multiple bruises in various stages of healing indicate the injuries were not inflicted at the same time and raise serious questions of repeated abuse. The color of bruises, indicated in Figure 13.4, can be used to determine approximately when the injury was inflicted. Coloration will also vary depending on the severity of the blow that caused the injury, how easily the person bruises, and whether the injury is located in soft tissue or over a bony area. Bruises may

indicate the type of object that caused them. For example, there may be an imprint of a hand, clothes hanger, or belt buckle; a beating with a belt may leave welts the width of the belt.

Other types of injuries may indicate possible abuse. External injuries to be aware of include first-, second-, and third-degree burns, cuts, bite marks, bald spots indicating severe hair pulling, and trauma to external genitalia or other portions of the body. Internal injuries or symptoms that may indicate abuse include broken bones, frequent complaints of soreness, awkward movements associated with pain, frequent urinary infections, and unexplained tenderness and/or swelling of the extremities, trunk, and cranial area.

Behavioral indicators of abuse. An adolescent's behavior may provide clues that physical abuse occurred. Symptoms may include overreacting to being touched in any way; provoking encounters of abusive treatment from adults as well as from peers; extremes in behavior—either great hostility and aggressiveness or withdrawal; assaultive, aggressive, or pugnacious behavior; appearing to be overly frightened of parents; and acting out continually or being incorrigible.

Investigating suspected abuse. Discovering that an adolescent has symptoms of abuse should trigger further investigation. Although injuries may have an innocent explanation, such as a skateboard accident, it is important to obtain statements from both the parent(s) and teen, and then determine if they are corroborated by the physical evidence. Inconsistencies, such as those in Figure 13.5, should alert you to possible physical abuse.

As critical as it is to treat any physical injury that may exist, it is equally important to try to determine what may have been the rationale for inflicting it. Valuable information can be gained by reading a social history of the family or, if that is unavailable, by speaking to indi-

Inconsistencies in the history obtained from parent(s) and teen
Discrepancy between parents' account of injuries and physical findings
Parent's reluctance to describe the circumstances surrounding the injury
Parent's denial of any knowledge of how injury occurred
Blame on sibling for the injury
Significant delay in seeking medical attention
Past history of numerous injuries
Parent's bypass of conveniently located hospitals to obtain emergency care for the teen at facility where the family is unknown
Inappropriate response to severity of injury by parent, such as underreacting or overreacting to teen's condition

Figure 13.5. Explanations of Injuries Consistent With Physical Abuse

SOURCE: Adapted from Kelley (1988).

Parent was abused as a child
Parent has unrealistic expectations regarding the teen
Parental stress including insufficient income, inadequate housing, loss of job
Social isolation
Role reversal
Poor self-image
Delay in maternal-infant bonding
Overpunishment
Lack of education or experience in child rearing
Rejection
Mirror image
Substance abuse
Family discord and/or broken family
Mental health problems
Spouse abuse
Police record (excluding traffic)
Lack of tolerance for teen's disobedience and provocation
Loss of control during discipline
Incapacity due to physical handicap or chronic illness
Authoritarian method of discipline

Figure 13.6. Family Factors Contributing to Physical Abuse, Neglect, and Incest

SOURCE: Adapted from Mead & Balch (1987).

vidual family members. Figure 13.6 identifies items that are potential contributors to physical abuse, neglect, and incest.

Incest

Incest is often identified as the last taboo. Refusing to talk about it, however, does not prevent it from occurring. Figures on the prevalence of incest vary widely, largely due to underreporting and the use of different definitions. In many cases, incest begins before the teen years and continues sporadically for a long period. Girls ages 8 to 12 are at highest risk, but boys are also victimized. Even if abuse has stopped before adolescence, emotional scars may result in mental health problems for the teens involved. Some will also suffer long-term medical problems as a result of pregnancy and/or STDs contracted during the incestuous relationship.

Numerous studies have tried to determine the prevalence of sexual abuse of children. Findings indicate that from 6% to 62% of females and 3% to 31% of males are sexually abused before the age of 18 (Finkelhor, 1986). These figures include incidents of incest as well as molestation by non-family members. The large variation in study findings is a result of differences in research design: how the sample was selected; definition of sexual abuse; how the questionnaire was administered; and the number, sequence, and specificity of questions asked.

Models explaining why people become incest perpetrators are rare. Finkelhor's *four preconditions model of sexual abuse* postulates that four preconditions must exist simultaneously before a person sexually abuses children: (a) motivation to sexually abuse, (b) overcoming of internal inhibitions against abusing, (c) overcoming of external obstacles against abusing, and (d) overcoming resistance by the child. If Preconditions 1 and 2 do not exist, the person will not sexually abuse children, even if Preconditions 3 and 4 are fulfilled (Finkelhor, 1986, pp. 86-87). Conversely, incest and other forms of sexual abuse of children can be deterred by making Precon-ditions 3 and 4 more difficult to achieve.

Numerous studies have been published that attempted to identify characteristics of people who sexually abuse children and teens. Several factors emerged: (a) sexual abusers show an unusual pattern of sexual arousal toward chil-dren, although no substantiated theory exists about why this is so; (b) molesters are blocked in their social and heterosexual relationships; (c) alcohol is well established as a disinhibiting factor that plays a role in a great many sexual abuse offenses; (d) children, because of their lack of dominance, have special meaning for pedophiles; and (e) many sexual abusers were themselves victims of abuse when they were children (Finkelhor, 1986, pp. 117-118). The most promising predictor, that abusers were themselves sexually abused as children, applies only to a small percentage of children (mostly boys) who have been molested. The larger question, why the majority of victims do not grow up to be abusers, remains unanswered.

The failure of research to isolate unique characteristics of this type of sexual predator has resulted in a focus on identifying children who are at greatest risk. Studies of sexually abused children indicate that preadolescent girls with few childhood friends are at greatest risk. Girls that are victimized are (a) more likely to have lived without their natural fa-thers, (b) more likely to have mothers who were employed outside the home, (c) more likely to have mothers who were disabled or ill, (d) more likely to witness conflict between their parents, and (e) more likely to report a poor relationship with one of their parents. Girls who lived with stepfathers were also at increased risk for abuse (Finkelhor, 1986, p. 79).

A number of studies agree that repeated in-cest experiences with the same perpetrator are more traumatic than single incidents. Abuse by fathers or stepfathers appears to be more traumatic than by other perpetrators. The use of physical force seems to clearly result in more trauma for the victim. Sexual abuse by

---

Physical appearance of teen

Torn, stained, or bloody underclothing

Pain or itching in the genital area

Bruises on or bleeding in external genitals, vaginal, anal, or oral regions

Swollen or red cervix, vulva, perineum, or anus

Semen about mouth, genitals, or on clothing

Pregnancy

Sexually transmitted disease

Behavior of teen

Withdrawn or engages in fantasy or infantile behavior

Poor peer relationships

Unwilling to participate in physical activities

Engages in delinquent acts or runs away

States he/she has been sexually assaulted by a parent or caretaker

Displays one or more of the following: anxiety, withdrawal, guilt, somatic complaints, sleep problems, substance abuse, suicide attempts, tics, aggression, acting-out disorders, or hostility

Low self-esteem

Figure 13.7. Indicators of Incest

SOURCE: Adapted from "Incest: The Last Taboo (Conclusion)." *FBI Law Enforcement Bulletin*, 53(2), February 1984); author credits Noreen M. Grella; Finkelhor (1986).

---

male adults was more traumatic than similar assaults by women or teenaged males. The prognosis was worse when the families were unsupportive of the victim and/or the victim was removed from his/her home (Finkelhor, 1986, p. 175).

Indicators of incest. Delayed reporting by victims of incest is common and frequently re-sults in a lack of evidence of recent violence, such as bleeding and torn clothing. Despite de-lays in reporting, bruises to the body as well as genitalia may be present in forced encoun-ters. Less violent encounters, such as cases where victims capitulate out of fear rather than physical violence, may result in less ob-vious evidence. A variety of other physical fac-tors, such as those in Figure 13.7, may be pre-sent. Characteristics of families where incest is most likely to occur were included in Figure 13.6. Individuals that are suspected of being the victims of incest should be monitored by both medical and mental health practitioners for an extended period of time. Aftermaths that may require intervention by professionals include STDs, pregnancy, and depression.

Teens who have been victims of sexual abuse frequently display some of the behavioral symptoms shown in Figure 13.7. One study of 7- to 13-year-olds who had been sexually abused found that 40% showed signs of serious mental disturbances in the 2 years following the incident; 36% showed signs of disturbed sexual behavior (Finkelhor, 1986, pp. 148, 151). Without therapy, these symptoms are likely to persist even though the abuse has stopped. Some symptoms, particularly arguing with parents and siblings, fear of the offender, and worry, may become worse over time. Adult women who were victimized as children but received no therapeutic intervention are likely to manifest depression, self-destructive behavior, anxiety, feelings of isolation and stigma, poor self-esteem, a tendency toward revictimization, and substance abuse (Finkelhor, 1986, p. 162).

Teens as Perpetrators

Many individuals contend that siblings in all families occasionally hit each other. The physical strength of teens increases the potential for injuries from such conduct; it also enables them to commit incest more easily. Both problems are compounded by the lower level of supervision afforded teens and the use of teens to watch younger siblings. Teenage parents, particularly those who were abused during their own childhoods, may be the perpetrators of child abuse.

Physical Abuse

Physical violence used between children living in the same home is sibling abuse. The 1975 Family Violence Survey indicated that teens between 15 and 17 committed at least one act of violence against a brother or sister during the previous year in 640 out of 1,000 households; 360 out of 1,000 households reported severe violence between these siblings (Straus & Gelles, 1988).

Incest

Studies have found that from 6% to 33% of sexual abuse cases are committed by another juvenile in the family. Although many incidents are mutual exploration and end when children realize their behavior is inappropriate, some involve one sibling forcing another to participate (Pierce & Pierce, 1990). Adolescents perpetrating the latter type of sexual activity are likely to continue as sexual abusers in adulthood unless there is therapeutic intervention.

An Illinois study of 43 juveniles who committed incest found 39% of the victims were sisters (including step-, adoptive, and foster sister) living in the home; 21% were brothers (including step-, adoptive, and foster brother) living in the home; and 40% were related to the perpetrator (such as a cousin) but not living in the household. A large majority (81%) of the abusers were male. The offender was usually the oldest child of his/her sex living in the home or an only child. Various patterns appeared: 30% involved only one known offense; 16% involved multiple incidents that occurred frequently; in 30% of the cases, the abuse occurred infrequently over a long period of time; and in 24% of the cases, there were several offenses occurring over a short period of time. Multiple offense cases involved older adolescents, who were described as more dysfunctional than the perpetrators in other categories. The victim was usually younger than the abuser, with a 5-year age difference observed in 46% of the cases and a 10-year difference seen in 13%. The majority of offenders were described as aggressive toward family members, involved in other delinquent acts, and having academic problems. Over one third had behavioral problems at school. Many had been sexually victimized themselves (Pierce & Pierce, 1990).

Another study described juveniles who commit incest as typically loners with little skill in negotiating emotionally intimate peer relationships. Low self-esteem, coupled with deep-seated feelings of inadequacy and emptiness, contribute to the juvenile's inability to handle life's demands (Groth & Loredo, 1981).

Child Abuse by Teenage Parents

Teenage parents may be immature and unprepared for parenthood. Unwanted pregnancies and lack of financial resources compound the problem. This increases the risk that they will abuse their children. The tendency to pattern parenting skills after those observed in the family of origin makes teens who grew up in abusive homes prime candidates for abusing their children. Educators, health care professionals, and others who deal with young parents must be especially alert for signs of abuse.

Every effort should be made to teach appropriate parenting skills and encourage teens to seek assistance from resources that are available in the community. These teens must learn to recognize signs of building anger and frustration and how to defuse volatile emotions before violence erupts. Programs for pregnant teens as well as those providing assistance after birth need to emphasize this.

Mandatory Reporting Laws

All 50 states mandate that most professionals who deal with children report suspected abuse. These *mandatory reporters* usually include teachers, day care workers, doctors, nurses, paramedics, dentists, mental health professionals, social workers, and public safety employees (including police officers and probation officers). Film processors are frequently required to report any evidence of child pornography. Facts that raise a suspicion that a child has been physically or sexually abused or is being neglected usually trigger a duty to file a formal report; probable cause to arrest is not required. Many states require that the report of suspected abuse be telephoned to a central registry immediately and a written report follow within a few days. There may be two local agencies designated to handle the reports: law enforcement processes the case in criminal court, while a social work agency evaluates the need for intervention, including removing the child from the home, and proceeds with civil action necessary to do so.

Most state laws cover all unemancipated juveniles: Cases involving suspected abuse of teens usually must be reported. Everyone who works with teens should review the local child abuse reporting laws and make all necessary reports in a timely manner. Failure to comply with mandatory reporting requirements is usually a misdemeanor. Most states provide immunity from civil suit to anyone who in good faith reports suspected abuse.

Prevention Strategies

Everyone needs to be aware of the problems associated with family violence and incest. Specific prevention strategies must be designed that relate to target populations. Examples include parent education designed to reduce physical violence, training to help teachers recognize signs of abuse and report them to appropriate authorities, courses for physicians and nurses on recognizing symptoms of abuse, sensitivity training dealing with cultural interaction, and appropriate intervention strategies for other groups. Clearly, aiding victims in discovering ways to stop the abuse in their current situation and seek assistance is important.

Many teens believe their problem is unique and no one else has ever been abused in a similar manner. Most teens are unaware of resources that are available to help them deal with problems stemming from family violence and incest. Brochures listing referral sources should be made readily available at locations frequented by teens. All teachers, youth workers, health care practitioners, and guidance counselors should be provided with copies to give teens. Peer counselors should have copies to distribute. Bulletin boards, student newspapers, and locker rooms should be used as potential distribution points.

Those interacting with teens must be sensitized, through various modalities, to problems relating to family violence. Cultural differences, both in disciplinary and other areas, need to be dealt with in a sensitive manner. To this end, parent/teacher meetings and cultural awareness programs are useful.

Physical abuse by parents is a result, in part, of inadequate parenting skills. Reliance on measures observed in the family of origin perpetuates abuse from generation to generation. Many parents are unaware that what they are doing is not appropriate or that other disciplinary techniques can be effective. Referrals to parenting classes, including those offered by adult schools and community colleges, are useful. Addressing contributing problems, such as substance abuse and spouse abuse in the parents' relationship, is important.

Prevention strategies can take one or all of the following directions: education, intervention, or treatment. Service providers with teen clients must acquaint themselves with warning signs leading to family violence as well as indicators that abuse has taken place. Once it is confirmed that family violence is the source of the symptoms, intervention strategies can be launched. Evaluation must be ongoing so that strategy changes can be made if the observed results indicate variations are needed.

Issues related to physical and sexual abuse of teens by family members are easily incorporated into existing curriculum on child development and family living. Factors that should be addressed include the importance of age-appropriate discipline and effective alternatives to corporal punishment. Environ-

ments should be established that will encourage students to share the unique aspects of their culture with their peers. Properly used, role playing may assist in creating an atmosphere in which individuals from many cultures can learn important facts about controlling family violence.

Discussions about sexual abuse of children, including incest, can be incorporated into sex education courses taught in middle schools, high schools, and colleges. Suggested topics include the boundaries of appropriate sexual conduct between adults and children and a teen's right to control his/her own body and reject unwanted sexual advances. The physical and emotional consequences of incest should be covered. Role playing is also appropriate to familiarize teens with techniques they can use to fend off inappropriate advances and seek help.

Dating Violence

Teens in dating relationships face threats from their intimate acquaintances similar to those experienced by some married couples. Physical violence occurs; so does sexual assault. Most of the incidents involve slapping and shoving without causing bruises; some result in serious injuries. Any physical force used against a dating partner without consent, except in self-defense, is considered dating violence. Date rape refers to unwanted sexual intercourse forced upon the victim by a dating partner.

Dating violence	Any physical force used against a dating partner without consent, except in self-defense
Date rape	Unwanted sexual intercourse (vaginal, oral, or anal, including penetration with objects other than the penis) by a date using force, threat of force, or alcohol or drugs to obtain the victim's cooperation

| Sexual coercion | Unwanted sexual intercourse occurring after psychological pressure or because the date used his/her position or authority |

Some studies indicate that teens who grew up in homes where one parent battered the other were more frequently involved in violent dating relationships than those from non-abusive households. This was true for both the violent partner and the victim (Smith & Williams, 1992). An even higher proportion of those studied who were in violent dating relationships, however, had previously been involved in a violent relationship with a romantic partner (Sugarman & Hotaling, 1989).

Teens as Victims

Physical assault can occur on a first date or any time during the relationship. The attack may occur whenever the couple are together; it could be at school or work rather than while on a date. Date rape can also occur at any stage of the relationship.

Physical Abuse by Dating Partner

Studies have produced a wide range of prevalence figures for dating violence. Most of the early studies were conducted on college campuses, but some of the more recent ones were administered at high schools (Anderson, 1994; Sugarman & Hotaling, 1989). From 10% to 40% of students involved in the high school studies reported being subjected to physical assault by a dating partner. Teens involved in dating violence generally attributed the assault to love, anger, confusion, and sexual jealousy (Anderson, 1994; Sugarman & Hotaling, 1989).

Overall there was little difference between the frequency of attacks by males and females against a dating partner. When attacks did occur, females usually received the most serious injuries. Victims reported suffering emotional trauma even when there were no serious injuries, but few sought assistance. Nearly one third of the female victims of dating violence reported major emotional trauma; 12% of the males who had been victimized also reported this type of problem (Sugarman & Hotaling, 1989, p. 13). It appeared that there may be two different scenarios represented by these statistics: violent first dates, which invariably led to termination of the relationship; and violence after a relationship was established, in which case the violence was not seen as a reason to break up (Makepeace, 1989, p. 103).

Date Rape

Date rape has become a common term used to describe forced sex on a date. A related problem is sexual coercion, which includes unwanted sexual intercourse occurring after psychological pressure or because the date used his/her position or authority. Both of these topics have been ignored until recently. Reliable statistics on the number of date rapes and instances of sexual coercion involving teens are not available.

Most studies on date rape have been conducted among college students. One recent study at a midsize southern university found that 14% (1 in 7) of the women had been victims of date rape or attempted date rape prior to beginning their freshman year. About 11% had been victims of sexual coercion; and 13% were recipients of other unwanted sexual contact (kissing, fondling, etc.). Questions about unwanted sexual contact outside dating relationships revealed even higher levels of abuse: 10% had witnessed exhibitionism, 19% had been sexually fondled against their will, 7% reported attempted rapes, and 14% indicated they had been raped (Vogel & Himelein, 1995).

Rape victims frequently exhibit symptoms that have been characterized as the rape trauma syndrome, which is a form of posttraumatic stress disorder. Three short-range reactions to the ordeal are common: repeated

A. Reexperiencing of the rape as evidenced by at least one of the following:
   Recurrent and intrusive recollections of the event
   Recurrent dreams of the event
   Sudden acting or feeling as if the rape were reoccurring because of an association with an environmental or ideational stimulus

B. Numbing of responsiveness to, or reduced involvement with, the external world, beginning sometime after the rape, as shown by at least one of the following:
   Markedly diminished interest in one or more significant activities
   Feeling of detachment or estrangement from others
   Constricted affect

C. Presence of at least two of the following symptoms that were not present before the rape:
   Hyperalertness or exaggerated startle response
   Sleep disturbance
   Guilt about surviving when others have not, or about behavior required for survival
   Memory impairment or trouble concentrating
   Avoidance of activities that arouse recollection of the rape
   Intensification of symptoms by exposure to events that symbolize or resemble the rape

Figure 13.8. Diagnostic Criteria—Posttraumatic Stress Disorder as Applied to Rape
SOURCE: Adapted from Foley & Davies (1983).

washing in an attempt to feel clean, withdrawal from contact with even closest friends without telling them what happened, and delayed reporting of the incident. Whether the perpetrator was a stranger or a date, the victim frequently experiences many of the following symptoms: emotional shock, disbelief, embarrassment, self-blame, anxiety, fear, guarded behaviors, anger, emotional numbness, compulsive repetition, psychosomatic reactions, and a need to master and control (Foley & Davies, 1983, p. 93).

As the name implies, posttraumatic stress syndrome occurs after a traumatic event. Behavioral symptoms indicated in Figure 13.8 may occur long after the victim was believed to have recovered. Ignoring or downplaying the trauma because the assailant was a "friend"

instead of a stranger is a mistake. The potential for long-range impact on the life of the date rape victim underscores the need for therapeutic intervention by mental health professionals trained to work with sexual assault victims.

Teens as Perpetrators

Teens are frequently the perpetrators of dating violence or date rape against their peers. This in no way diminishes the seriousness of the problem. The paucity of research in this area, coupled with the fact that most offenses remain unreported, has made it hard to develop good profiles of teenage perpetrators.

Dating Violence

Sugarman and Hotaling (1989) reviewed published research on dating violence looking for risk markers that were found to be statistically significant in more than one study. Three risk markers appeared consistently in both dating violence and spouse abuse: high levels of male sexual aggression, high stress levels, and low income levels. Three factors associated with spouse abuse, however, were not found to be related to dating violence: low educational attainment, greater religious incompatibility, and witnessing marital violence as a child. Caution should be used before discounting educational attainment as a risk marker for dating violence, however, because most of the studies were conducted using college students and therefore were not representative samples.

Some, but not all, characteristics of dating relationships are similar to those found in marital situations. Riggs and O'Leary (1989) believe this necessitates a separate model to explain dating violence. Two separate components must be considered: factors that will cause a person to behave aggressively toward any dating partner in any situation and factors contributing to a person becoming aggressive

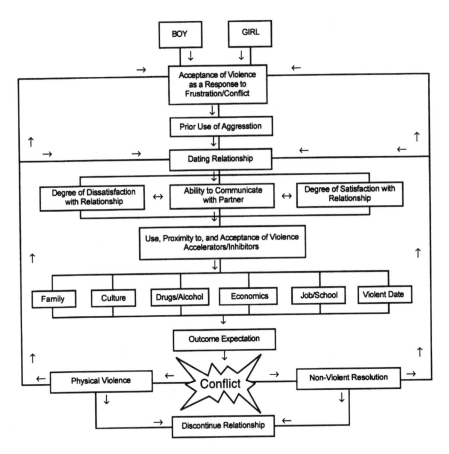

Figure 13.9. A Model of Potential Precipitators of Dating Violence

toward a partner in a specific situation. Potential contributors to violent behavior that practitioners should be aware of include

- Exposure to aggression in intimate relationships, particularly in the form of parents or other role models, increases the likelihood that a person will use aggressive means to solve conflict in a relationship.
- Parental aggression toward the child is thought to directly increase the likelihood of aggression in dating relationships and indirectly influence it through other constructs such as personality, acceptance of aggression, and general use of aggression.
- Acceptance of aggression as an appropriate response to conflict, frustration, or threat results in the person being more likely to be-

have aggressively both in general and in dating relationships.

- Psychopathology or neuropathology, although inadequately studied in the context of dating violence, have been shown to be causative factors in some forms of aggressions.
- Arousability and emotionality contribute to the occurrence of dating violence directly and by increasing the likelihood that aggression will be used more generally.
- Personality serves as a mediating variable between the historical constructs and the current use of aggression in the dating relationship.
- Prior use of aggression and coercion, whether against siblings, friends, or others, influences the frequency with which an individual acts aggressively toward a dating partner. (Riggs & O'Leary, 1989, pp. 58-63)

1 Factors that enhance motivation to sexually abuse	2 Factors that reduce internal inhibitions	3 Factors that reduce external inhibitions	4 Factors that reduce victim resistance
a. power and control needs b. miscommu- nication about sex c. sexual arousal d. emotional incongruence e. imbalance in power differential	a. attitudes □ traditional sex roles □ acceptance of violence □ endorsement of rape myths □ adversarial relationships b. prior abuse	a. date location b. mode of transportation c. date activity d. use of alcohol or drugs	a. passivity b. poor self defense technique/ strategy c. history of sexual abuse d. traditional attitudes e. poor sexual knowledge

Figure 13.10. Four Preconditions Model of Date Rape

SOURCE: Based on Paula Lundberg-Love & Robert Geffner (1989), "Date Rape: Prevalence, Risk Factors, and a Proposed Model," in M. A. Pirog-Good & Jan E. Stets (Eds.), *Violence in Dating Relationships* (pp. 169-184), New York: Praeger, an imprint of Greenwood Publishing Group, Inc., Westport, CT. Reprinted with permission.

Events associated with a current situation can be the catalyst that sets off the violent confrontation. Past experiences may have taught a person that aggressive behavior is an effective way to get what he/she wants. High stress levels also contribute. Being under the influence of alcohol or drugs during the argument increases the potential for a violent outburst. Dissatisfaction with the quality of the current relationship further lessens inhibitions against violence. Aggressive conduct by the partner cannot be ignored as a contributing factor. Figure 13.9 shows how all of these elements interact in a dating relationship.

Date Rape

Lundberg-Love and Geffner (1989) constructed a model to explain why individuals commit date rape. It starts with the rapist's motivations, both conscious and subconscious, and adds factors that reduce internal inhibitions against rape. The likelihood of rape escalates if two types of events occur simultaneously: a reduction in external inhibitions, such as being alone with the victim in an isolated location or the victim's intoxication; and fac-

tors that reduce the victim's ability to resist, such as lack of self-defense skills. Figure 13.10 depicts this model.

Mandatory Reporting Laws

Mentioning child abuse reporting laws triggers images of parents hitting small children. Many states, however, define child abuse to include all physical and sexual abuse of people under 18 years of age. When this is true, incidents of dating violence and date rape involving most teens must be reported. It is important to check local laws to determine if reports must be made when it is suspected that a teen has been victimized.

Prevention Strategies

Prevention programs for dating violence and date rape must focus on increasing the level of awareness of the problem. Any segment of the community that interacts with teens can be a vehicle. Existing programs should be reviewed to determine whether or not their information is current and appropriate for the age groups that will use it.

Interdependence of the various agencies and groups involved in these complex issues cannot be overemphasized. No single institution can adequately approach this problem independently. A task force composed of representatives from many local agencies is needed. Resources should be identified and achievable goals established.

Awareness campaigns can be staged on several fronts. Special events, such as Rape Awareness Week, can use posters, speakers from the community, and films. The local rape crisis hotline will be able to provide invaluable assistance. One of the strongest ingredients in a successful program for teens is peer involvement. Student organizations can sponsor many of the events. When constructing these programs it is important to have both males and females involved: Allowing it to be a "women's issue" will seriously diminish the program's effectiveness.

Teens are more likely to tell a friend about being abused than they are to report the incident to an adult. For this reason, it is important to make all teens aware of the issues of dating violence and date rape and not merely target suspected victims and abusers. Those who do seek adult assistance frequently pose the problem as if they are seeking help for a friend. Responses to all questions must display sensitivity to the potential needs of the abused teen.

Most teens are unaware of resources that are available to deal with problems stemming from dating violence and date rape. Brochures listing referral sources should be made readily available at locations frequented by teens. Many local merchants are willing to help defray the cost of printing these materials. All teachers, youth workers, health care practitioners, and guidance counselors should have copies to give teens. Peer counselors must have resource information readily available. Bulletin boards, student newspapers, and locker rooms are effective distribution points. Family planning clinics should also provide information on these topics.

Teachers and others who work with teens need to be alert for both physical and behavioral indicators of abuse. Issues of dating violence and date rape can be piggybacked onto training that is conducted about mandatory reporting of child abuse. Additional training should focus on making referrals for therapeutic intervention for the teens involved. Incorporating family and dating violence into the middle school and high school curriculum is crucial. Family living classes should include segments on dating violence and date rape. Date rape should be included as a topic in sex education courses. The physical, emotional, and legal consequences of date rape should be covered. "No means no" is an important idea to stress. Role playing and techniques to give teens experience in defusing violent situations and deflecting unwanted sexual advances are important to reinforce didactic explanations.

Communication and mutual respect in a relationship are important topics related to dating violence and date rape. Strategies to assist teens in acquiring and using a variety of skills for both verbal and nonverbal communication need to be emphasized. Improving communication skills by articulating one's own thoughts and listening to what the other person is saying will help deescalate situations that lead to physical violence. The "time out" technique, which allows a participant to call for a cooling off period when arguments become heated, and other similar measures should be included.

It is critical that prevention programs reflect the fact that both males and females need to understand the consequences of initiating violence. Teenage girls slap and otherwise abuse their dates at a rate equal to or greater than boys. This sets the stage for a violent response that may be particularly hazardous to girls who are smaller and/or weaker than the boys involved.

Self-defense classes need to address appropriate techniques for dating situations: a fear of strangers without awareness of the threat by intimates builds a false sense of security. Other crime prevention programs, such as those emphasizing installation of better locks in homes, also need to be revised for this reason.

Conclusions

Family and dating violence against teens may be difficult to spot and even harder to investigate. Nonetheless, the potential damage to the mental and physical health of the victims makes it imperative that action be taken. The issue must be approached from two directions: treating the victims and preventing future abuse.

Victims seldom report the abuse; in fact, many will deny it. The first step in intervention is to recognize symptoms of abuse. Many physical and behavioral indicators have been covered in this chapter to alert you to the problem. Referrals need to be made for appropriate professional treatment in order to prevent long-term physical and mental health problems. Strategies need to be developed to prevent reoccurrence of violence by the perpetrator. Therapy is frequently needed by the perpetrator to address root causes of violence and prevent future attacks. The fact that the couple has broken up does not eliminate the need for treatment: The violence is likely to surface again during future relationships.

"Tea and sympathy" for the victims will not solve the problem of family and dating violence. People must stop denying that family and dating violence exists and take action to stop it. Awareness campaigns are the first step in attacking underlying causes. All segments of the target population—teens, parents, and professionals who deal with them—must understand the issues involved. Awareness comes first, then changes in attitudes and finally modification of behavior. No "quick fix" will work. Commitment to long-range efforts is a key to reducing the prevalence of violent behavior in the family and dating relationships.

Resources

Many organizations can be called on to provide brochures, speakers, and films. Check your local telephone directory for organizations that can provide materials on physical and sexual abuse of teens:

Children's Protective Services
Parents Anonymous
For Kids Sake, Inc.
Parents United
Parental Stress Hotlines
Child Abuse Control Council
Junior League
National Center on Child Abuse and Neglect (NCCAN)
National Committee for the Prevention of Child Abuse (NCPCA)
The American Professional Society on the Abuse of Children (APSAC)
National Center for the Prosecution of Child Abuse

Local police officers, prosecutors, probation officers, and social workers who handle abused juveniles are also valuable resources. Battered women's shelters and counseling centers with programs for batterers provide excellent materials on dating violence. Rape hotlines and counseling centers are good resources for materials on date rape. Therapists who specialize in treating these cases are frequently eager to speak to groups.

References

Anderson, E. M. (1994). *Knowledge of and attitudes toward dating violence among college freshman.* Master's thesis at California State University, Long Beach.
Bartol, C. R. (1991). *Criminal behavior a psychosocial approach* (3rd ed.). Englewood Cliffs, NJ: Prentice Hall.
Biden, J. R., Jr. (1994). *Vital speeches of the day.* Mount Pleasant, SC: City News Publishing Co.

Christoffel, K. K. (1994). Editorial: Reducing violence—how do we proceed? *American Journal of Public Health, 84*(4), 539-541.

Finkelhor, D. (1986). *A sourcebook on child sexual abuse.* Beverly Hills, CA: Sage.

Foley, T. S., & Davies, M. A. (1983). *Rape: Nursing care of victims.* St. Louis: C. V. Mosby.

Garbarino, J., Kostelny, K., & Dubrow, N. (1991). What children can tell us about living in danger. *American Psychologist, 46*(4), 376-383.

Gelles, R. J. (1973, July). Child abuse as psychopathology: A sociological critiques and reformulation. *American Journal of Orthopsychiatry, 43,* 611-621.

Gelles, R. J. (1987). *Family violence* (2nd ed.). Newbury Park, CA: Sage.

Gelles, R. J., & Straus, M. (1979). Determinants of violence in the family: Toward a theoretical integration. In W. R. Burr et al. (Eds.), *Contemporary theories about the family* (Vol. 1, pp. 549-581). New York: Free Press.

Glazer, S. (1993). Violence against women–is the problem more serious than statistics indicate? *C Q Researcher, 3*(8), 171-190.

Groth, N., & Loredo, C. (1981). Juvenile sexual offenders: Guidelines for assessment. *International Journal of Offender Therapy and Comparative Criminology, 25,* 31-39.

Hawkins, J. D. (1995). *Controlling crime before it happens: Risk-focused prevention.* Rockville, MD: National Institute of Justice.

Lundberg-Love, P., & Geffner, R. (1989). Date rape: Prevalence, risk factors, and a proposed model. In M. A. Pirog-Good & J. E. Stets (Eds.), *Violence in dating relationships* (pp. 169-184). New York: Praeger.

Makepeace, J. (1989). Dating, living together, and courtship violence. In M. A. Pirog-Good & J. E. Stets (Eds.), *Violence in dating relationships: Emerging social issues* (pp. 94-107). New York: Praeger.

Mead, J. J., & Balch, G. M., Jr. (1987). *Child abuse and the church* (pp. 31-35). Costa Mesa, CA: HDL Publishing Co.

Mead, J. J., Balch, G. M., Jr., & Maggio, E. (1985). *Investigating child abuse.* Brea, CA: Volunteers For Kids Sake.

Office of Juvenile Justice and Delinquency Prevention. (1995). *Juvenile offenders and victims: A focus on violence* (NCJJ Publication No. 90-JN-CX-K003). Pittsburg, PA: National Center for Juvenile Justice.

Oreskovich, J., & ten Bensel, R. W. (1991). Maltreatment of adolescents. In W. R. Hendee (Ed.), *The health of adolescents: Understanding and facilitating biological, behavioral, and social development* (pp. 347-376). San Francisco: Jossey-Bass.

Pierce, L. H., & Pierce, R. L. (1990). Adolescent/sibling incest perpetrators. In A. L. Horton, B. L. Johnson, L. M. Roundy, & D. Williams (Eds.), *The incest perpetrator: A family member no one wants to treat* (pp. 99-107). Newbury Park, CA: Sage.

Riggs, D. S., & O'Leary, K. D. (1989). A theoretical model of courtship aggression. In M. A. Pirog-Good & J. E. Stets (Eds.), *Violence in dating relationships: Emerging social issues* (pp. 3-32). New York: Praeger.

Roth, J. A. (1994). *Understanding and preventing violence* (NCJ 145645). Washington, DC: U.S. Department of Justice, National Institute of Justice.

Smith, J. P., & Williams, J. G. (1992). From abusive household to dating violence. *Journal of Family Violence, 7,* 153-165.

Straus, M. A., & Gelles, R. J. (1988). How violent are American families? Estimates from the National Family Violence Resurvey and other studies. In G. T. Hotaling, D. Finkelhor, J. T. Kirkpatrick, & M. S. Straus (Eds.), *Family abuse and its consequences: New directions in research* (pp. 14-36). Newbury Park, CA: Sage.

Sugarman, D. B., & Hotaling, G. T. (1989). Dating violence: Prevalence, context, and risk markers. In M. A. Pirog-Good & J. E. Stets (Eds.), *Violence in dating relationships: Emerging social issues* (pp. 3-32). New York: Praeger.

Vogel, R. E., & Himelein, M. J. (1995). Dating and sexual victimization: An analysis of risk factors among pre-college women. *Journal of Criminal Justice, 23*(2), 153-162.

Wood, G. S. (1993). Founding of a nation 1786-1787. In Arthur M. Schlesinger (Ed.), *The almanac of American history* (pp. 16-21). Greenwich, CT: Brompton Books.

14

Selected Factors Associated
With Demonstrating Success
in Health Education Programs

Gail C. Farmer
Pamela C. Krochalk
Malinee Silverman

The purpose of this chapter is to identify crucial factors associated with the evaluation of health education programs that target adolescent populations. Program evaluation is both an essential and a positive component of program development and implementation. Basically, evaluation employs research methods to obtain information about the program for purposes of clarifying goals and objectives, identifying outcomes, monitoring implementation and direction, adjusting to the needs of the target population, and measuring success. Thus, evaluation and the program itself must be totally integrated, beginning at the time of conceptualization and continuing throughout the life of the program.

Program evaluation is an ongoing systematic means of answering key questions about program process and outcomes. Weiss (1972) suggests that failure to demonstrate success typically results when a program, in its entirety or individual components, does not achieve its desired outcomes. Another problem, which Patton (1986) identifies, is when a program appears to have achieved its stated outcomes, however, success is not statistically supported due to an inadequate research design and/or inappropriate measurement tools (p. 35). Both of these problems relate to the initial task in program evaluation of achieving consensus among program planners, evaluators, recipients, and funding agencies as to what the outcomes should be (Fink, 1993, p. 3). Thus, four critical operations identified with program success are addressed in this chapter:

1. Verifying the needs of the adolescent population being served as a means of formulating measurable outcomes
2. Establishing linkages among program goals, objectives, and outcomes
3. Monitoring program implementation
4. Measuring the program's effect upon the target population

Verifying the Needs of
the Adolescent Being Served

Health educators significantly improve the probability of their program's success when decisions are founded upon information gained from an extensive knowledge of the target population. Windsor, Baranowski, Clark, and Cutter (1994) suggest that this knowledge is typically accrued through a systematic assessment of need (pp. 32-37). This assessment provides the health educator with the following information: (a) a description of the adolescent community and the problem being addressed; (b) an enumeration of the desired outcomes, for example, the ideal adolescent behavior(s) to resolve or manage the problem; (c) the identification of instrumental behaviors expected of the adolescent that would remedy the problem; (d) the specification of information and skills that health education staff and adolescent must learn in order for the program to succeed; and (e) a delineation of factors outside the health education program or adolescent that will most inhibit and enable the desired change to take place, including personal and material resources. Thus, a successful program is one that is based upon a thorough understanding of the problem and concentrates its efforts upon a target population (Van Vugt, 1994, pp. 2-3).

Identify the Target Population

The intent of most adolescent health education programs is to intervene (to incur some change) in the lives of a program's participants. Change may take the form of one or more elements, such as knowledge, perceptions, attitudes, behavior, biology, or environment (Smith, 1981). The promotion of change and the measurement of outcomes (Babbie, 1994, Chapter 5) is usually targeted at one of the following categories: (a) individual (e.g., persuade an adolescent to stop smoking ciga-

rettes, to wear seat belts, to stop abusing alcohol or other drugs), (b) organization (e.g., persuade a school district to serve lunches that are low in saturated fats), or (c) society (e.g., persuade state legislators to adopt laws restricting the placement of billboard advertisement of cigarettes within a mile of elementary or secondary schools).

Successful adolescent health programs are those having targeted a particular category (individual, organization, or society) in which to evince a change. A single program that simultaneously promotes change in more than one category risks confusion over who is the target population. This confusion may dilute limited resources and reduce the magnitude of change as a result of the program's intervention (Windsor et al., 1994, pp. 66-69).

Systematically Describe
the Problem and Population

Information obtained from a needs assessment enables service providers to examine systematically the adolescent problem under consideration, including the community in which the problem occurs and the availability of services. This information is often acquired through answers derived from questions posed about the nature of the problem and the affected population (Fink, 1993, p. 5). For example, a needs assessment of adolescent suicide should answer the following questions: What is the nature of suicide among adolescents? What is the rate of attempted and completed suicide (the number of adolescents affected)? Among which adolescent groups does suicide predominate? What are the risk factors associated with teen suicide? Where is teen suicide distributed geographically? How has attempted suicide among adolescents been treated in the past? How do community agencies and school districts currently address the problem of adolescent suicide? In addition to describing the problem and target population, information obtained from a needs assessment is vital to (a) guiding changes in existing programs, (b) developing new programs, and (c) providing baseline comparisons for subsequent evaluation studies of program outcomes (Bell, Warheit, & Schwab, 1977, p. 69).

There are several methods available for assessing a population's needs, which can be applied to adolescent health. Each method has inherent strengths and limitations associated with formulating a precise description of a community and its problems. Thus, the application of more than one method to assess need yields greater accuracy in describing (a) the type, extent, and intensity of the problem under consideration; (b) the unique qualities of the adolescent population being served; and (c) the nature of the potential solutions. Basic needs assessment methodologies include utilization of services, health and social indicators, key informant, community forum, and field survey. During the previous two decades, these methods have been developed and refined (Bell et al., 1977; Posavac & Carey, 1992; Rossi & Freeman, 1993; Siegal, Attkisson, & Carson, 1978; Windsor et al., 1994).

Utilization of Services Method

The utilization of services method is a means of assessing adolescent needs based on data obtained from private and public agencies as well as school districts. This method consists of collecting agency and school records to develop a profile of the adolescents using their services. The profile should provide information relevant to program planning and implementation. Conclusions are drawn about the larger adolescent population based upon information from records of those adolescents who received services. The utilization of services method is most useful when included as the component of a more comprehensive assessment that combines other methods of determining needs, such as the commu-

nity forum or field survey (Windsor et al., 1994, pp. 72-74).

Ease and low cost are the chief advantages of the service utilization method. In addition, there is a high degree of reliability and accuracy as to the verification of the problem (Bell, Nguyen, Warheit, & Buhl, 1978, p. 261). Adolescents using the program have been evaluated by professionals, for example, a physician, public health nurse, educator, or social worker. This methodology is often applied by agencies or school districts, which use data from their own records as a basis for drawing conclusions about their current programs and planning future projects (Bell et al., 1977, pp. 73-74).

There are two major disadvantages associated with the utilization method. First, it is difficult, if not impossible, to obtain information from such sources as physicians, psychologists, and school districts. Ethical and legal issues related to patient, client, or student confidentiality are of major concern (Bell et al., 1977, p. 73; Posavac & Carey, 1992, p. 64). As a consequence, the available data are limited to governmental sources that periodically release their information for analytic purposes. Findings from governmental sources represent only those adolescents who receive services by meeting qualifying criteria, for example, socioeconomic status or location of residence (Siegal et al., 1978, pp. 234-237).

The lack of information about adolescents who do not use services is a second disadvantage of the utilization method of determining need. Information is missing on those who encounter barriers to service associated with issues of accessibility and acceptability (Rossi & Freeman, 1993, p. 75). Conclusions drawn from these data are based upon adolescents and their families who possess sufficient knowledge of service availability, transportation, and personal skills in coping with bureaucratic regulations. Data germane to adolescents in need of help who have not used services are excluded with this method of assessment, and, consequently, their needs are not taken into account.

Health and Social Indicators Method

The health and social indicators method of needs assessment obtains information about adolescents from two primary sources: the Census and the Vital Statistics Reports. The Census, conducted once each decade, provides a demographic profile of all geographic regions in the United States, for example, age, gender, race/ethnicity, education, income, and housing. The Vital Statistics Reports routinely compile data on topics such as number of births, number of marriages and divorces, morbidity (the prevalence of acute and chronic diseases), and mortality. Applying the health and social indicators method of assessment to the adolescent population is based upon the assumption that particular community descriptors represent adolescent health service needs. This method is valuable as an initial source of information about the general population within a given geographic area (Rossi & Freeman, 1993, pp. 68-71).

The ease of data access and quality of the data are the leading advantages of the health and social indicators method of needs assessment. Data relevant to adolescents from the U.S. Census and the Vital Statistics Reports are available in local libraries, on computer data tapes, and on CD-ROMs. The information from these sources is relatively inexpensive, standardized nationwide, and geographically comprehensive (Bell et al., 1977, pp. 74-75).

The major disadvantage of the health and social indicators method is that it provides only an indirect assessment of adolescent needs. For example, high rates of teen pregnancy, low socioeconomic status, high divorce rates, and high suicide rates may accurately reflect low self-esteem for a particular segment of adolescents. The generalization to an individual adolescent's need based upon demographic characteristics may result in ecological fallacy.

Research has shown that correlations between rates or averages for areas often do not reflect the characteristics of individuals within the area. Consequently, needs assessment studies based on health and social indicators are most useful when a general overview of a community is desired or when they are used as one component of a more comprehensive assessment program that includes more specific measures of needs and care pattern. (Bell et al., 1977, p. 75)

Key Informant Method

The key informant method obtains information about adolescent health and psychosocial needs from "experts" who possess knowledge of the problems and knowledge of service accessibility and acceptability. Informants on adolescent health concerns include parents, teachers, physicians, school health nurses, social workers, counselors, religious leaders, and adolescent leaders within school and community organizations. Key informants usually provide a description of the nature and extent of the problem from their perspective. In addition, these experts can identify and prioritize the range of possible interventions that may be successful in the adolescent population. Informants can also identify potentially successful outreach methods to recruit program participants. Finally, key informants can recommend how to implement the suggested interventions in the target community (Rossi & Freeman, 1993, pp. 71-75; Windsor et al., 1994, pp. 69-70).

There are several advantages associated with the key informant method (Bell et al., 1977, p. 71). It is simple, inexpensive, and provides an opportunity for experts on adolescent health to meet and discuss critical issues. Linkages among diverse professionals working with the adolescent population can be established such as school, health, and police. Finally, the key informant method provides a comprehensive view of adolescent needs and the necessary coordination of services to meet a community's adolescent physical and mental health problems.

A significant disadvantage associated with the key informant method arises from the inclination of each expert to represent his or her organization's particular interests, especially when competition for limited resources exists. "Vested interests may prevent the informants from an honest, open appraisal of what services are needed and which agencies should be responsible for delivering them" (Bell et al., 1977, p. 71). When recruiting key persons to take part in a needs assessment, one must verify their area of expertise and identify their organizational affiliation (Rossi & Freeman, 1993, pp. 73-74).

Community Forum Method

The community forum method of needs assessment consists of a series of public meetings at which members of the community are invited to express their experiences and opinions. The concept of *community* can refer to a geopolitical designation (e.g., neighborhood, city, county, state), an attribute (e.g., race, ethnicity, gender, disability), and a style of life (e.g., occupation, gang membership, sexual orientation). The community forum method is similar to the key informant method, but it differs by augmenting the group of informants to include all people (professional and nonprofessional) who have knowledge regarding the physical and mental health issues of adolescents. The perspectives shared by the participants provide valuable insight "concerning the accessibility, availability, acceptability, and organization of services" (Siegal et al., 1978, p. 239).

The advantages of the community forum method for assessing adolescent needs center on its versatility, inclusiveness, and relatively low cost. According to Bell and associates (1977),

this method has the potential to bring into public consciousness areas of unmet needs. In addition, forum participants include those most interested in dealing with their community's problems. Frequently, they can be recruited for membership on program advisory boards that provide guidance on the development and implementation of intervention programs (pp. 71-72).

The disadvantages associated with the community forum method involve issues of availability for participation. Often, it is difficult to set a meeting time and location that facilitates broad-based representation from the community. Lack of transportation, child care responsibilities, and fears associated with a particular neighborhood frequently inhibit full participation in community forums. In addition, individuals who feel isolated are not likely to participate, for example, people who are very shy, ethnic minority, disabled, or socially isolated. Thus, adolescents with severe problems may remain isolated and unnoticed; consequently, plans to meet their needs are not formulated. Without a valid representation of the population under study, only a partial view of the community's needs and services is gained (Windsor et al., 1994, pp. 74-75).

Also, community forums can become grievance sessions instead of a positive means of information gathering, particularly when a small vocal group gains control over the discussion (Bell et al., 1977, pp. 72-73). Forums tend to heighten expectations in the community that all identified adolescent problems will be treated. This leads to pessimism, skepticism, and conflict when these expectations are not satisfied. Thus, community forum leaders must consistently guide the discussion to clarify problems and prioritize potential solutions.

Field Survey Method

The field survey method to assess need is based on the collection of information from members of the target population (Bell et al., 1977, p. 75). For example, information can be obtained from a sample of adolescents and their families about the nature of their problems and patterns of service (program) use. Surveys can be conducted in households or at other locations where members of the target population tend to congregate. Data collection techniques include face-to-face interviews, telephone interviews, and mailed questionnaires (Windsor et al., 1994, pp. 75-76). Scientific research procedures require designed instruments that accurately assess need, a representative sample of members from a defined population, trained data collectors to yield valid and reliable data, and appropriate statistical tests to determine significant trends (Bell et al., 1978, pp. 278-287; Rossi & Freeman, 1993, pp. 76-81).

The chief advantage of the field survey method is the identification of a population's unmet needs. For example, the data include adolescents who have accessed services as well as those who have not. In addition, this method uses scientific sampling procedures that enable the findings to be generalized to the entire target population and their problems (Windsor et al., 1994, p. 75).

There are several disadvantages associated with the field survey method (Bell et al., 1977, p. 76). The implementation requires a considerable investment of financial resources and time. Special attention must focus upon procedures that minimize the refusal rate and mechanisms that enhance recall and truthfulness among adolescents reporting on sensitive issues. In addition, this method typically relies upon self-reports with no verification by professional assessment; the development of valid and reliable questionnaire items is crucial to the integrity of the findings (Bell et al., 1978, pp. 287-288; Rossi & Freeman, 1993, p. 78).

Establishing Linkages Among Program Goals, Objectives, and Outcomes

Establish a Program Based on Behavioral Science Principles

The components of a health education program should stem from theory-based principles derived from the behavioral sciences (Windsor et al., 1994, pp. 85-89). This provides a framework for developing and implementing the program and assessing outcomes. Theory provides the justification as to why the intervention should result in the desired behavior change (outcomes). Effective programs link theory-based content with the following: the models of behavior change, the extent of program participation, and the measurement of outcomes (Posavac & Carey, 1992, pp. 54-57).

Theory-based programs are also cost-effective. An explanation of why the components of a program function in the predicted manner facilitates the application of the program to other populations (portability). This reduces the development costs associated with new programs. In addition, understanding the dynamics associated with program failure can become the foundation for implementing changes that have a higher probability of improvement (Meacham, 1993).

Develop a Consensus on the Goals and Objectives of the Program

For a program to be successful, there must be agreement on the goals and objectives (Weiss, 1972, pp. 30-32). There may be a discrepancy between the written goals and objectives of the program and those to which the organization holds itself accountable. This discrepancy is often a function of the varying perspectives and the vested interests of primary program constituents. Such constituents include the board of directors, program managers, service providers (staff), clients, and the community at-large (Windsor et al., 1994, pp. 36-44). These constituents have particular perspectives, depending on their function in the organization and the program components to which they are held accountable. Each of these perspectives can dramatically influence definitions of programmatic goals and objectives. Thus, the issue becomes whose objectives and whose goals should the program focus upon (Posavac & Carey, 1992, pp. 46-49).

Conflict over program goals and objectives may arise when domains of power and expertise are challenged (Windsor et al., 1994, pp. 45-47). To the extent that an individual functions in one domain or area of control, he or she may become "insensitive" to the goals and objectives of constituents in other domains. To prevent conflict and mistrust from becoming dysfunctional to the program, each constituent's function and sphere of influence must be understood and taken into account if consensus is to be achieved in goal setting. Consensus about goals and objectives becomes important in specifying the outcomes to be measured in program evaluation and enacting changes in how the program is implemented (Berk & Rossi, 1990, p. 75).

In addition, one must be aware of subtle sources of informal control when identifying the goals and objectives (Rossi & Freeman, 1993, pp. 110-111). *Informal* (latent) refers to those sources of control that are not formally stated but are important to the functioning of the organization or program. Examples include a secretary, a member of the PTA, or a gang member. These may represent a *self-appointed gatekeeper*. The self-appointed gatekeeper refers to an activist who is well-networked within the target population and unofficially defines the nature of the problem, determines the range of acceptable solutions, and influences access to the population. Although the true extent of gatekeepers' influ-

ence in the target community may be difficult to discern, it is nonetheless important to include them in the consensus building process relative to programmatic goals and objectives.

Consensus over program goals and objectives is crucial in deciding which health behaviors are feasible to change. This often involves narrowing the health problem(s) and scope of work in terms of what can be accomplished (Windsor et al., 1994, p. 58). For example, selecting a portion of the problem and identifying a limited number of behaviors for change may be necessary given restricted resources such as time, money, and expertise. Because the demonstration of program success is based on achieving the stated objectives, it is important to designate realistic objectives for program accountability.

Link Program Goals and Objectives to Measurable Outcomes

To demonstrate success, what is meant by success must be clearly and objectively defined. The program's goals and objectives must be operationalized into measurable outcomes. As Weiss (1972, pp. 26-30) suggests, a successful program is designed by starting at the end, that is, by addressing what one wants to be able to say about the program when it is over. The major purpose of health programs is to promote primary, secondary, and tertiary prevention. In primary prevention, the goal is to reduce the incidence of a disease by developing and implementing programs that promote behavior change in order to reduce risk factors, for example, reducing the number of new cases of lung cancer through health education programs designed to prevent the start of smoking and smoking relapse among adolescents.

Through secondary prevention, the negative impact of a disease or condition is reduced by early identification to deter more serious consequences. This may be accomplished through health education programs designed to promote the use of screening for diseases or conditions that can be detected in their early stages. Examples include the dissemination of knowledge about the existence of the disease, its seriousness, degree of individual vulnerability, and access to health screening services.

Tertiary prevention refers to treatment of the disease or condition and the reduction of premature mortality or disability. The focus is on the development and implementation of health education programs that facilitate the treatment process. This may be accomplished in three ways:

1. Informing adolescents on how to access needed health care, for example, by giving guidance on where and how to obtain appropriate services
2. Teaching patients about the importance of compliance with medication and other treatment regimens, for example, by ensuring that adolescents with diabetes understand dietary guidelines
3. Training adolescent caregivers in the support of the ill person, for example, by educating significant others in home care skills and stress reduction

Once the expected program outcomes have been specified, decisions must be made as to which outcomes will be measured. This involves specifying the full range of behavior changes associated with reducing the health problem (Windsor et al., 1994, p. 83). Remember that all problems are multidimensional and should not be reduced to a single measurement. For example, the rate of STDs among adolescents is a continuing problem (Zabin & Hirsch, 1988). Program outcomes depend to some extent on the dissemination of information and the accessibility and acceptability of screening as well as treatment services. Thus, each of the program's components affects outcomes and must be measured in terms of the range of behaviors associated with reducing the infections. Such behaviors might include abstinence, monogamy, condom use, early detection, and early treatment.

Deciding the criteria for program success becomes the next task. What level of achievement will be considered successful involves anticipating the magnitude of the results expected based on each program goal and objective (Patton, 1986, pp. 96-100). For example, it might be decided that an intervention program for early detection of testicular cancer among 15- to 33-year-old males (the highest risk group) is "successful" if it achieves a 25% increase in the number of males participating in an early detection program. Note that specifying the criteria for success defines the outcomes to which the program will be held accountable.

Monitoring Program Implementation

Foster a Sense of Ownership Among Those Administering the Program

A conviction held by those administering the program that the outcomes are important to the population being served is a primary ingredient in the success of any program. Programs that promote behavior change in adolescents are dependent upon the functioning of a team, usually consisting of members from the organizational staff, school, and community. To the extent that individuals responsible for the program's implementation lack adequate training, experience time constraints, or doubt the merits of the program, the probability of achieving program success is diminished (Scheirer, 1981, pp. 130-132). Thus, it is imperative to have all those responsible for the program's implementation to champion the entire program, including its goals, objectives, outcomes, program components, and methods of operation.

Establishing a milieu of sensitivity toward diversity within an organization facilitates the sense of ownership among those administering the program. Respect for different perspectives on the methods of implementation, different cultural orientations, different managerial techniques, and different styles of communication conveys the impression that all the individuals responsible for implementation are important to the ultimate success of the program. A milieu of sensitivity can be encouraged by conducting periodic focus groups and surveys within the organization, among the recipients of service, and in the target community from which the recipients of service originate (King, Morris, & Fitz-Gibbon, 1987). Data obtained from these activities can provide knowledge of the program's perceived progress and sources of conflict as well as satisfaction. This information can become the basis for instituting the necessary changes to promote the successful attainment of programmatic goals and objectives.

Train Staff in Program Implementation and Monitoring

Monitoring the implementation of adolescent health programs is directed at three key points: (a) the extent to which a program is reaching the appropriate adolescent population, (b) the extent to which the delivery of program services is consistent with program design specifications, and (c) the extent to which resources are expended as allocated. Program monitoring is always an essential activity in the achievement of desired program outcomes. When a program demonstrates little or no impact, often its implementation was faulty or incomplete (Rossi & Freeman, 1993, pp. 167-168; Windsor et al., 1994, pp. 103-104).

Without adequate quality control procedures (monitoring), it is impossible to estimate whether a program's intervention is efficacious. Furthermore, to estimate the benefits or effectiveness of a program relative to its costs, information on resources expended by the

program must be available (Berk & Rossi, 1990, pp. 66-69).

Program monitoring usually includes the collection of such information as number of programs developed, amount of time each employee devotes to tasks, number of sessions provided, number of adolescents recruited, number of adolescents participating in the program, number of adolescents completing the program, estimated proportion of adolescent population reached, and documentation of staff performance. Thus, the overall function of program monitoring is to document the amount of program or session exposure, that is, who among the participants received what, how much, and when (King et al., 1987, pp. 115-127).

Measuring the Program's Effect on the Target Population

Measurement of program effectiveness requires the same methodological rigor as other types of research studies. This section considers issues most critical to evaluating program impact. There are five essential procedures to measure the impact of a program upon the target population: (a) the formation of an intervention group (which receives the program) and a comparison group (which receives a placebo program); (b) the selection of a sample from the target population using probability methods and their assignment into the intervention and comparison groups; (c) the pretesting of both groups on the desired program outcomes, as well as other factors important to the demonstration of the program's effect; (d) the implementation of the program within the intervention group and a placebo program within the comparison group; and (e) the posttesting of both the intervention and comparison groups, using the same measurement criteria as in the pretest, to assess the amount of change that has occurred.

Procedure 1: Formation of Intervention and Comparison Groups

To ensure that the amount of change observed in the intervention group is a result of the health education program alone and not due to other factors, the control of possible sources of bias and error must be established. Random or matched assignment of members of the target population into the intervention and comparison groups increases the probability that these two groups are similar in all aspects other than exposure to the health education intervention program (Fink, 1993, pp. 50-51). The intervention group receives the health education program under investigation, whereas the comparison group receives the status quo or placebo program.

Procedure 2: Selection of Sample

An accurate assessment of the impact of a program on the target population assumes that unbiased recruitment procedures for participation were followed. The number of individuals assigned to the intervention and comparison groups refers to the sample size. The size of the sample is critical to the magnitude of change necessary to demonstrate statistical significance (Posavac & Carey, 1992, pp. 240-242). With a smaller sample, a greater magnitude of difference between the intervention and comparison groups is required to achieve statistical significance.

Four factors are involved in determining the appropriate sample size: identification of the amount of change that would occur without an intervention, selection of the alpha error, specification of the beta error, and identification of the amount of change that is expected as a result of the intervention program (Langbein, 1980, p. 164; Patton, 1986, pp. 205-207; Rossi & Freeman, 1993, p. 228; Windsor et al., 1994, pp. 159-161).

Procedure 3: Pretesting of Intervention and Comparison Groups

Assessment of program impact is accomplished through a research design that permits the measurement of change and controls the sources of bias and error (Posavac & Carey, 1992, pp. 140-169). The measurement of change requires a comparison of two or more assessments (tests) over time. The adolescent participants are assessed on the desired outcomes before the introduction of the health education/placebo programs (pretest) and after the completion of the health education/placebo programs (posttest). The pretest provides baseline information for comparisons with posttest data to reveal the amount of change that has taken place as a result of the intervention.

Procedure 4: Implementation of Intervention and Placebo Programs

While the intervention group receives the health education program under study, the comparison group (e.g., placebo group/control group) receives what is considered the "usual" health education program. For ethical reasons, services cannot be withheld from the comparison group in health education research. For example, when examining the effects of a new AIDS education program upon an intervention group, it would be unethical to withhold all forms of AIDS education from adolescents in the comparison group.

Procedure 5: Posttesting Intervention and Comparison Groups

In assessing program impact, one must demonstrate through a posttest that the desired outcomes are present in adolescents who received the health education program under study (the intervention group) and that these same desired outcomes are absent in those adolescents who did not receive the health education program (the comparison group).

In reality, the extent to which the desired outcomes may be present or absent in either the intervention or comparison groups is a matter of degree. Statistical testing determines whether the magnitude of the difference observed between these groups is significant or likely due to chance (Langbein, 1980).

Conclusion

Evaluation research is a mandatory component of intervention programs. It is a means of facilitating program planning and development, providing feedback for ongoing program decision making, monitoring activities related to program implementation, and demonstrating program effectiveness. To ensure that these functions are accomplished with scientific rigor, adherence to the following elements that underlie the evaluation process is essential:

1. The program evaluator must have demonstrated expertise in research methods with specialized training in program evaluation.
2. Sufficient resources such as time, money, and staff must be allocated to support the program evaluation function.
3. A program advisory board must be established that includes professional and community representatives with specialized knowledge about the intervention and the adolescent population targeted.
4. Overall community support must be established with special interest groups and leaders and maintained throughout all phases of the program, including the evaluation. Adherence to the methods of successful program evaluation discussed throughout this chapter and commitment to the elements of effective evaluation listed above ensure that the evaluation process is responsive to the needs and values of the adolescent community.

References

Babbie, E. (1994). *The practice of social research*. Belmont, CA: Wadsworth.

Bell, R. A., Nguyen, T. D., Warheit, G. J., & Buhl, J. M. (1978). Service utilization, social indicator, and citizen survey approach to need assessment. In C. C. Attkisson, W. A. Hargreaves, M. J. Horowitz, & J. E. Sorensen (Eds.), *Evaluation of human service programs*. New York: Academic Press.

Bell, R. A., Warheit, G. J., & Schwab, J. J. (1977). Needs assessment: A strategy for structuring change. In R. D. Coursey, G. A. Spector, S. A. Murrell, & B. H. Hunt (Eds.), *Program evaluation for mental health*. New York: Grune & Stratton.

Berk, R. A., & Rossi, P. H. (1990). *Thinking about program evaluation*. Newbury Park, CA: Sage.

Fink, A. (1993). *Evaluation fundamentals: Guiding health programs, research, and policy*. Newbury Park, CA: Sage.

King, J. A., Morris, L. L., & Fitz-Gibbon, C. T. (1987). *How to assess program implementation*. Newbury Park, CA: Sage.

Langbein, L. I. (1980). *Discovering whether programs work: A statistical method for program evaluation*. Santa Monica, CA: Goodyear.

Meacham, C. E. (1993). State of New York minority internship program: Avenue to gaining access in the public policy arena. In P. D. McClain (Ed.), *Minority group influence: Agenda setting, formulation, and public policy*. Westport, CT: Greenwood.

Patton, M. Q. (1986). *Utilization-focused evaluation*. Newbury Park, CA: Sage.

Posavac, E. J., & Carey, R. G. (1992). *Program evaluation: Methods and case studies*. Englewood Cliffs, NJ: Prentice Hall.

Rossi, P. H., & Freeman, H. E. (1993). *Evaluation: A systematic approach*. Newbury Park, CA: Sage.

Scheirer, M. A. (1981). *Program implementation: The organizational context*. Beverly Hills, CA: Sage.

Siegal, L. M., Attkisson, C. C., & Carson, L. G. (1978). Need identification and program planning in the community context. In C. C. Attkisson, W. A. Hargreaves, M. J. Horowitz, & J. E. Sorensen (Eds.), *Evaluation of human service programs*. New York: Academic Press.

Smith, N. L. (1981). Creating alternative methods for educational evaluation. In N. L. Smith (Eds.), *Federal efforts to develop new evaluation methods*. San Francisco: Jossey-Bass.

Van Vugt, J. P. (1994). The effectiveness of community-based organizations in the medical social sciences: A case study of a gay community's response to the AIDS crisis. In J. P. Van Vugt (Ed.), *AIDS prevention and services: Community-based research*. Westport, CT: Bergin & Garvey.

Weiss, C. H. (1972). *Evaluation research: Methods for assessing program effectiveness*. Englewood Cliffs, NJ: Prentice Hall.

Windsor, R. A., Baranowski, T., Clark, N., & Cutter, G. (1994). *Evaluation of health promotion, health education, and disease prevention programs*. Mountain View, CA: Mayfield.

Zabin, L. S., & Hirsch, M. B. (1988). *Evaluation of pregnancy prevention programs in the school context*. Lexington, MA: D. C. Heath.

15

Project CUFFS (Communities for United Fullerton Safety)

Daria Waetjen

Background

A model, multiagency, grant-funded program is positively affecting gang violence in Fullerton, California. It is largely responsible for the renewal of hope for many youth and their families in this community.

In the early 1990s, the city of Fullerton experienced a marked increase in youth violence as related to gang activity. The escalation of crimes such as drug trafficking, graffiti, vandalism, home invasion robberies, drive-by shootings, and the well-publicized brutal bludgeoning murder of an honor student by other honor students brought a new level of fear and concern to community members. With proximity to Los Angeles, easy freeway access, and mobility of gang associates, Fullerton was fertile ground for problems to escalate.

Fullerton, located in north Orange County, has experienced a tremendous influx of new residents, much like other southwestern metropolitan areas. Immigrants from Mexico, South America, Southeast Asia, and Korea have contributed to overcrowding, an increased demand for social services, and social

problems that often accompany increased demands on social services with the assimilation of new cultures. This demographic transformation of a community of about 114,000 created new challenges. South Fullerton was affected by traditional territorial and multi-generational Hispanic gangs, whereas north Fullerton was affected by less territorial Asian, mostly Korean gangs. Several programs, as well as city and county agencies, were already independently addressing these concerns. Yet, schools and neighborhoods continued to experience the impact of gang-related violence and were seeking available assistance. It became clear that a coordinated, proactive effort was necessary to effectively address the issue of gangs and youth violence in Fullerton.

Created in 1991, Project CUFFS (Communities United for Fullerton Safety), the multi-faceted plan of a group of established agencies involved with the concerns of youth, was developed to provide integrated prevention, intervention, and suppression services to youth already involved or easily lured to the gang lifestyle. The Orange County Department of Education, two local school districts, the police and probation departments, and the District Attorney's office, along with 13 community-based organizations (CBOs), were awarded a grant to fund Project CUFFS. The goals of this comprehensive prevention, intervention, and suppression program are to

1. Reduce the level of violence in the city of Fullerton and divert potentially dangerous gang activity of youth into positive and constructive alternative activities
2. Enhance communication between law enforcement agencies, the district attorney's office, CBOs, the probation department, schools, the community, and family members of active or potential gang members
3. Promote factors that protect young people from experimentation with drugs and involvement with gangs. These include promoting bonding to family, school, and positive peer groups through opportunities for active participation; defining clear social norms and teaching skills necessary to live these norms, and providing recognition, rewards, and reinforcement for newly learned skills.

Program Description

Since 1992, Project CUFFS has provided coordinated services to over 2,200 youth from 12 to 18 years old in the city of Fullerton. The program targets student populations who exhibit signs of high need, based on the presence of high-risk behaviors relative to drug use, violence, or gang activity and who attend three targeted high schools and their three feeder middle schools in the city of Fullerton. A local coordinating committee representing members of the community, as well as all project affiliates, meets bimonthly to coordinate project activity, review progress, and serve as an advisory and resource body.

Project activities are funded through a grant awarded by the California Governor's Office of Criminal Justice Planning. This funding allows services to be provided to youth and families with no fees involved.

Thirteen agencies provide social services, including individual and family counseling, focus groups, and alternative youth activities. A gang prevention specialist works with six school-site facilitators to implement prevention and intervention strategies. These facilitators are responsible for referring students and monitoring the progress of services rendered. Multilingual services are provided to families in nonthreatening settings to encourage participation. Youth services are provided at the school site, alternative educational locations, the Fullerton Boys and Girls Club, and the Orange Korean Church.

Professional educators, counselors, gang prevention specialists, community agency workers, and volunteer mentors all provide direct and/or indirect services to identified youth. All staff members are acquainted with the grant goals and objectives and attend local coordinating committee meetings.

Community Collaboration

Project CUFFS is a model of collaboration bringing together the expertise of staff from schools, law enforcement, and community organizations in the type of public-private partnership necessary to achieve real solutions to local problems. The commitment of the participating individuals and agencies involved in this collaboration is evident in their diligent work to effectively break down territorial boundaries. Striving for results based on group action has become the norm. CUFFS' agencies support one another in meeting all identified objectives.

The role of each of the partners is critical. Law enforcement provides a Gang Violence Suppression (GVS) officer to help track gang-related criminal activity and work with the district attorney assigned to the project. Two full-time resource officers are assigned to the targeted school sites and act as liaisons to the

GVS officer. These officers conduct classes and community and parent meetings and maintain a record of activities. An assigned probation officer facilitates daily communication with the officers, schools, and families of all targeted youth with a supervision or probationary standard.

The school supports the educational process by including a curriculum about gang violence and drug prevention in classroom content. The curriculum addresses anger management, conflict resolution strategies, and alternatives to gang membership and substance abuse. In addition, the school refers the highest-risk youth and families to individual counseling services. The school climate also supports the building of resilient youth by providing services to any child in need. All named agencies collaboratively provide educational and awareness opportunities for families, staff, and students. The Department of Education coordinates the ongoing reporting, staffing, and management of the project and acts as the liaison to the funding agency.

Thirteen CBOs provide critical services to youth. The lead prevention agency, the Boys and Girls Club, coordinates all activities of the CBOs, provides free club membership for high-risk youth, and offers a mandatory evening program for youth with a truancy history. An after-school student center for junior high youth provides incentives for youth participation. Summer employment, volunteer activities, community service assignments, and parent education classes are also provided at the club.

The YWCA provides conflict resolution training, sponsors a trip to the Museum of Tolerance, and coordinates a cross-age pen pal program. Tough-love parent support groups at the high schools stress parent behavioral management strategies and the legal ramifications of youth behavior. The Coalition for Children, Adolescents, and Parents (CCAP) provides parenting classes in multiple languages created to address at-risk youth behavior at a variety of locations accessible to families. AVALON/ACTION offers daytime counseling and teen support groups. STOP GAP, a theater-based action group, delivers two educational presentations annually to each school on topics such as AIDS, sexual assault, racial prejudice, alcoholism, and self-esteem building.

Additional services are provided by the Orange Korean Church, which hosts a conference dealing with gang violence awareness and offers after school and summer programs, basketball leagues and clinics, camping trips, and mentors provided by church staff. Shortstop, an intervention program for first-time offenders, takes school referrals and provides a presentation annually. The Fullerton Museum provides art classes and a summer art workshop. The Orange County Human Relations Council provides curriculum and presentations to increase positive interpersonal relations among youth and adults.

The city of Fullerton coordinates a mentoring program, recruiting adult role models from the community and matching them with "mentees" from the junior high schools. The city also provides a graffiti coordinator to sponsor community education, and to conduct volunteer-run graffiti paintouts. KOCE public television supports this project with broadcasts of public service announcements and the distribution of parent education booklets entitled *Act Against Violence.*

Western Youth Services supports CUFFS' youth with the provision of individual and group counseling provided by licensed counselors and clinical interns; a licensed counselor also is available for individual counseling. The Victim Offender Reconciliation Program provides mediation services between victims and offenders to help reach accord following the commission of a crime, as well as training in conflict resolution for volunteers. This skilled ensemble supports youth who are recommended for services by the program specialist and/or site-based facilitators.

Evaluation and Indicators of Program Success

Project CUFFS has served hundreds of youths and their families over a 5-year period. Beyond the number directly served by the project, testimonials offered by parents and educators indicate that the school, home, and community climates have also been indirectly affected by the reduction of gang activity and violent behavior. In addition, truancy rates have decreased, and many students have returned to school or to an alternative placement after previously dropping out. Suspension and expulsion rates have also decreased at the project schools.

Many of the strongest indicators of the success of this project include the spontaneous emergence of new project components striving to meet the same objectives as CUFFS. These include the city's commitment to assume leadership of the mentor program, which provides "life coaches" for youth involved in the project. Additional evidence includes plans for the institutionalization of the prevention content taught in project schools, the continuation of the intervention programs in the community, and the increase of student participation in project activities.

Keys to Success

As a gang-violence prevention and intervention program, Project CUFFS is a model for other communities. This project is renowned for its ability to attract youth to positive alternatives and assist them in the transition to positive lifestyle choices.

Key components of the program's successes include:

- Common goal: Law enforcement, educators, parents, and community agencies are united in a common goal to promote a safer generation of youth.
- Interagency collaboration: Agencies with clearly defined goals work harmoniously to meet common objectives.
- Trust and understanding: Time and commitment focused on youth allow participants involved in the project to work, demonstrating respect and trust in one another's contributions.
- Mentoring: Caring adult mentors for youth build resiliency.
- Skill building: The emphasis is on teaching coping strategies, skills to resolve conflict, and activities that build self-esteem and prosocial life skills.

Client Example

Bonnie is a 14-year-old 8th-grade student, one of six female siblings. She grew up in a family with multigenerational gang involvement, where violence was the norm, not the exception. Her father was abusive, often exposing his children to the gang lifestyle. Two of Bonnie's older sisters were in trouble with the law and were experiencing school failure. They both later enrolled in the district's continuation school.

Bonnie too was beginning to act out in school. She was angry and often exhibited this anger through verbal aggression, lying, and stealing. She was perceived as unpleasant by both peers and teachers, had few friends, and was often antagonistic.

In 7th grade, Bonnie was referred to Project CUFFS as an intervention. She joined the "Get a Life" pre-job training program and the girls' afterschool group at the Boys and Girls Club, and she was assigned a life coach mentor who was a local community member. Bonnie is in her second year of intervention. She is currently experiencing a new kind of personal and school success. She has non-gang friends, is getting along with her peers and teachers, and is quick to smile. She has encouraged her two older sisters to also seek CUFFS intervention services at the continuation school.

Very significant is the changing family dynamic, as related by observers. Dad is attending CUFFS-sponsored parenting classes, occasionally bringing mom along, and Bonnie is a top achiever in her classes at school. Such coordinated intervention with one child has dramatically affected her family as well as those who interact with Bonnie on a daily basis. Her prognosis is positive. Prevention and intervention truly made a difference in this child's life.

Program Information

Program Title: Project CUFFS
(Communities United for Fullerton Safety)
Contact Person: Nina Winn, Ed.D
Agency: Orange County Department
 of Education
200 Kalmus Drive
Costa Mesa, CA 92628

16

Peer Education . . . a Little Help From Your Friends

Jan Lunquist

Background

"Peer Education . . . a Little Help From Your Friends" was initiated in 1982 by Planned Parenthood Centers of West Michigan in order to capitalize on the fact that kids talk to kids. Knowing that uninformed young people often pass on myths and misinformation about critical but sensitive issues, the agency set up a paid training experience in which teens would learn and disseminate information on teen issues; demonstrate communication, decision-making, and assertiveness skills; provide facts and referrals to friends and family; and participate in school and community projects.

Program Description

Adolescents ages 14 to 17 are recruited through schools, agencies, faith communities, and word-of-mouth; they are interviewed and then trained in a 40-hour series. Topics include substance use, self-esteem, relationships, sexuality, sexual orientation and sex roles, anatomy and physiology, suicide, decision making, violence prevention, eating disorders, sexual abuse, diversity, contraception,

sexually transmissible infections, and communication. Teens are paid a stipend midway through and at the completion of the training if they meet attendance and other agreed-upon criteria. All the responsibilities inherent in a job including a job application, references, and interview, as well as the need to be on time and accurately fill out time sheets, are expected to be fulfilled. Trained teens log each contact made on a form and turn the log in with their time sheets. A contact may be defined as answering a question, providing a pamphlet, making an appropriate referral to a community resource, delivering a formal presentation, or otherwise providing guidance to another person.

Ten teens participated in the first training in 1982. In 1995, over 200 teens completed the 40-hour program. Numbers have varied over the years according to funding. Private foundations, public monies from health and human service providers, and donations have supported Peer Education. The approximate cost per teen for the 40 hours of training is $660. This includes stipends ($170), materials, refreshment, and staff hours. Experienced education specialists with strong presentation skills and a major enthusiasm for young people facilitate the program from recruitment through evaluation. Although most sessions have been held at the Planned Parenthood headquarters in downtown Grand Rapids, several trainings have been completed in neighborhood settings including other youth-serving agencies and community service centers.

Community Collaborations

Collaboration has been demonstrated in multiple ways throughout the history of the program. Other agencies and institutions have provided educational sessions and consultations on their areas of expertise during the training. Individuals and businesses have donated refreshments, audiovisual equipment, and subsidies for teen stipends. Schools and other youth-serving entities have spread the word to young people about the peer education experience and made applications available. This model has been adopted in various locations throughout the nation with the help of the manual and in Michigan through onsite training.

Evaluation

Overall, 95% of posttests show an increase in knowledge. Role playing demonstrates that trained teens know how to answer questions, find community resources, and make better decisions. Body language shows a marked increase in self-confidence. Feedback from presentations done by peer educators indicates that messages about healthy behavior are heard more readily when given by peers.

A specially funded 3-year (1992-1995) project with a peer education component was more intensively evaluated. The 50 peer educators trained during 3 years were between the ages of 14 and 17 and were a mix of African American, Caucasian, Hispanic, Native American, and Asian American students. About one

third of the trained peers were male. Each of the 50 peer educators completed pre- and posttests and an extensive feedback form. Of the 50 peer educators who were trained, 98% improved on the posttest. Feedback concerning the most important aspect of the training included the following responses: "Now I feel prepared to help my sisters and friends stay out of trouble." "I feel very comfortable with people of different colors and with different beliefs." "Peer education opened up my eyes to the pressures I face and the facts I can get to stay safe and healthy." "It's helped me in making the right choice in my life—without peer ed I'd probably not be a virgin right now." Comments from adults who watched peer educators present programs or speak on panels indicated that they felt peer educators provided a bridge to family planning services and sexuality education. Teachers reported that students who had contact with a peer educator were more likely to reach out to community resources than those who did not have contact with a peer educator.

In early 1995, a confidential survey was administered to 25 peer educators ages 14 to 21 who had been out of peer education for at least a year. These individuals completed demographic information and reported on contraceptive use, family situations, and pregnancy status; knowledge of anatomy, HIV, and STDs, and shared opinions on substance use, the value of peer education, and what young people need from adults.

Results from the survey indicated that three females and one male are parents (one was 13 at first paternity, two were 14 at first pregnancy, one was 19 at first pregnancy). Three of the four pregnancies occurred before peer education training. All parenting teens reported having teen parents in their immediate families. Of the 25 former peer educators, 77% reported consistent use of a contraceptive method including abstinence, and 32% reported that they were sexually active. Three reported having had an STD. The mean number of sexual partners for the group was 5.57. The majority saw substance use as a primary factor in risky sexual behavior. All reported that peer education was a must for teens and probably would be worthwhile for people of all ages. This survey and the follow-up discussion validated what daily life is like for many young people: dysfunctional family situations; basic needs neglected; poor or no role models; pressures from the media, friends, and siblings; unstimulating classrooms; "no one person who really cares what happens to me"; confusing messages regarding sexuality; diminished self-esteem; and environments of risk. Peer educators made 6,271 logged contacts with peers, siblings, and parents over the 3 years.

Keys to Success

- This program is intensive, not a "one-shot" event.
- This program is separate from school and therefore not subject to topic "bans" in the curriculum.
- This is a first job experience for many young teens. Stipends are critical.
- The curriculum thoroughly involves participants through active learning methods.
- A companion parent program called "Parents as Peers" provides parents with information and practice related to talking with their kids about sensitive topics.
- A detailed, user-friendly manual, *Peer Education . . . a Little Help From Your Friends,* and a supplement, *Teens in Action,* provide a framework for consistency in implementation as staff change.

Client Example

William was encouraged by his principal to fill out an application for peer education training. As an 8th grader in a public school, William would turn 14 during the first week of training. His application was filled out, complete with three nonfamily references, and signed by his father.

An interview was scheduled and conducted by a staff educator. William had obviously been coached by a caring adult, and he came prepared and dressed appropriately for a job interview. His reserved demeanor changed to a whoop of satisfaction when he was hired on the spot. He proudly went to the reception area to assure his buddy that "it wasn't so bad."

A follow-up letter to William described the training schedule and attendance expectations. He was offered a free physical exam and encouraged to keep his family informed as he went through the program.

Guidelines for group interaction were developed by the 12 teens in the first session, paperwork was completed, and warm-up activities began the group growth process. Each 2-hour block of training after school on Mondays and Wednesdays may include videos, demonstrations, guest speakers, and/or discussions on a designated topic. Thank you notes to guests are required and evaluations of sessions are done verbally or in writing.

Outside of training time, William was making and logging contacts with his older sister, younger brother, neighborhood friends, and classmates. He brought in a question about menstrual cramps from his sister during the third session and provoked a long discussion about periods. He said that his father "pumps" him for news every night about what he learned and asks if he has any pamphlets. During a health class at school, he challenged the instructor on some facts about HIV and was asked to do a presentation on AIDS.

William wrote on his final feedback form that the two sessions that impressed him most were the ones on violence prevention and gay/lesbian/bisexual youth. He said he now feels much smarter about how to avoid fights and much more accepting and appreciative of differences. William really wants to stay connected with peer education and decided to audition for Stages, the teen theater component of the program. He was selected for roles in the sexual harassment and teen esteem skits and did seven presentations in 3 months. He also filled in when needed in the "How to Say Later" series for middle school students and helps with the student-produced newsletter. He recruited two friends for the next peer education training and promoted the program at a community breakfast for legislators.

Although William seemed pretty know-it-all before peer education started, he now exhibits a solid self-confidence backed up by facts, communication skills, and many successful experiences.

Program Information

Program Title: Peer Education . . .
A Little Help From Your Friends
Contact Person: Jan Lunquist,
   Vice President of Education
Agency: Planned Parenthood Centers
   of West Michigan
425 Cherry Street SE, Grand Rapids MI, 49503
(616) 774-7005 FAX: (616) 774-0516

17

—— ✆ ——

Baile de Vida: The Dance of Life

Donna Lloyd-Kolkin

Background

Baile de Vida, the Dance of Life project, seeks to reduce the risk for cardiovascular disease, cancer, and diabetes among Latinos in Santa Paula, California, by promoting "life-long" good eating habits and regular aerobic exercise to low-income Latino youth, ages 10 to 14. Conducted by Ventura County Public Health Services in co-operation with the Santa Paula Health Action Coalition, the project is funded by the California Adolescent Nutrition and Fitness Program (CANFit), which seeks to improve the nutritional status, including physical fitness, of low-income African American, Latino, Asian, and Native American youth 10 to 14 years old.

Santa Paula is an agricultural town of 25,000 people in Ventura County, about a half-hour drive from the city of Ventura. About 60% of Santa Paula's population is Latino, representing a mixture of new monolingual immigrants and acculturated bilingual Mexican Americans. Because the community is geographically discrete, the agricultural and food processing workers and their families who live there tend to have less access to services than their counterparts in more urban areas of the county.

In 1993, Ventura County Public Health Services conducted the Santa Paula Community Health Needs Assessment Survey in collaboration with the Santa Paula Health Action Coalition. In the survey, diabetes was identified as the most important health concern to the respondents; almost one half (48%) indicated that they or a family member had diabetes. Local hospital discharge records indicated a rate of diabetes among Latinos in 1992 that was twice that of the non-Latino white population.

One of the major risk factors for diabetes is obesity. A pediatric surveillance study conducted by the Child Health and Disability Prevention program reported a 15.5% rate of obesity among Latino youth under the age of 21 in Ventura County, exceeding the statewide rate of 13% and the U.S. rate of 9.3%. The Health Department identified a lack of nutrition and fitness programs for youth as a contributing factor to this pattern in Santa Paula. No community-based programs to encourage positive diet and activity patterns in young Latinos existed in the community at the time the project was proposed.

The Santa Paula Health Action Coalition was formed in 1992 to identify and address the health needs of the Santa Paula Latino community and to improve the quality of life by empowering, educating, and advocating for healthy lifestyles. The coalition comprises concerned community members and representatives from local schools, community-based organizations, churches, and the local police department. Coalition members proposed responding to the CANFit grant opportunity with afterschool Mexican *Quebradita* dancing classes for 10- to 14-year-old youths who have nothing to do after school. *La Quebradita,* the newest rhythm among Latinos in Southern California at the time, resembles Brazil's Lambada and is a combination of metropolitan Mexico's soft rock, Caribbean-Mexican tropical music, and northern Mexico's country music. A dance event sponsored by another health promotion project had attracted over 300 Santa Paulans. Thus, the appeal of *La Quebradita* was thought to provide an avenue to attract teens who avoid traditional aerobic exercise, teens with poor body images who do not perceive of themselves as exercisers, and teens who are not involved in team sports.

Program Description

Baile de Vida began in September 1994 and was funded through August 1996. Socorro Lopez-Hanson, a former teacher, coordinated *Baile de Vida* with assistance from Silvia Navarro, a bilingual nutritionist within the Health Department, and a local *Quebradita* dance teacher.

Specific components of *Baile de Vida's* initial plan included culturally appropriate aerobic exercise centered around *La Quebradita;* formal and informal nutrition and fitness education at the dance sessions; parent education; and the "Lean Team," a group of young adults who would become community experts, or resource people, on nutrition and fitness.

First-Year Activities

During the first year of the project, afterschool classes 1½ hours in length were conducted on a biweekly basis. Attendance was low at the beginning, ranging from 1 participant at the first session to 15. Recruitment and retention of participants remained an issue throughout the year. Coalition members called program participants to invite them to come to classes. The project sent out mailings, reminding students to come and listing incentives available for participation. These incentives included gift certificates, class credit, Isbell School Dance Passes, and passes to local amusement parks. By the end of the school year, participation was up to 57 youngsters in the target age group, plus an additional 23 children outside the 10- to 14-year-old program guidelines. Ethnic distribution among participants was primarily Latino (83%), with some Anglo (14%) and African American (3%) participation.

Within a few months, the project developed a class structure that worked for participants. Snack became the first item on the agenda. As the participants ate, the project coordinator discussed what they were eating, and they planned the next snack. An emphasis was placed on trying new foods, such as low-fat granola bars and crackers, dried fruit, and string cheese.

A parent workshop was offered about 6 months after the start of the project. Eleven parents, one grandparent, and various siblings attended, along with the assistant director of food services for the Santa Paula Elementary School District and the Isbell cafeteria manager, for a total of 20 people. Tostadas Primaveras were served, with baked tortillas, browned ground turkey simmered in salsa, lettuce, tomatoes, chopped green onions, 98% fat-free refried beans, and grated mozzarella cheese. Dessert consisted of *arroz con leche* (rice pudding) made with skim milk. Youngsters participating in *Baile de Vida* planned and helped prepare, cook, and serve the meal.

In addition to dinner, the evening featured a nutrition presentation by Navarro and games and appetizers. The games included *Una Comida Balanceada*/A Balanced Diet (connect the dots), *La Comida y la Salud*/Food and Your Health (sentence completion), and *Piramide de Nutricion*/Food Guide Pyramid (crossword puzzle). Prizes were given to the first five people who completed each game.

Three community-wide events occurred during the year to promote healthy eating among Latino families in the community. One, for example, was a Family Night Out cosponsored by the Santa Paula Happy Families Project. About 100 people attended. Dinner included turkey chili nachos, friendship fruit salad, raspberry iced tea, and orange juice.

By the fourth quarter of the project, *Baile de Vida* expanded to become incorporated into Santa Paula's Boys and Girls Club '95 summer session. Because the club has kitchen facilities, cooking classes could be offered in addition to dance and nutrition games/information. The program was planned for Monday and Thursday from June through mid-August for 1½ hours each day. Forty-six young people participated.

Challenges

One of the first problems encountered by the project was lack of transportation between Isbell Middle School, which most students in the target population attended, and the Casa de Mexicano community center, where the afterschool classes were to be held. Therefore, the project sought and received permission to conduct the classes at Isbell, resulting in a higher level of participation.

The passage of Proposition 187 in November 1994, which was designed to limit services to noncitizens of California, also resulted in a drop in attendance. The project coordinator called all parents to reassure them that this need not be a concern.

Finally, some parents (particularly fathers) did not want their daughters involved in a dance activity in which they would be in physical contact with young men.

Another problem was recruiting the Lean Team. Lack of a social security number deterred some young people from participating, because the county could not hire an individual who lacked one. In the end, two older students from Isbell Middle School participated as unpaid volunteers.

Because of the difficulty of conducting the afterschool classes, discussions were under way by the middle of the project's first year about incorporating *Baile de Vida* into the Isbell School physical education curriculum for 1995-1996. The school was short a unit in its physical education program. The school planned to hire two new physical education teachers who would work with the project. By the end of the school year, the school principal committed to allowing *Baile de Vida* staff to conduct the program in all 6th-grade physical education classes during the 1995-1996 school year. The physical education teachers would observe the teaching and learn how to incorporate it into their own curriculum. In this way, *Baile de Vida* has an opportunity to become institutionalized within the Santa Paula community.

Community Collaborations and Linkages

As noted above, the Santa Paula Health Action Coalition was the creative force behind the design of *Baile de Vida*. The project also linked with the school district to incorporate its activities into the middle school's physical education program. Finally, the project linked with the Santa Paula Boys and Girls Club to include the dance and nutrition components of the program into their summer session.

These linkages were highly successful, and Lopez-Hanson notes a number of things that contributed to their success. First, she worked hard to expand the Health Action Coalition to include more community *members* in addition to community leaders. Second, she discovered that it takes a long time to build credibility within the Latino community. It took a lot of face-to-face interaction to convince the Latinos in Santa Paula to accept her and the *Baile de Vida* program.

Evaluation

A case study of the *Baile de Vida* project will be developed by a team of independent evaluators hired by the CANFit Program Office. In addition, *Baile de Vida* administered some pre- and posttest surveys to youngsters who participated in the program. Among their findings:

- An increased consumption of whole grain products, even though the number of servings in the Breads and Cereal group remained inadequate
- An increased consumption of milk, especially with female participants, and a consistent reported switch from whole milk to 2% low-fat milk
- An increased consumption of red meats and poultry from rarely to daily, although the increase was mostly for female participants
- Increased physical activity both during school days and on the weekend
- Changes in attitudes in the way the participants viewed their body size from dissatisfied at the beginning of the program to satisfied at the end, even though their perception of body weight did not change

In addition, there were some unanticipated impacts of the project. The Isbell School Cafeteria planned to install a salad bar, with nonfat dressings, at the request of students participating in *Baile de Vida*. The Santa Paula Health Action Coalition is on the verge of becoming a nonprofit organization, due in large part to the team spirit required to move the project forward.

Keys to Success

- Project staff were bicultural as well as bilingual and could therefore relate to the population being served.
- The involvement of a community coalition made the project credible and allowed creative trouble-shooting when problems arose.
- Program planning was driven by the interests and participation of the youth involved.
- Community feedback was very positive and translated into community support in the form of financial and in-kind contributions.
- The message was straightforward and effective: Good nutrition and fitness are within everyone's reach and not merely something that only rich people can achieve.

Client Example

When Pedro first came to the *Baile de Vida* afterschool program, he was an angry and frustrated young man. He was very irritable and would hit others in the class. Pedro was tall, overweight, and, by far, the largest program participant. Project leader Socorro Lopez-Hanson began on building his self-esteem, and Pedro persisted with the program. Little by little, he came to realize that being big was not all bad. One day, he asked if moderation applied to drinking beer. It turned out that his father was consuming up to two 6-packs a night. Pedro brought his mother in one day and asked if they could talk about "too much of anything." The project appeared to make a big impact on the entire family. Pedro now makes sure that all family members, including his father, attend all *Baile de Vida* events.

18

The Vermont School and Mass Media Project

Megan Wiston

Background

The Vermont School and Mass Media Project began as an initiative to reduce the numbers of schoolchildren adopting cigarette-smoking practices and to keep these numbers down throughout adolescence. Previous smoking prevention programs targeting middle school students have been unsuccessful in the long term. These programs have delayed smoking behavior by only a few years (Flynn et al., 1992). This study's goal was to see if a mass media intervention could achieve an additional impact. When used in conjunction with a school cigarette-smoking prevention program, mass media intervention should help to reduce smoking initiation among middle schoolers (Flynn et al., 1992).

The researchers' hypothesis was that the initiation of cigarette smoking would increase less among adolescents receiving a mass media intervention and a school smoking-prevention program than among those receiving a school program only (Flynn et al., 1992). Through the combination of these two intervention programs, the researchers could advance their objectives, which would promote positive behavior outcomes. As a result of these educa-

tional interventions, the students would also have:

- A more positive view of nonsmoking
- A more negative view of smoking
- Improved skills for refusing cigarettes
- A better understanding that most people their age do not smoke cigarettes (Flynn, Worden, Secker-Walker, Badger, & Geller, 1995)

Together, the school program and the mass media intervention should reduce the number of students who begin smoking.

Program Description

The researchers developed a school smoking-prevention program based on the four common educational objectives of the project. This program ran concurrently in four study communities. The program contained grade-specific materials for Grades 5 to 10, and the classroom teachers were trained annually in daylong workshops (Flynn et al., 1992). Through the different teaching units, the students explored various issues regarding smoking, including health effects, social influences and pressures, and social policy concerns. The students also engaged in decision making and refusal skills (Worden et al., 1988). For Grades 5 to 8, four class periods were required per year; for Grades 9 and 10, the curriculum required three class periods annually (Flynn et al., 1992).

Mass media have been shown to have a huge impact on adolescents and the greatest impact when they are combined with educational interventions. For these reasons, the researchers decided to produce smoking prevention television spots targeted at adolescents. Their goal was to target students who were at high risk of becoming habitual smokers. Through initial focus groups and surveys, the researchers explored the ideas and concepts for the media spots. Their results found a decrease in television watching and an increase in radio listening as the students aged. From this information, the researchers concluded that they would produce both television and radio spots and that they would need different campaigns and a variety of formats for different age groups (Worden et al., 1988).

Once the media spots were produced, the researchers developed a media plan by (a) determining the number of exposures per week for adequate saturation, (b) assigning these exposures to specific time slots in television programs, and (c) assigning specific television messages to these time slots (Worden et al., 1988). The researchers asked the students about specific programming and times of the day when they watch television and listen to the radio. The researchers then figured out the best times to air each spot.

The study was established in the spring of 1985. The first school curriculum units were taught in the fall of 1985. The first television and radio campaigns ran from January through May 1986. The program continued for 3 additional years (Flynn et al., 1992).

The researchers located two pairs of sample groups for their study. Selection criteria included (a) an independent media market; (b) populations between 50,000 and 400,000; and (c) matched demographic characteristics for each group, including education, income, and ethnicity (Flynn et al., 1992). Vermont and south-central New York State were the first sample pair. The other pair was located in Montana. Within each pair, one district became the media-and-school group while the other became the school-only group. All four groups received the smoking prevention curriculum, and one group from each pair also received the mass media intervention.

The total sample size equaled 5,458 students. The students were surveyed at baseline while in Grades 4, 5, and 6. They were followed for 4 years and surveyed annually. The curriculum and media messages continued throughout this entire period. The smoking prevention curriculum was taught in the schools by the usual classroom teachers. The mass media component ran through television and radio spots.

Funding was awarded by the National Cancer Institute and the National Heart, Lung, and Blood Institute (Flynn et al., 1992). Both institutes awarded the grants with the hope that students would not adopt cigarette-smoking behaviors and that these effects would be maintained into young adulthood (B. S. Flynn, personal communication, April 12, 1996).

Production and development costs of television advertisements averaged $10,369 per message. Average broadcast cost in the two markets equaled $25,000 per market annually (Flynn et al., 1992). The researchers requested public service announcement time whenever possible; however, paid advertising was often necessary to have the advertisements run during requested slots (Worden et al., 1988).

Community Collaborators

For the Vermont School and Mass Media Project to be successful, the researchers needed the support of two distinct organizations—the schools and the media. The school systems in all four communities showed approval for the program. The school system requested the support of the individual schools and teachers. The local television and radio stations in the two school-and-media communities were paid for their airtime. As requested, they ran the media spots during selected times and television shows. Therefore, one obstacle in the replication of this study would be the compliance of the school systems in providing the time to train the teachers and teach the materials. The other main obstacle would be the expense of producing and airing television and radio spots.

Evaluation

Because the objective of this program was to test the ability of mass media intervention to enhance the efficacy of school cigarette smoking-prevention programs, the program has been evaluated for its effectiveness. The researchers compared the annual surveys of the school-and-media groups to the school-only groups to assess if there were significant differences in the behavior and attitudes between the two groups.

The results showed that the interventions had an impact on cigarette smoking behavior. A difference in cigarette smoking rates existed between the school-only group and school-and-media group, with significant differences found in the final 2 years. In the school-and-media group, fewer students were smoking, and fewer cigarettes were smoked per week. The annual surveys measured the number of cigarettes smoked per week, and the Smoking Behavior Index represented the average number of cigarettes smoked per week. In the fifth year of the project, the school-only group reported smoking 4.4 cigarettes per week, whereas the school-and-media group re-

ported smoking 2.6 cigarettes per week (Flynn et al., 1992).

The data also showed an impact on the educational objectives of the program. Perceived peer smoking, attitudes toward smoking, advantages of smoking, and disadvantages of smoking were all analyzed for the purposes of this study. Although the groups were equivalent at baseline, they showed significant differences in the second through fifth years in each variable (Flynn et al., 1992).

The most impressive findings come from a 2-year follow-up of the study. Flynn et al. (1994) assessed the long-term cigarette smoking prevention effects of mass media and school interventions. The researchers attempted to contact the entire sample, including those who failed to answer all of the annual surveys. The percentage of weekly smokers in the school-only group was significantly higher than the percentage of weekly smokers in the school-and-media group (24.0% and 16.5%, respectively) (Flynn et al., 1995). These results extend to earlier findings of the interventions' effects and find that the effects persisted 2 years after the interventions ended.

An additional follow-up study, targeting only the girls in the cohort, has recently been completed. This follow-up study was conducted because the national smoking rates for girls are higher than boys. The results show that the girls in the school-and-media community smoke less and have more positive views toward nonsmoking than the girls in the school-only group (Worden et al., in press).

Keys to Success

The Vermont School and Mass Media Project owes its success to several elements. First, the media messages were supplemented with an annual school education program. The classroom education enhanced the learning objectives of the media spots, teaching the students information that cannot be obtained from 30- or 60-second advertisements. Second, the media spots all used peers and role models as their social basis of power because they are most effective in persuading behavior change in junior high and high school students. Adolescents and role models for adolescents starred in each television and radio spot. Third, the interventions maintained a high level of intensity throughout the critical years of smoking adoption. Finally, the project presented the media spots frequently during the school year and increased the radio spots and decreased the television spots as the cohort aged.

Client Example

In 1985, Julia Cole was 10 years old and had just begun 5th grade at Burlington Middle School in Burlington, Vermont. In her fall semester, Julia's class learned about the dangers of cigarette smoking and the peer pressure that they might encounter. This segment was taught as a 1-week curriculum with one class period per day for 4 days.

In late winter and early spring of 1986, Julia began to see media spots about smoking while she was watching television after school and in the early evening. For example, Julia was watching *Scooby Doo* one afternoon when a commercial aired showing a girl named Mindy who was worried about an upcoming party. She was afraid that her friends would pressure her into smoking a cigarette, and she did not want to start smoking. The spot ended with Mindy refusing the cigarette at the party, and it all works out fine. On another occasion, Julia was watching the *Cosby Show* and saw a spot where three older teenagers tell why they do not smoke. Julia remembered learning about the dangers of cigarette smoking from her science teacher and decided she would not smoke cigarettes either. At the end of the school year, Julia was given a survey to fill out,

and she wrote that she does not smoke and that she perceives it as a bad habit.

Throughout 6th, 7th, and 8th grades, Julia continued to learn about the effects of cigarette smoking and how to combat social pressures. She also continued to see spots about smoking during her favorite television shows. By 8th grade, Julia was listening to her radio after dinner every night. On occasion, she heard radio spots about smoking prevention. She tried a cigarette at a friend's house one afternoon in 7th grade and did not like it. Some of her friends have started smoking, but Julia has decided that she does not like it and since it is bad for her, she will not smoke in the future. During the annual survey, Julia wrote that she does not smoke and thinks there are many more disadvantages than advantages to smoking.

In 10th grade, Julia's class was asked to fill out the survey again. Julia continued to be a nonsmoker and indicated this on her form. By 12th grade, about 15% of Julia's friends smoke. Julia cannot understand why some of her friends smoke if they know it is bad for them. Julia thinks back to the smoking education she obtained through her teachers and the media spots she has seen and heard. These influences helped her to make the decision not to smoke cigarettes.

Program Information

Program title: The Vermont School and Mass Media Project
Contact person/Title: Brian S. Flynn, ScD–Associate Director of the Office of Health Promotion Research
Agency: College of Medicine, University of Vermont
One South Prospect Street
Burlington, VT 05401
(802) 656-4187 (Phone)
(802) 656-8826 (Fax)

References

Flynn, B. S., Worden, J. K., Secker-Walker, R. H., Badger, G. J., & Geller, B. M. (1995). Cigarette smoking prevention effects of mass media and school interventions targeted to gender and age groups. *Journal of Health Education, 26*(2), S45-S51.

Flynn, B. S., Worden, J. K., Secker-Walker, R. H., Badger, G. J., Geller, B. M., & Costanza, M. C. (1992). Prevention of cigarette smoking through mass media intervention and school programs. *American Journal of Public Health, 82,* 827-834.

Flynn, B. S., Worden, J. K., Secker-Walker, R. H., Pirie, P. L., Badger, G. J., Carpenter, J. H., & Geller, B. M. (1994). Mass media and school interventions for cigarette smoking prevention: Effects 2 years after completion. *American Journal of Public Health, 84,* 1148-1150.

Worden, J. K., Flynn, B. S., Geller, B. M., Chen, M., Shelton, L. G., Secker-Walker, R. H., Solomon, D. S., Solomon, L. J., Couchey, S., & Costanza, M. C. (1988). Development of a smoking prevention mass media program using diagnostic and formative research. *Preventive Medicine, 17*(5), 531-558.

Worden, J. K., Flynn, B. S., Solomon, L. J., Secker-Walker, R. H., Badger, G. J., & Carpenter, J. H. (in press). Preventing cigarette smoking among adolescent girls using mass media. *Health Education Quarterly.*

19

Postponing Sexual Involvement

Lori Friedman

Background

Grady Hospital's Teen Services Program was established in 1970 to address the problem of teenage pregnancy. The staff members at the family planning clinic discovered that they were seeing a significant number of teenagers who were coming into the clinic for pregnancy and STD tests. To address this situation, the Postponing Sexual Involvement (PSI) program was developed for the 1984-1985 school year to reach youth before they became sexually active rather than waiting until they came to the clinic for disease and pregnancy testing. Although the major goal of the program was to help young adults make the decision to postpone sexual involvement, it also provided information on birth control options for those participants who were already sexually active (Moore, 1996).

The PSI program is unique in its use of teenage leaders. The creators of the program found that adult-driven lectures have a limited effect on young people. Younger students look up to the high school leaders and tend to mimic their behavior. This presents an opportunity for the leaders to tell younger teenagers that it is OK to postpone having sex (Howard & McCabe, 1990). Who better to stimulate dis-

cussion of the social and peer pressures associated with becoming sexually active than teenage leaders only a few years older than the participants themselves?

Program Description

PSI is a skills-based program facilitated by both adult counselors and teenage staff members. Participants practice techniques to help them resist succumbing to peer pressures. Sessions focus on why young people are having sex and how they might avoid it rather than on the consequences of this type of behavior (Howard, 1991).

The program supplements the regular health education curriculum with a sex education focus. It is geared for both boys and girls and comprises six sessions lasting 1 to 1 1/2 hours each (Collomb & Howard, 1988).

The program was first developed for the 1984-1985 school year. It has been, and will continue to be, an ongoing program. The program serves the greater metropolitan Atlanta area. There are 4,000 eighth graders from 16 middle schools who participate in the program each year.

The first session is designed to provide basic information on topics such as how and why puberty affects the body. Discussions also focus on the risks of unsafe sexual involvement, such as contracting a disease and/or becoming pregnant. Participants are asked to think about the importance of delaying sexual activity until they feel physically and emotionally ready.

The second session discusses the social pressures surrounding the issue of sex. Slides and a live-action video are used to portray sexual images commonly depicted in the media. This session talks about how sex is perceived as a rite of passage to adulthood and emphasizes that the sexual scenarios depicted in the movies and on television are not always indicative of reality.

The third session deals with peer pressure. It addresses the importance of having both male and female friends and describes the advantages of bonding to people in a nonsexual manner. It also emphasizes the importance of belonging to a group without caving into peer pressures to participate in activities that go beyond a teenager's comfort level.

The fourth session deals with assertiveness training. It provides the participants with the skills to say no and to discuss with others how they feel about and deal with pressure, and it reinforces newly learned behaviors through role playing. This type of modeling is designed to give teenagers time to practice their responses. It equips them with appropriate comebacks so they will be prepared for uncomfortable situations as they arise.

The fifth session focuses on reinforcement skills. Using a game show format, the participants are asked their perceptions about how other teenagers would respond to a variety of questions dealing with sexual issues. This technique enables teenagers to practice delivering responses in a slightly different way.

The sixth and final session involves more role playing and skits. These activities are de-signed to simulate situations where the teenagers come face-to-face with peer pressure and date pressure. For example, a young man might be presented with a situation in which he is playing basketball with a group of friends who start giving him a hard time because he has not yet slept with his girlfriend. This role-playing situation enables the young man to think about how this might make him feel and equips him with appropriate responses. Another scenario may involve a young woman who is being pressured by her date to participate in a sexual activity she feels she is not ready for.

The PSI program has changed over the past 11 years in response to changing societal attitudes and participants' needs. For example, whereas pregnancy prevention was the big issue in the late 1980s, AIDS now receives a lot of attention. New components have been added to the program to address this issue (Rey, personal communication, March 25, 1996). New slides replace older, outdated ones, and some aspects of the program have been shortened to make the sessions flow more smoothly.

Due to the success of the program for 8th graders, funds are being sought to develop a program for 5th and 6th graders. It has been suggested that this age group could benefit from a similar program adapted with age-appropriate materials.

The budget for the school outreach program, which includes peer counseling and human sexuality sessions, is about $120,000 annually. On average, the school system pays half, and Grady Hospital pays the remainder (Moore, 1996).

There are 54 sophomores, juniors, and seniors from the Atlanta area who serve as peer leaders. These teenage leaders are selected on the basis of recommendations from past leaders as well as principals, counselors, and teachers. Interested students must submit an application and are interviewed both over the phone and in person. During the in-person interview, the applicant is placed in a group with four or five other applicants and is presented with a scenario that he or she must act out. This process enables the selection committee (a staff of seven nurses and counselors from Grady Hospital) to observe the applicants' communication and problem-solving skills. In addition to the teenage leaders, there are six adult leaders, who are nurses and counselors. A counselor is always present with the teenage leaders (Rey, personal communication, March 25, 1996).

The teenage leaders spend 20 hours in initial training and participate in a 2-hour in-service training each month throughout the year. They are paid by the session. In addition to the financial gains, the teenage leaders benefit from the program by developing leadership and presentation skills and increasing their self-esteem (Howard, 1991).

The teenage leaders have to miss some of their own classes to facilitate the PSI sessions. Therefore, they must make arrangements with their teachers to make up any missed classwork, and they are not permitted to miss more than two classes in a week. As the teenagers facilitate only five to six classroom sessions per school year, this is not much of a problem.

Community Collaboration and Linkages

The PSI program was developed by Grady Hospital in conjunction with Emory University. The program's creators made arrangements with the Atlanta public school system to supplement its health education curriculum with the PSI program (Moore, 1996).

Although the program was designed to be used primarily in schools, other organizations such as youth agencies, boys and girls clubs, and churches can take advantage of a condensed version of the program. When this type of request is made, staff volunteers and available teenager leaders will present a one-time session (Collomb & Howard, 1988).

Evaluation

An evaluation of the program was funded by the Ford Foundation. Results from the evaluation were published in 1992. They revealed that students who participated in the PSI program were significantly more likely to continue to postpone sexual activity through the end of 9th grade than were students who did not participate in the program. Due to their lower rate of sexual activity, PSI program students were less likely to become pregnant or cause a pregnancy than their non-PSI student counterparts (Howard & McCabe, 1990). In fact, by the end of the 8th grade, students who had not participated in the program were five times more likely to have begun having sex than those who participated in the program. The study found that the program participants were 33% less likely to become sexually active than peers who did not participate. In addition, results from the study revealed that even though the program was offered only to 8th-grade students, reported sexual activity of both 8th- and 9th-grade female students had decreased (Collomb & Howard, 1988).

Informal tests given to participants before and after the program showed positive results. Most participants reported that they would recommend the program to a friend. About 95% of the students who participated in the program felt that the skills they learned would be helpful in delaying sexual activity. Unfortunately, the program did not affect the behavior of sexually active participants. These students did not reduce their sexual activity or increase their use of birth control (Howard & McCabe, 1990). This program is being replicated by a number of cities and states, including the Cincinnati school system and state health departments of Kentucky and North Carolina.

Keys to Success

Program managers believe the key to the success of the program is primarily the teenage leaders. They feel that younger teenagers are more likely to identify with and listen to older teenage peers rather than adults. They reason that the teenage leaders are more effective because they are recent survivors of the 8th grade and can relate to the pressures of being that age. They can tell program participants how having or not having sex can affect their lives (Moore, 1996).

For other organizations considering developing a similar program, PSI program managers have some suggestions. Determine who the key stakeholders are; they could be school systems, local government agencies (such as the health department), or hospitals. Once it is determined which stakeholder(s) is most likely to cooperate, get a commitment from them. Look for partners in the community, such as religious groups, boys and girls clubs, and the YMCA. Any organization with young members may be willing to help manage the program.

Finally, be sure to find someone to take charge of the program and coordinate all the details. This is critical to the success of the program.

Client Example

Vivian Smith is an 8th grader at an Atlanta middle school. She is enrolled in a required health education class. As part of this class, she participated in the PSI program. The following description is what the program is like from her perspective.

During the first session of this program, I learned how and why my body has been changing. I've already started menstruating, so that information was old news. But the only sexually transmitted disease I'd ever heard about was AIDS. In this session, I learned about a number of other STDs. This session also reminded me of ways to prevent pregnancy and disease.

I really liked the second session. We watched clips of popular commercials and my favorite show, *Beverly Hills 90210*. The teenage leaders and Mrs. Thomas (the PSI counselor) talked with us about how sex is always glamorized in the media. They told us to remember that those images are just that . . . images. I'll have to remember that.

During the third session, we learned that it is good to have both girl and boy friends who you are comfortable with. I already knew that. I mean, me, Glen, and Marcy—we've been best friends ever since I can remember. They would never make me do something I didn't want to. But my friend Prill, she's been acting different lately. She's wearing more makeup, coming late to school, and hanging out with kids who smoke. She never used to be like that.

The fourth session made me think about how I could comfortably express myself physically without going too far. They taught us ways to stop if things got out of control. Me and Billy haven't even kissed yet, but I'll be prepared if he ever tries something I'm not ready for.

We played a game in the fifth session. It was kinda like *Wheel of Fortune*. The teen leaders would pick a scenario out of a hat and read it out loud. The contestants had to yell out how they would respond.

The last session, we did role playing. The scenario I acted out was about me going to a dance with a boy I liked (of course, I imagined Billy) and another couple. The other couple snuck outside to fool around. Billy wanted to, too, but I didn't want to. He tried to make me feel bad by saying I was no fun. To respond to this, I told him if he wanted that kind of fun, he should've taken someone else to the dance. And that was that! Everyone clapped, but down inside, I hope this never happens.

Program Information

Program Title: Postponing Sexual Involvement
Contact Person: Marie Mitchell,
     Program Manager

Agency: Emory/Grady Hospital Teen
Services Program
Teen Services Program–Grady Health
System
P.O. Box 26158
80 Butler Street, S.E.
Atlanta, GA 30335
(404) 616-3513
(404) 616-3717 (fax)

References

Collomb, K., & Howard, M. (1988, April). Georgia schools help teens postpone sexual involvement. *Journal of the Medical Association of Georgia*, 230-232.

Howard, M. (1991, November-December). Evaluation: It makes a difference. *Bulletin of the New York Academy of Medicine, 67*(6), 595-605.

Howard, M., & McCabe, J. B. (1990, January/February). Helping teenagers postpone sexual involvement. *Family Planning Perspectives, 22*(1), 21-26.

Moore, L. M. (1996, February). Show and tell, peer counselors teach young teens to say "no" to sex. *Trustee, 49*(2), 8-12.

20

Class of 1989 Study

Rebecca Miller

Background

The Class of 1989 Study was created to test a community-wide smoking prevention program that is aimed at reducing heart disease among adolescents in the study community. The Class of 1989 Study is a part of the larger Minnesota Heart Health Program (MHHP). The MHHP is a research program designed to decrease cardiovascular disease. The MHHP originated in 1980, with the Class of 1989 Study starting in 1983.

The specific purpose of the Class of 1989 Study was to evaluate the youth component of the MHHP. The goal of the study was to investigate the efficacy of a school-based smoking prevention program maintained over a 6-year period. It was hypothesized that the following might be characteristics of a successful smoking prevention program for adolescents: (a) adults are involved, (b) new smoking ordinances are proposed at school and in the community, and (c) a number of complementary programs are instituted at school and in the community (Perry, Kelder, Murray, & Klepp, 1992).

In the past, cigarette smoking interventions have largely targeted individual adolescents. The Class of 1989 Study has an intervention component related to preventing smoking among adolescents, as well as having an intervention component that addresses changing the environment to provide support for remaining a nonsmoker.

Program Description

The MHHP was originally funded for 13 years, 1980-1993. The MHHP was intact in six communities in Minnesota, North Dakota, and South Dakota. The Class of 1989 Study began in April 1983 in two of the six MHHP communities. All 6th-grade students in the public schools of the two communities were invited to participate in the study. A baseline survey was conducted and that cohort was followed annually until graduation from high school in 1989. The survey administration was every April (Kelder, Perry, Klepp, & Lytle, 1994). The number of students who participated in the study from the baseline is 2,401. At the end of the study, 45% of the cohort was still involved in the study (Perry et al., 1992).

Three matched pairs of communities in Minnesota, North Dakota, and South Dakota participated in the MHHP. In each area, one community was the control group and the other the experimental group (Perry, Hearn, Kelder, & Klepp, 1990). The Class of 1989 Study involved two of the six communities. The Fargo, South Dakota-Moorhead, Minnesota, area was the intervention community, and the Sioux Falls, South Dakota, community was the control site.

The population in the Class of 1989 Study was established on a quasi-experimental premise. In the first 4 years of the study, students from 13 grade schools were part of the sample. For the last 2 years of the study, students attending seven high schools were eligible for the study. The selection of the cohort was not dependent on attending one of the sample schools throughout the entire study. Students could enter the program at any point in time, regardless of their prior participation. A cross-sectional sample of students can be analyzed from the annual surveys. A cohort sample, those involved in the study from the baseline, allows for analysis of the continuous effect of the Class of 1989 Study. Due to the addition of the cross-sectional sample in the study, the Class of 1989 Study was able to maintain a larger sample size than if only the cohort was involved in the study (Perry et al., 1992).

The Class of 1989 Study is a school-based behavioral intervention. The intervention, however, does not solely take place in the classroom. It is the community involvement in the intervention that makes this school-based study a community-wide effort.

The funding source for the Class of 1989 Study was the National Heart, Lung, and Blood Institute. There was no program fee for the study. The staff makeup consisted of Masters of Public Health students, faculty, and research staff from the University of Minnesota. The field staff included teachers and other people from the community. These individuals were trained to administer the annual survey (M. Davis, personal communication, April 2, 1996). The teachers received a 1-day training for each year of the study.

Community Collaborators and Linkages

The Class of 1989 Study is based upon a partnership with the community. The previous research demonstrates the need for smoking prevention programs to target the environment surrounding adolescents. In addition to the school-based intervention, the students are receiving an indirect intervention from their community. There are seven strategies to the community-wide intervention of the MHHP: risk factor screening, heart healthy food labeling in restaurants and food stores, citizen task forces to develop risk factor education campaigns, continuing education of health professionals, mass media education, worksite adult education, and youth education (Perry et al., 1992). The Class of 1989 Study and the MHHP are innovative in their link between the school environment and the community. The community-wide approval of the intervention creates a supportive environment for the teenagers in the study area (Perry et al., 1992).

Evaluation

Outcome evaluation was the method of evaluation used for the Class of 1989 Study. The evaluation was conducted on an annual basis in all of the schools participating in the study from April 1983 to April 1989. A self-report survey was used to conduct the assessment. The survey was administered to all of the students who were present in the classroom on the day of the administration, regardless of previous enrollment in the study (Perry et al., 1992).

The instrument measured many different variables associated with tobacco use, including weekly smoking, daily smoking, and smoking history. Prevalence of weekly smoking assessed the impact of the intervention.

Smoking intensity was a score created from the self-report instrument that was representative of the number of times per week a cigarette was smoked by each student (Perry et al., 1992).

The National Heart, Lung, and Blood Institute also funded three other projects at the time of the MHHP to investigate cardiovascular disease prevention. These projects took place at Stanford, in Rhode Island, and in Pennsylvania (Perry et al., 1990). At the completion of the National Heart, Lung, and Blood Institute grant, the communities involved in the intervention decided to undertake the expense of the program (M. Davis, personal communication, April 2, 1996).

Keys to Success

The Class of 1989 Study proved to be successful in many capacities. At the baseline survey, there was no significant difference between the control and intervention communities. In all of the subsequent analyses, the intervention group had lower rates of tobacco use when measured by weekly smoking prevalence or smoking intensity. This is true for the cohort group followed for the 6 years, as well as for the cross-sectional samples in all of the grades. The Class of 1989 Study is innovative in its use of the school and community together. Sustaining its effects may require behavioral education at school, booster programs to reinforce training, and complementary changes in the community (Perry et al., 1992). The complete package of the smoking prevention program is what makes the Class of 1989 Study a success.

The involvement of the adult community in the program was beneficial for the youth in the communities. The adoption of tobacco use behaviors is often a direct influence of adult role modeling. With a concerted community effort and interest, the delay of tobacco use was evident in the intervention community.

All of the community members had a role in the intervention. The credibility of the Class of 1989 Study among the students in the community must have been high due to the active participation among educators, parents, and community leaders.

Due to the positive outcomes of the Class of 1989 Study in terms of delaying tobacco use, the model is applicable to other health behaviors. The design and methods used for this study could possibly be transferable to other high-risk health behavior interventions for adolescents (Perry et al., 1992). Changing health behaviors among adolescents is a difficult task. The Class of 1989 Study shows the importance of creating a supportive environment and an involved community.

Client Example

Scott Anderson was a 6th-grade adolescent living in the intervention community of Moorhead, Minnesota, on the baseline date of the Class of 1989 Study, April 1983. Scott would be introduced to the intervention in the fall of 7th grade. The school-based curriculum would include the Minnesota Smoking Prevention Program. The purpose of this program is to discourage the onset of tobacco use during adolescence. Within the Class of 1989 Study, there are several different components. The program follows a systematic time sequence of events.

First, Scott would learn the short-term consequences of smoking. This is done in an age-appropriate discussion format. Second, Scott and his classmates would discuss smoking as a habit that should not be considered normal for teenagers. This part of the curriculum addresses teenagers' expectations about who smokes compared to the true prevalence of smoking. Third, reasons why adolescents smoke are discussed. Fourth, Scott would learn about the connection between tobacco use and advertising.

Students are taught the methods advertisers employ to target adolescents. Fifth, Scott and his classmates would learn ways to resist peer pressure. This is done by role playing and skits. This is one of the most fundamental lessons of the intervention. The sixth component of the program would involve Scott making a public pledge to abstain from smoking (Perry et al., 1992).

In addition to the school-based component of the study, Scott would receive many antitobacco messages from the surrounding community. The program makes a deliberate attempt to reorganize the environment into a health community. Reinforcers for smoking prevention would abound in the community.

Program Information

Program Title: The Class of 1989 Study
Contact Person: Dr. Cheryl Perry,
    Epidemiologist

Agency: School of Public Health,
    University of Minnesota
School of Public Health
University of Minnesota
1300 S. Second Street
Minneapolis, MN 55454-1015
(612) 624-1818

References

Kelder, S. H., Perry, C. L., Klepp, K. I., & Lytle, L. L. (1994). Longitudinal tracking of adolescent smoking, physical activity, and food choice behaviors. *American Journal of Public Health, 84*(7), 1121-1126.

Perry, C. L., Hearn, M. D., Kelder, S. H., & Klepp, K. I. (1990). The Minnesota Heart Health Program Youth Program. In D. Nutbeam (Ed.), *Youth health promotion: From theory to practice in school and community* (pp. 254-276). London: Forbes.

Perry, C. L., Kelder, S. H., Murray, D. M., & Klepp, K. I. (1992). Communitywide smoking prevention: Long-term outcomes of the Minnesota Heart Health Program and the Class of 1989 Study. *American Journal of Public Health, 82*(9), 1210-1216.

21

Adolescent Family Life Program

Marguerite Mills

Background

In the mid-1970s, adolescent pregnancy was recognized as a major social problem. By the 1980s, programs were being developed to help adolescent girls who were pregnant or who were already young parents (Miller & Dyk, 1990). The Adolescent Family Life Program (AFLP), one of the earliest programs to assist pregnant and parent teens, began as a pilot program in 1983 and was sponsored by the Kennedy Foundation for its first 4 years. The program's goals were to increase healthy birth outcomes, to increase adolescent responsibility and improve skills to cope with the stresses of parenthood, and to prevent subsequent teen pregnancies within a year of delivery (La Clinica de Familia, 1994).

Program Description

The AFLP comprises several comprehensive classes addressing health, educational, and psychosocial issues. The AFLP integrates the following components and services:

• Prenatal/parenting component: This includes referrals and follow-up for early/adequate prenatal care. Educational classes are provided by a health educator once a week for 24 weeks, covering topics such as breastfeeding, nutrition, physical body changes, and emotional aspects of pregnancy. After birth, a lactation consultant visits the teen mother to encourage breastfeeding and provide instructions and support. Social workers visit the teen mother/father for 1 year after the birth of the child and assess current needs. Clients (teen mother/father) and babies return for ongoing classes in infant first aid, newborn care, immunization information/reminders, and child safety.

• Breastfeeding—education and support: Teens are provided with education on breastfeeding. Teen mothers who choose to breastfeed are given additional educational sessions on successful breastfeeding and problem resolutions regarding difficulty in breastfeeding. Clients who are high risk are encouraged to breast-feed to enhance bonding with their child. Further information is provided on mother/infant bonding and breaking the cycle of abuse and neglect. Visits are conducted in the hospital and at home.

• Male involvement component: This component actually promotes male responsibility throughout the pregnancy for the first year of parenting and during the child's life. Fathers are expected to attend prenatal/parenting class and support groups. The coordinator for this component is a male who serves as a role model and assists clients with issues that may arise and supports them in their new role as parents.

• Job placement component: This program helps clients with job research skills, job referrals, resume development, and practice in job interviewing. This component also assists clients in finding access to job training and education programs.

• Social services component: Social workers complete an intake/assessment on all female and male clients. Required income status eligibility is verified for Income Support Division programs such as Medicaid, food stamps, and WIC. Social workers counsel clients in need of short-term therapeutic services.

• Domestic Violence Component: At intake, clients are assessed for history of domestic violence, sexual abuse, and verbal abuse. Those possessing an abuse history are immediately referred to counseling. Clients participate in support groups that deal with many issues such as responsibility for pregnancy, change in family relationships, conflict resolution, discipline, and equity in relationships.

• Outreach support and educational services for grandparents: This component was designed to give support and assist parents of the teens. They are given information in the areas of domestic violence, conflict resolution with teens, adolescent development, and com-

munications skills (*La Clinica de Familia*, 1994).

At this time, the AFLP serves the community of Dona Ana, New Mexico, with sites in the cities of Las Cruces and Sunland Park. AFLP serves about 1,500 square miles of rural/semirural areas that border Mexico (*La Clinica de Familia*, 1994). One of the AFLP areas served is southern Dona Ana County, which has a population that is largely young, poor, and 80% minority. The satellite area, Sunland Park, is 98% Mexican American; 49% of its residents are under the age of 20 (*La Clinica de Familia*, 1994).

When the program first started, it served the 13- to 18-year-old group. Because early experimentation with sex is on the rise, the program has served clients as young as 11 and up to 19 years of age. The Sunland Park site serves teens from 13 to 19 years of age due to the lack of resources available in the rural area (*La Clinica de Familia*, 1994).

Currently, AFLP serves about 702 clients, who include pregnant and parenting teens (separate figures for each group were not provided). In fiscal year July 1, 1995, through June 30, 1996, AFLP enrolled 331 new clients. This figure includes both female and male teens (*La Clinica de Familia*, 1994).

The programs are located in two local county school districts and community agencies in Dona Ana County and Sunland Park. These sites receive funding from the following sources: La Clinica's operations; New Mexico Department of Health; Department of Children, Youth, and Families; and various local service organizations (Civitan International, Sertoma, United Way, and March of Dimes) (*La Clinica de Familia*, 1994). AFLP was originally funded by the Kennedy Foundation Community of Caring. At this time, teens (clients) who participate in the AFLP programs do so free of charge.

The Las Cruces Center employs the following: administrative assistant, social workers, outreach worker, lactation consultant R.N., health educator, and a client and community educator (responsible for male clients). the Sunland Park satellite center has: client and community educator (responsible for male clients), social worker, community education specialist, receptionist, and health educator (*La Clinica de Familia*, 1994).

Community Collaborators and Linkages

AFLP social workers have established a network of many community agencies with which they work to provide linkage between teens and services. The following agencies work with AFLP in a variety of capacities:

- The Children, Youth, and Families Department of Social Services provides funding for client services.
- The Income Support Division provides adolescents with Medicaid services, AFDC, and food stamps.
- First Step OB clinic of Memorial Medical Center provides prenatal, labor, and delivery services once clients have been approved for Medicaid.
- Dona Ana County Public Health Office provides teens with WIC certification and insurance vouchers.
- Southwest Counseling provides long-term counseling based on a sliding fee scale. This counseling center also provides free group counseling to AFLP clients.
- La Casa Domestic Violence program trains AFLP staff in the area of domestic violence and is another resource for counseling.
- Maternal Child Health Task Force and New Mexico Breastfeeding Task Force are organizations that promote prenatal and postpartum care and breastfeeding in the community (*La Clinica de Familia*, 1994).

Evaluation

AFLP receives funds from the W. K. Kellogg Foundation to replicate its Las Cruces program in Sunland Park. Funds from the W. K. Kellogg Foundation are also used to conduct evaluations of existing programs. AFLP contracted with the staff from the Department of Anthropology and Health Sciences at New Mexico State University to assess current (and proposed) programs and to provide AFLP with appropriate tools for future evaluation (*La Clinica de Familia*, 1994).

The breastfeeding component of the program has been recognized as a success by the state of New Mexico in a state newsletter (*La Clinica de Familia*, 1994). This component encourages teen mothers to breast-feed in order to enhance mother-child bonding (*La Clinica de Familia*, 1994). In the fiscal year between July 1, 1995, and June 30, 1996, the program had 101 teen mothers breastfeeding and 51 who chose not to (*La Clinica de Familia*, 1996).

Although a formal evaluation component is not yet completed, there are many indicators of the program's success: its replication in Sunland Park; its continuation to serve people since its inception in 1983, while many other programs have come and gone; and the support (financial and service) it receives from community and governmental agencies. All these reflect the program's value and importance to the community.

Keys to Success

Many innovative community programs fail because they do not establish relationships with community agencies and governmental departments. AFLP has been successful because its leaders established strong ties with the surrounding community, ensuring that their program would survive after the initial Kennedy Foundation funding ran out. Many factors have contributed to AFLP's success.

- Over the years AFLP has built and established many relationships.
- AFLP has gained support from surrounding community agencies and governmental departments.
- AFLP has acquired funding that targets preteens and adolescents directly in middle and high schools so that they better understand the consequences of teen pregnancy (*La Clinica de Familia,* 1994).
- The community educator component aims at preventing first pregnancies among southern Dona Ana County's teen populations through public school and community-wide presentations on health, sexuality, and healthy responsible sexual behavior.

Client Example

A pregnant teen may have first contact with AFLP through several channels. The teen might have been recommended by the school counselor, nurse, Planned Parenthood, First Step OB client, or may come in on her own. To be eligible for these services, the pregnant teen must be under the age of 18 and pregnant for the first time (La Clinica de Familia, 1994).

Mary, a 15-year-old who lives in the Las Cruces area of New Mexico, became pregnant for the first time. Confused and uncertain about what to do, she sought help from her school counselor. The counselor suggested that Mary contact AFLP. Mary's counselor told her that AFLP would provide her with information and help in making decisions concerning her pregnancy.

After Mary's initial contact with AFLP, an appointment was scheduled by the receptionist for Mary to meet with a social worker who would begin the intake process. Because Mary was still living at home, it was recommended that she bring one of her parents to the intake appointment.

At this first meeting, it was determined that Mary would enroll in the prenatal/parenting classes. Her parents agreed to seek help with the outreach support group for grandparents. Through talking to the social worker, Mary's parents realized that communication with their daughter had been poor, and they agreed to try different communication tactics in the months ahead.

Mary as of yet has not applied for any social services. She receives assistance in applying for Medicaid and other benefits from the AFLP social worker. Appointments are scheduled with Memorial Medical Center for prenatal care. It has also been determined through the intake process that Mary will not be using all the program components. Her boyfriend has decided not to participate in the program. But if he should change his mind he will be able to attend the prenatal/parenting classes and enroll in other support components.

In the months ahead, up to the time that Mary delivers, she will receive education on issues such as health, nutrition, prenatal care, and self-esteem. If at any time during the pregnancy Mary needs counseling for any reason, she will be eligible for group or individual help. AFLP will encourage Mary to stay in school as long as possible during the pregnancy.

After delivery, AFLP will send a lactation consultant out to the hospital to visit Mary and provide instruction and support for breastfeeding. With the birth of the child, a social worker will continue to visit Mary at home and to work with the grandparents for up to 1 year.

Within 3 to 6 weeks, when Mary is ready to return to AFLP, she and the baby will attend classes on newborn care, immunization, child safety, infant first aid, and breastfeeding. During this time, Mary will be encouraged to continue to pursue her educational goals and access the job placement component to help further define her future plans.

Program Information

Program Title: Adolescent Family Life Program
Contact Person: Nancy Tafoya
La Clinica de Familia
Las Cruces, NM
(505) 523-2042
(505) 526-9650 (fax)

References

La Clinica de Familia. (1996, July). *Evaluative data*. Las Cruces, NM: Author.

La Clinica de Familia. (1994, June). *Adolescent Family Life Program (W. C. Kellogg, Grant)*. Las Cruces, NM: Author.

Miller, B. C., & Dyke, P. A. H. (1990). Adolescent fertility-related behavior in the 1990s: Risking the future continued. *Journal of Family Issues, 11*, 235-238.

22

New Jersey School-Based
Youth Services Program

Robin Ziman

Background

The School Based Youth Services Program (SBYSP) was developed in 1988, because of a need seen by both educators and human services agencies. The originators of the program believed that common family disarray, violence, poverty, and personal health issues combined with the typical issues surrounding childhood and adolescence, strongly affected a child's capacity to learn, complete schoolwork, and behave appropriately in a school or community setting (Knowlton & Tetelmen, 1994). By linking the education system with human services agencies, health systems, and employment systems, the state of New Jersey would be able to more effectively deal with these social issues. Uniting governmental agencies, such as the Department of Education and the Department of Human Services, with local initiatives and community resources allows this program to provide a comprehensive set of services in a "one-stop shopping" setting to New Jersey's youth. The program meets the local needs of each community it serves by

augmenting and coordinating necessary services in that community. It does not impose a statewide model to be used by all communities and does not duplicate or replace currently existing services (Knowlton & Tetelmen, 1994).

The goal of this program is to give adolescents and children, particularly those with problems, the opportunity to finish their education, obtain skills that lead to employment or additional education, and enjoy a mentally and physically healthy life (U.S. Department of Education [USDE], 1995). Its objective is to decrease violence, adolescent pregnancy, school dropout and suspension, and unemployment for youth throughout New Jersey.

Program Description

Program Beginnings

The SBYSP was first endorsed by New Jersey Governor Tom Kean in 1987. Cooperation and collaboration with the Departments of Labor, Health, and Education led to the de-

AUTHOR'S NOTE: All information not referenced in this article was obtained from the New Jersey SBYSP information packet. Materials did not list authors and were not dated as they were not prepared for publication. Any clarification of information should be obtained directly from the program.

velopment of a request for proposal in 1987. Communities interested in starting a SBYSP in their area were asked to submit a proposal for working with the school system and local agencies. In January 1988, 29 sites were selected, including at least one in each county of the state. Therefore, youth throughout the entire state of New Jersey have access to the SBYSP. By April 1988, several sites had begun serving adolescents. This program is now a line item on the state budget, and there are no plans to discontinue the project in the future. The continuity of funding played a major role in the acceptance of this program by the school systems. Often subjected to temporary programming, which leaves schools without funding for the program after its end date, schools in New Jersey are wary of introducing new programs to their students. By assuring schools that funding would remain available and that the program was not merely a pilot, acceptance of these services increased.

Services Provided

Each program site is required to provide a set of core services to youth in the area, including youth both in school and out of school. The core services include primary and preventive health services, mental health and family counseling, job and employment training, substance abuse counseling, and crisis intervention. In addition, all sites offer recreation, information, and referral services. Sites may subsidize their program with additional services, if necessary or desired. Additional services currently being implemented include teen parenting education, transportation, day care, tutoring, family planning, hotlines, and special vocational programs.

Program Setting and Geography

Twenty-nine high school sites throughout New Jersey, a northeastern state, provide services at a public secondary school or at a site located near a school. Settings include urban, suburban, and rural areas. The sites run programs before, during, and after school, and in the summer months. Some sites also run programs on weekends. When possible, programs run in rooms designated by the school for services. Those not run in a school provide services at a local site, in close proximity to the school.

Population Served

The 29 original SBYSP sites serve adolescents ages 13 to 19 years old and their families. Additional sites now serve elementary school-age children. All adolescents in an area may use the program's services, regardless of student status. Although program services are available for all youth, services target those at risk for dropping out of school, becoming pregnant, using drugs, developing mental illness, or becoming unemployed. Data from 1991 suggest that an equal number of males and females use the program. African Americans are most likely to use the services, followed by Caucasians. Hispanics are least likely to make use of these services. Students in the 9th and 10th grades most often access program services.

In 1992, more than 20,000 adolescents used services of the SBYSP. One of every three eligible teens is reached by some program component. High-risk teens made up about 45% of these program users, or about 9,000 people. Of the 20,000 people accessing services, about 16,000 used individual care services.

Program Funding

The largest portion of funding for the SBYSP is provided by the state. The state allocates about $6 million each year to its operation. An average site receives about $200,000 a year from this fund. In addition, each host community must contribute either money or in-kind services to cover part of the operating costs of the program. Also, the Department of

Human Resources (DHR) coordinates existing services (such as Medicaid well-child care) with the program's services, enabling the department to augment the program with money generated through these other services.

Several grants have been obtained to pay for operating costs, including staff costs, materials, liability coverage, and renovations to some rooms or buildings. In addition, contractual agreements for special services provide funding for these non-core services. A federal Youth 2000 grant has been given to the program to help cover the costs of technical assistance and to better link the educational system with the human services system.

Staff Makeup

The entire SBYSP is overseen by the state, through the Department of Human Services. Locally, each program site is managed by involved public and nonprofit agencies and the school systems, under the direction of a program director. Usually a nonprofit or public agency serves as the managing agent in an area.

Program staff include counselors, nurses, social workers, teachers, and school administrators, as well as teens and parents. Staff provide the core services and additional services where available and are invited to participate in school activities (such as faculty meetings). This allows for more collaboration between the program staff and the school staff. A local advisory committee, consisting of school staff, professionals, parents, and community representatives, makes decisions about programming issues. Each month, all program directors meet with the Department of Human Services to discuss progress, problems, and ideas.

Community Collaborators and Linkages

The success of the NJSBYSP is based on the collaboration of state departments, local school boards, and community agencies. For a community to be offered a grant as a program site, it must show shared support and participation of a wide range of groups, including local community groups, teachers, parents, businesses, public and nonprofit agencies, students, and local school district administration. Each school district was required to apply for the grant jointly with one or more local agencies. At present, most sites work with an average of 12 agencies in the community. A feedback system between these groups allows for open communication, cooperation, and more effective follow-up with students in the program.

Community service agencies not involved in the program from its inception may join the program and add their services. However, schools involved and the local managing agency must first approve the addition of an agency and a new service.

Evaluation

Each program site throughout New Jersey has a unique blend of services in combination with the core services. Therefore, each site may also choose to evaluate success in certain programs or within their site as a whole. There are a multitude of evaluation types and results gathered from these different sites and programs. In addition, the Annie E. Casey Foundation is the sponsor of a statewide, comprehensive evaluation project. The School and Community Services Department of the Academy for Educational Development (AED) is responsible for the design, implementation, and analysis of the evaluation.

The goals of the evaluation are to conduct a cross-site analysis of the 29 program sites, comparing the organization, staffing, services, management, and collaboration efforts between the sites. In addition, a sample of program sites will allow for a study of student outcomes.

Preliminary data provided by the Department of Human Services shows that over 90% of school personnel believe that the SBYSP has a positive effect on both students and the school as a whole. Personnel also believe that the services have had a positive effect on social problems, including school attendance, dropout rates, and graduation rates. The most positive effects are believed to be seen in substance abuse and academic performance rates.

Since its inception, the SBYSP has been expanded in the state of New Jersey to include several elementary and middle school sites. In addition, both Iowa and Kentucky are now replicating the program. Replication of the program indicates that this program concept is admired and considered successful in other areas of the country.

The overall evaluation of this program is funded by the Annie E. Casey Foundation. This generous contribution has allowed program sites to focus on materials and services and to conduct mini-evaluations of individual programs without depleting money allotted to the program as a whole. No fee is charged to any of the clients who use program services.

Keys to Success

"SBYSP brings integrated services to interrelated problems" (Knowlton and Tetelmen, 1994, p. 107). This program fills the need for a "one-stop shopping" place for youth services, which is essential to its ongoing success with teens, parents, schools, and the community.

Several structural elements and activities enhance the SBYSP. First, the program was conceived as a permanent program, not a temporary pilot study. This was essential for school approval. Because many programs are started and then left to the school for future funding and operation, schools are hesitant to start new programs. Permanent funding allayed any fears of this occurrence.

Second, a broad base of support from the state level to local groups was secured prior to implementation. Local organizations have power and responsibility toward site functioning. Parents participate on an advisory board regarding program development. Teens participated in focus groups before the program began to determine what activities they wanted in the program. Adjustments to services were made based on teens' concerns and suggestions. Collaboration between groups and the schools allows for more effective interactions and support for students. This combination of group involvement has ensured positive responses from the multiple groups affected by the program.

A third factor in the SBYSP's success is the provision of recreation services at all sites. This service gives all students an opportunity to participate in the program, thus introducing them to other available services. Most important, it protects the confidentiality of teens using the counseling services. Other teens remain unaware of who is using the program for which services, minimizing the stigma associated with the program and maximizing its potential to help students. Additional confidentiality is ensured because program staff are not school staff. Therefore, they are not required to release records of participating students to school faculty. Faculty members know only that a teen is attending the program and are given only the information the student wishes to share.

Client Example

A student may enter the SBYSP through several channels. All students are welcome to come to the site programs on their own and request services. In addition, they may be referred to the program by school administrators, teachers, or guidance counselors. The collaboration between the program and the schools allows for easy interaction between the groups. Therefore, if a student is having a problem or requests help from a particular person (such as a counselor or teacher), this person will work with program staff to help find appropriate resources for the student.

Due to the numerous and varied services available at each site, it is difficult to examine the process which a teen would encounter in this program. For example, some may enter the program for its recreational activities, enjoying games and social events with teens their age and a program staff member. Others take part in the program's counseling services. A teen has the opportunity to approach a staff member and to build a relationship of trust with an individual. He or she may then choose to disclose issues of concern and to work with a counselor to find solutions. Many teens, especially those at high risk, enter the program, either on their own or through referral, and use multiple services. The flexibility of this program to accommodate student needs is key to its popularity in the schools. When accessing services in this program, students have the opportunity to make their own connections to program staff and to decide what they would like to gain from using the program.

Overall, the wide array of services offered by the New Jersey SBYSP is a welcome addition to the school systems throughout the state. Rather than having to seek out services on their own or having to be referred to outside agencies, students now have the opportunity to make contacts and to seek counseling, health services, and employment training all within their school area. In addition, recreational services provide an alternative for teens who have been unable to participate in productive activities after school or in the summer prior to implementation of this program.

Program Information

Program Title: The School Based Youth Services Program
Contact Person: Roberta Knowlton, MSW, LCSW Director,
New Jersey Department of Human Services, (609) 292-7901
Capital Place One
222 South Warren Street
CN 700
Trenton, NJ 08625-0700
(609) 292-7816
(609) 984-7380 (Fax)

References

Knowlton, R., & Tetelmen, E. (1994). Educators respond to New Jersey's "one-stop shopping" program. In R. A. Levin (Ed.), *Greater than the sum: Professionals in a comprehensive services model* (pp. 103-114). Washington, DC: ERIC Clearinghouse on Teacher Education.

U.S. Department of Education. (1995). *School-linked comprehensive services for children and families: Services for children and families* (SAI 95-3025). Washington, DC: Author.

23

Archway: Treating Adolescent Substance Abusers

Madeline Zevon

Background

Getting an adolescent substance abuser into treatment is a difficult job. In fact, getting any substance abuser into treatment is difficult. The stigma causes denial and renders the person virtually blind to what is happening to him or her. With young people who are in the early stages of the disease of chemical dependency or "only experimenting," the serious consequences are only beginning to show and denial is very strong for both the adolescent and his family. The model described in this chapter illustrates how several different systems have coordinated their efforts to deal with this difficult population.

The Setting and Community

The setting is a comprehensive outpatient drug and alcohol treatment center in Mount Vernon, New York. Mount Vernon is located in Westchester County, a suburban area north of New York City just over the Bronx borderline. Although technically a suburban area, Mount Vernon has many inner-city problems due to family, social, and environmental characteristics such as homelessness, chemical dependency, crime, drug dealing, assaultive behavior, unemployment, illiteracy, and disintegrated family life.

The city has one of the highest concentrations of poverty and single female-headed families in Westchester County. There is a high youth dropout rate and extremely high pregnancy rates for females ages 10 to 16 years. Mount Vernon's population density is the highest in the county, with the highest concentration of African Americans per capita.

The Program

Archway's Outpatient Program is a division of Yonkers General Hospital, which has a comprehensive network of services for people who have drug or alcohol problems and their families. Services include two detoxification units, a crisis center, inpatient rehabilitation, a methadone program, three outpatient programs, and several satellite clinics in homeless shelters. There are also programs in the jail and an alternative high school.

Archway has a day rehabilitation program for adults; individual and group counseling sessions in the evening, including family groups; and a uniquely large program for children of alcoholics/addicts between the ages of 5 and 18 years old.

Treatment is reimbursed primarily through Medicaid; a small number of clients have private insurance (usually with very limited benefits) or pay a fee on a sliding scale. Archway receives deficit funding from the state through Westchester County to compensate for services rendered to adolescents and families who cannot afford to pay for treatment.

Archway has a special state license to operate an Intensive Adolescent Treatment Program. This is a 3-day-a-week program meeting from 4 p.m. to 7 p.m. for a total of 9 hours a week. Group therapy sessions are held from 4 p.m. to 5:30 p.m., and a hot dinner is served from 5:30 p.m. to 6 p.m. The program activities include a recreation session at the YMCA gym once a week from 6 p.m. to 7 p.m. and attendance at a Narcotics Anonymous meeting once a week at our facility. The major focus is on group therapy. The program is culturally sensitive, and we have actively sought out African American speakers from various walks of life. Special events include trips to the National Black Theater in Harlem to see plays. Our treatment films are varied and appropriate for people of color and adolescents.

The counselors are considered role models the kids look to, identify with, and respect. They are not afraid to set limits, and there have been no significant behavior problems. Most staff members are credentialed alcoholism counselors or social workers.

There are three phases to treatment: Phase 1 consists of engagement and education. Phase 2 is identification of treatment issues and development of strategies for remaining abstinent. Phase 3 is an advanced group, centered

on completing treatment goals. Urine tests are conducted randomly and treatment plans are reviewed every 3 weeks. The average adolescent is in treatment for 6 months. Every effort is made to engage the family in treatment, despite a great deal of resistance. Adolescents unable to maintain abstinence in the outpatient setting are referred to inpatient rehabs and return to Archway after they complete their stay (usually 28 days).

Collaboration and Community Linkages

Because of the nature of denial, leverage is nearly always necessary to get a person into treatment. The following three programs illustrate how this was accomplished through collaboration with state and local health, law enforcement, and other government agencies.

Youth Prevention and Treatment

There was a great need in Mount Vernon to address the problem of teenage substance abusers appearing in the Mount Vernon Criminal Court. To meet this need, a program was developed called Youth Prevention and Treatment (YPAT). Archway received a grant from the Westchester County Department of Community Mental Health and the City of Mount Vernon Recreation Department to facilitate staffing. This grant allows a caseworker assigned to the YPAT program to be present in the Mount Vernon Criminal Court 5 mornings a week.

The Westchester County Department of Community Mental Health, Alcohol and Drug Abuse Services, serves as a regulatory body, monitoring funding and ensuring effective delivery of treatment services and compliance with state guidelines as stipulated by the New York State Office of Alcohol and Substance Abuse Services. The county has been working toward linking various service providers to improve treatment collaborations.

In the YPAT program, adolescents between the ages of 16 and 21, usually charged with a misdemeanor, such as disorderly conduct or possession of a controlled substance, find their charges reduced to a noncriminal violation when they are assigned to the YPAT program in an effort to refer them to treatment. The YPAT caseworker facilitates a chemical dependency evaluation at Archway. Youth are referred to the Intensive Adolescent Treatment Program for alcohol/drug treatment and may receive other services, including mental health treatment at specialty programs. Educational and vocational needs are addressed by the Archway clinic. Clients are strongly encouraged to complete high school education and pursue higher education or vocational training. Youth who are employed and unable to attend treatment during the 4 p.m. to 7 p.m. time period attend services at other times.

The YPAT worker reports issues of noncompliance to the court. The youth will receive a violation which usually motivates them to return to treatment. If not, their conditional discharge is rescinded. Adolescents enrolled in the program are monitored for 1 year by the YPAT caseworker.

An important element in the success of YPAT has been the cooperation and commitment of the local judges and other governmental/agency officials. In fact, one of the judges initiated this program. All of the judges have individually visited our agency and have participated in the groups with our adolescents, as has the mayor and representatives from each of the sponsoring agencies. These visitors provide the clients with examples of some of the positive role models in the community. The clients interact well with these guests, and the guests have the opportunity to see firsthand how the program works. Each guest gives an informative talk followed by a rap session with the adolescents. There is a tremendous attitude of caring and concern.

Gang-Related Intensive Programming

Gang-Related Intensive Programming (GRIP) is part of the Department of Probation and is for adolescents convicted of a misdemeanor or a more serious charge. Probation officers have relatively small caseloads (20) and are able to devote time and effort to seeing the youth often, making school and home visits when necessary. Once again, the Westchester County Department of Community Mental Health, Alcohol and Substance Abuse Services, was instrumental in linking our agency with GRIP. Currently, almost half of the adolescents in our program are referred through GRIP. We conduct assessments on all GRIP clients. Our team of counselors meets once a month with the GRIP probation officers. This process has been one of mutual education and understanding; we review cases during this meeting and work cooperatively. The line of communication is open and effective.

Nelson Mandela Community High School

The Mandela school is an alternative high school in Mount Vernon. Due to concerns related to substance abuse, the school district requested our assistance in that facility. As a result, a part-time clinic has been established with an adolescent counselor providing services 4 half-days per week. The counselor provides on-site assessment and conducts early educational/engagement groups. Often, after this process is started, some adolescents will attend treatment at Archway. With the encouragement of the school and their parents, these teens have had some success in the program. For those who are resistant, our counselor continues to see them in the school. The

Westchester County Department of Community Mental Health, Alcohol and Drug Abuse Services, has been instrumental in facilitating this program.

Keys to Success

The keys to our success have been leverage and linkage. Because denial is so strong for substance abusers, leverage is critical in getting the abuser into treatment. The linkages Archways has with other agencies and systems, particularly law enforcement, provide the necessary leverage. Linking health departments, law enforcement, schools, and other agencies in the pursuit of a common goal creates a stronger, more efficient, and more effective program by allowing each entity to do what it does best.

Collaboration among the agencies involved is essential. Collaboration is attained by getting the commitment and cooperation of stakeholders early in the planning process, such as the judge who initiated the YPAT program. Collaboration is maintained through open and effective lines of communication, which requires an ongoing process of mutual education and cooperation.

Communication with the client population is also essential. This means choosing an appropriate team of counselors to work with this population. The program's counselors are people the clients can identify with, yet provide positive role models.

Client Example

Guy, an 18-year-old black male, was referred to Archway through the YPAT program in January. His charge was possession of a controlled substance. A native of Jamaica, he came to the United States when he was a child, with his mother and younger sister. He was

attending the 12th grade at Mount Vernon High School at the time he was referred here.

Guy admitted he was 14 when he began smoking marijuana and drinking alcohol. When he was a teenager, he began to sell crack. He dropped out of treatment after five sessions and did not respond to our outreaches. He was discharged from treatment 1 month after his admission date. The court was notified of his noncompliance, and he was incarcerated for 3 months. He returned in April, now under the GRIP (probation) mandate. His attitude had changed considerably. He actively participated in the program and interacted well with other clients. Areas of concerns were relationship with mother, separation from his father, peer pressure, and feelings of anger and hopelessness. He progressed through the levels of treatment and took a leadership role in group. He graduated from high school by attending the summer session and has been successfully discharged from treatment.

Currently, Guy is working at a supermarket; he is involved with the College Careers program and is planning to attend college. He visits the group from time to time, telling group members how the program has helped him. The following is a paper he presented to the group shortly before he left treatment:

Drugs were always a way of life for me. I grew weed in Jamaica even when I didn't know how to smoke. I was mixing weed and dry leaves following my older brother and cousins. Then as I grew, I didn't have to smoke it. I could walk through the field and be high without knowing I was high.

My aggression grew. Then I came to America, and before long, I was sparking Phillies, only once in a while not on a regular basis. That stopped when I started selling crack and seeing pregnant mothers coming still smoking twisted out the frame, and I was like, I ain't smoking or drinking 'cause I can't see myself like that, although I didn't know the definition for it, I know crack heads started somewhere.

Before long, I got caught and put in this program. I felt I didn't belong here, but if you open your ears and keep an open mind, you'll identify with the group, and you'll see that you do belong here and just use this to your advantage as a stepping stone.

Conclusion

When the adolescent initially comes into treatment, we have had little success with engaging the parent in our family program or persuading them to pay our fee. However, sometimes after they see positive changes in their children, they do respond and become supportive to treatment.

There are two adolescents in our program who were referred here by their parents. One parent, in recovery for many years, was very aware. When she saw her son begin to use drugs, she moved swiftly to get him into treatment. The other parent is paying her son to attend. But these adolescents are the exception. In this community, it was necessary for various service agencies to come together to meet the needs of substance-abusing adolescents. Treatment with this population can be successful if there is a coordinated effort. The earlier a young person comes into treatment, the better the chances are of avoiding more serious consequences of substance abuse.

Program Information

Program Title: Archway Outpatient Treatment Center
Contact Person: Madeline Zevon, ACSW, CASAC, Assistant Coordinator
Agency: Yonkers General Hospital
100 East First Street, 6th Floor
Mount Vernon, NY 10550
(914) 668-1450

24

In Context:
The Future for Adolescent Health

Alan Henderson

It is tempting to conclude from the chapters in this volume that adolescent health needs are overwhelming and that, in the future, considerable resources need to be allocated to cope with each of these complex and difficult issues. In fact, that has been the approach taken with adolescent health needs at least since the beginning of the "war on drugs" in the 1960s. The pattern of sudden attention and identification of a health problem, diagnosis of who is involved and who is at risk, and development of programs to address the issue(s) has been well developed. These programs have been complemented by our increasing technological capacity to gather and analyze greater and diverse amounts of data to help address adolescent health needs.

Far from being future-oriented, the recognition-problem definition-program approach to health problems has been a staple of American life for decades. We now possess more and better tools to apply to this well-used strategy, giving health professionals and policymakers hope that this time we can really get a handle on teenage health issues.

An underlying assumption of our methods is that we can eradicate these problems and allow teenagers to return to their development

from children into adults unfettered by the dangers of alcohol and other drugs, premature sexual activity and resulting pregnancies and STDs, and intentional and unintentional injuries. Underscoring the desire to eradicate these problems is selective remembrance of our own adolescent lives and applying our experiences to guide our responses to current challenges facing teenagers. Although the developmental process of making the transition from a child to an adult is continuous, the context for today's youth is substantially different from the past generation.

Part of our assumption that we can do something about teenage health problems is based on our social development, where life span continues to expand, the nation's economy grows richer, and our ability to generate and use new knowledge and technology continues to increase at a geometric pace. This assumption is also based, in part, on our societal belief in the value of individual endeavor and self-determination where individuals have the opportunity, by dint of their own personal efforts, to overcome whatever barriers or problems they might face. Yet, another facet of this assumption is our expectation that the family will function as the crucible for rearing children, helping them to acquire the values, ethics, morals, codes of conduct, and motivation to become adults who fully participate in society.

In sum, we have an expectation that the future for adolescents will be better than it was in the preceding generation. Differences between the realities facing adolescents of today and tomorrow and our expectations challenge our beliefs and assumptions. It is crucial that we use our concern for youth as a guide to develop different approaches to close gaps between expectations and realities and, potentially, change our expectations about adolescent health problems and our expectations of adolescence itself.

Essential Issues

The future for adolescents is unknowable, except that it will be different, negating the temptation to predict what will occur. As Toffler (1990) pointed out, data from media, publications of analyses, and lists of trends lead to disjointed and fragmented views of the future. It is possible, however, to use available resources to project the future with an understanding that underlying perspectives and assumptions have to be explicitly spelled out:

• Adolescent health problems cannot be eradicated. They may be reduced to their lowest level, which may be difficult to determine. Adolescent health problems, as we have seen from the chapters in this volume, continue to change.

• Individual effort on the part of adolescents to adopt healthy behavior is necessary, but we cannot solely rely on them to help themselves. The period of adolescence requires assistance and guidance by caring and reliable adults.

• American families are under enormous social and economic stress resulting in funda-

mental changes in family structure and the context for child rearing (National Research Council, 1993), making it difficult, if not impossible, for families to assume the sole responsibility expected by society for helping adolescents.

• Youth health issues reflect the context of their environments:

— Adolescents are physically less healthy than their parents' generation.
— Social environments affect successful transition to adulthood: family, school, neighborhood, economic opportunity, bias, and prejudice.
— Emotional vulnerability is reflected by increasing rates of youth suicide and homicide, among other indicators.

• The period of adolescence has grown. Children begin the process at younger ages and remain in this role into young adulthood, particularly for those who remain in postsecondary education environments, increasing their vulnerability.

Demographic Changes

Expectations and assumptions about adolescence are affected not only by future projections about the changing dynamics of society, but also by demographic changes occurring in society. For example, despite the fact that half of the world's population is under the age of 25 years (Friedman, 1993), the proportion of the U.S. population age 20 years and under was 32% in 1980 and is projected to shrink to 23% by 2080, if 1980 trends remain the same (Vaupel & Gowan, 1986). In turn, life expectancy is continuing to steadily increase, leading to an increase in those age 65 years and over from 11% to almost 20%, given the same population scenario.

Demographic changes affect adolescents in significant ways. An aging population relying on social insurance for retirement, along with a shrinking base of young adults, may well result in the need for workers to stay on the job for many years past age 65. Thus, youth will be kept out of many economic opportunities occupied by older Americans. Similarly, the health needs of older Americans already command a disproportionate share of health services resources. Older Americans are effective competitors for scarce resources, whereas youth require others to advocate for their needs.

The population will continue to diversify, with substantial increases in Latino and Asian groups and a proportionate decline in whites. The changing diversity of the population challenges us to develop opportunities for equitable inclusion of all groups in society, an issue keenly felt by adolescents. Adolescents need a sense of inclusion and hopefulness about the future if they are to become contributing and participative adults.

To anticipate changes in the population affecting youth, long-term strategies focusing on the needs of youth in the context of broader social changes due to a growing, aging population need to be initiated. The opportunities for considering population change need to be taken out of the academic environment of population studies and injected in public policy forums for debate, discussion, planning, and action. This is difficult to accomplish in a society with an orientation to a short-term, bottom-line approach to issues.

Crisis-Oriented Topical Programs

For many reasons, our society has approached adolescent health issues as a response to a perceived crisis. Individual programs have been developed to address particular categories of health issues, such as the war on drugs. Most programs have been developed in isolation, as if the targeted behavior or problem existed in isolation from the other facets of life. Using this approach it has been possible to design episodic, fragmented, and ineffective programs with the hope that by "doing something," the problem

will be resolved so that other issues may take center stage. As we have learned from the chapter on alcohol and other drugs, the problems do not go away: They change and evolve but remain present among our youth. Furthermore, although they are taken in isolation, these topical issues are more often related to other facets of the lives of youth than programmers imagine. Our societal concern about HIV/AIDS reveals that many have become infected during adolescence and that alcohol and other drugs are often involved in youth engaging in high-risk behaviors. Alcohol and other drugs are also associated with intentional and unintentional injuries.

Topical crisis-oriented programs also have a way of labeling young people as those at risk. Certain factors present in the lives of youth increase the probability of developing health problems. Resulting efforts have focused on identifying those at risk and devoting program resources to address their needs. The unintended effect of these programs has been to divide the youth population in a segregation-like fashion, rather than looking for collective solutions to issues.

Recognition of connections of topical health issues is the beginning of developing opportunities for collective solutions to problems. There is no question that pressing adolescent issues demand action to be taken. At the same time, thoughtful collaborative efforts need to be developed to promote coordinated efforts to improve opportunities for all adolescents. Furthermore, it must be understood that adolescent health problems cannot be eradicated. Therefore, we need to take a developmental approach to help adolescents cope and to mitigate the problems they face as best as possible.

Adolescence: A Turbulent Time

The transition from child to adult is fraught with difficulties as youth undergo physical, emotional, and social changes. Changing beliefs, thoughts, values, emotions, decisions, and actions combine to make growth and development processes vulnerable to many health-compromising behaviors. Adolescents need a stable context for their development (Pittman & Cahill, 1992):

- They need to feel physically and emotionally safe at home, at school, and in the neighborhood.
- They need a social structure for their lives to enable them to develop their personal, social, and intellectual skills.
- They need meaningful relationships with their peers and with reliable, caring adults.
- They need opportunities to contribute at home, at school, and in the community to gain a sense of self-worth.
- They need opportunities to gain control over important aspects of their lives by participating in decision making and establishing independence.

Rather than focusing on health issues that cannot be eradicated, providing a stable context for adolescent development and focusing on skills adolescents need to participate in society as adults are essential where home, school, and community can contribute:

- Health-promoting behaviors, such as lifelong fitness, rather than problem prevention or self-treatment
- Personal and social skills
- Cognitive and creative development
- Vocational skills
- Citizenship, including ethics and participation (Pittman & Cahill, 1992)

Where Do We Go?

The focus of this volume on adolescent health concerns requires those involved in the lives of teenagers to reevaluate current approaches to youth. Many programs are funded on a categorical basis and offered through agencies and social services that form the fabric of social support for society: schools, medical care facilities, public health departments, social service and voluntary agencies, recreational groups, and the like. Professionals are educated and oriented toward working in these settings and providing services from the agency context. Working with adolescents as a target population requires a change in perspective. Adolescent lives are not cleanly divided among health topics and agencies. Rather, their lives represent a continuum of home, school, and community environments. Virtually all facets of society are affected by the well-being of youth, either now or in the future.

Investment in the future is required, but not in the traditional manner. It is evident from the chapters in this volume that a different kind of approach is called for if the health of youth is to be conserved and promoted. Collaboration is needed to help young people prepare for their futures as adults. The emphasis for such collaboration is to help youth through the growth and development process. Because of the complexities of society currently, it is virtually impossible for any one individual or agency to facilitate the growth and development of adolescents. Youth need help. Families need help. Alone, the school cannot provide the necessary support and services that youth require. Community agencies and policymakers cannot guide youth through this process, but they can develop opportunities to help youth in collaboration with other elements of society.

If we are to help youth develop the skills to resist and work through the numerous challenges that confront them and prepare them for their roles as adults, we are required to change the episodic, individualistic approaches that we have tried in the past. Although some of these have been successful, the opportunity for all to work together to promote the well-being of adolescents is at hand. We need to take up this challenge.

References

Friedman, H. L. (1993). Promoting the health of adolescents in the United States: A global perspective. *Journal of Adolescent Health, 14*(7), 509-519.

National Research Council. (1993). *Losing generations: Adolescents in high-risk settings.* Washington, DC: National Academy Press.

Pittman, K. J., & Cahill, J. (1992). *Pushing the boundaries of education: The implications of a youth development approach to education policies, structures, and collaborations.* Washington, DC: Council of Chief State School Officers.

Toffler, A. (1990). *Power shift.* New York: Bantam.

Vaupel, J. W., & Gowan, A. E. (1986). Passage to Methuselah: Some demographic consequences of continued progress against mortality. *American Journal of Public Health, 76*(4), 430-433.

Name Index

Abraham, S., 38, 43
Abramo, D. M., 117, 130
Abramowitz, A., 123, 130
Adams, C. M., 153, 157, 164
Adams, G. R., 153, 157, 164
Adams, H. G., 102, 115
Advocates for Youth, 141, 149
Aggleton, P., 142, 143, 149
Ahia, R. N., 129, 130
Alan Guttmacher Institute, 100,
    102, 103, 105, 115, 135,
    136, 137, 138, 140, 143
Allensworth, D., 68, 76
Allensworth, D. D., 39, 43
American Dietetic Association, 37,
    43
American Medical Association, 1,
    6, 13, 21, 41, 43, 177, 179
American Psychiatric Association,
    36, 43
American School Food Service
    Association, 40, 43
Anderson, B., 73, 76
Anderson, E. M., 192, 197
Anderson, G., 74, 76
Anderson, K., 134, 149
Anglin, T. M., 117, 131
Apter, S. J., 170, 179
Arbeit, M. L., 35, 43
Armstrong, D., 127, 130
Armstrong, J., 73, 76
Arno, P. S., 101, 116
Ary, D., 5, 6, 123, 130
Attkisson, C. C., 201, 203, 209
Austin, G., 49, 50, 53, 57, 60, 64,
    69, 76

Babbie, E., 200, 209
Bachman, J., 58, 60, 62, 63, 77

Bachman, J. G., 34, 43, 57, 60, 76
Badger, G. J., 223, 224, 225, 227
Bagnall, G., 124, 130
Bagwell, M., 36, 45
Baizerman, M., 64, 76
Balch, G. M. Jr., 182, 186, 198
Baldo, M., 142, 143, 149
Balentine, M., 37, 43
Bandura, A., 129, 130
Banton, J. G., 168, 180
Baranowski, T., 200, 201, 202,
    203, 204, 205, 206, 207,
    208, 209
Barth, R., 141, 149
Barth, R. P., 108, 115, 122, 131
Bartlett, J. G., 117, 130
Bartol, C. R., 182, 197
Bastian, L. D., 172, 179
Battaglia, J., 153, 164
Behrens, R., 151, 153, 164
Bell, R. A., 201, 202, 203, 204, 209
Benard, B., 75, 76
Bennett, S., 67, 76
Bensel, R. W., 181, 190, 198
Berenson, G. S., 28, 30, 31, 35, 39,
    43, 44, 45
Berk, R. A., 205, 207, 209
Berlin, B., 139, 149
Berlin, B. M., 122, 131
Berliner, B., 172, 180
Bessinger, C., 40, 41, 43
Bibeau, D., 171, 180
Bickel, A., 67, 76
Bickel, S., 67, 68, 77
Biden, J. R., Jr. 183, 197
Bidgood, B. A., 32, 43
Biglan, A., 5, 6, 123, 130
Billy, J. O. G., 105, 115
Black, D., 123, 130
Black, T., 171, 179

Blank, M. J., 68, 77
Blanken, A. J., 2, 6
Blonde, C. V., 28, 30, 43
Blumenthal, B. A., 143, 150
Blythe, B. J., 173, 179
Bonner, J., 37, 43
Borra, S. T., 35, 45
Botvin, G. J., 108, 115
Boyer, C. B., 122, 130
Boyer, D., 139, 149
Brechenmaker, L. C., 143, 150
Brindis, C., 100, 101, 102, 103,
    104, 105, 113, 114, 116
Brookmeyer, R., 117, 130
Brown, C. R., 171, 179
Brown, J., 64, 66, 76, 77
Brown, L., 123, 130
Brown, S., 133, 149
Brown, Z. A., 102, 115
Buchta, R. M., 122, 130
Buehler, J., 125, 130
Buhl, J. M., 201, 204, 209
Bunch, D. L., 117, 131
Burghardt, J., 33, 43
Bush, G. B., 179
Bushlong, C., 153, 164
Butterfield, B. D., 8, 21
Byers, R. H., 117, 118, 131
Byler, R. V., 108, 115

Cahill, J., 255, 256
California Department of Justice,
    167, 173, 174, 179
California Vital Statistics Section,
    139, 149
Callahan, C. M., 168, 179
Camburn, D., 105, 116
Cameron, G., 32, 43
Camp, B., 144, 149

Subject Index